DEVELOPING A FORENSIC
PRACTICE

Developing a forensic practice can be confusing and intimidating. Dr. William Reid, a highly experienced forensic psychiatrist, has written a practical, straightforward guide for clinicians interested in doing it right and increasing their opportunities for a successful transition to forensic work. This book, which will be of interest to many attorneys as well, provides straightforward details, along with many case examples, of lawyer–expert communications and relationships, case assessment, record review, evaluations, reports, deposition and trial testimony, fees and billing, office operations, marketing, liability, and professional ethics. A bonus chapter by a successful malpractice attorney gives a unique and valuable "lawyer's perspective" on the content and mental health experts in general. The huge appendix provides over 40 highly useful examples in the appendices of common office forms, letters, reports, and affidavits.

Any mental health professional who currently practices, or wants to practice, at the interface of mental health and the law will find this an indispensible practice resource.

William H. Reid, M.D., M.P.H., past president of the American Academy of Psychiatry and the Law, has practiced forensic psychiatry for over 35 years in private settings, medical schools, and the public sector.

Other Books by
William H. Reid

The Psychopath: A Comprehensive Study or Antisocial Disorders and Behaviors
(editor) (1978)
Psychiatry for the House Officer (1979)
Basic Intensive Psychotherapy (1980)
The Treatment of Antisocial Syndromes (editor) (1981)
Terrorism: Interdisciplinary Perspectives (co-editor) (1983)
Treatment of the DSM-III Psychiatric Disorders (1983)
Assaults Within Psychiatric Facilities (co-editor) (1983)
Unmasking the Psychopath (co-editor) (1986)
DSM-III-R Training Guide (co-author) (1989)
The Treatment of Psychiatric Disorders (1989, co-author 1997)
DSM-IV Training Guide (co-author) (1995)
A Clinician's Guide to Legal Issues in Psychotherapy (1999)
Treating Adult and Juvenile Offenders with Special Needs (co-editor) (2001)
Handbook of Mental Health Administration (co-editor) (2003)

DEVELOPING A FORENSIC PRACTICE

Operations and Ethics for Experts

William H. Reid

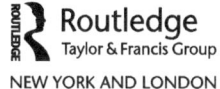

NEW YORK AND LONDON

First published 2013
by Routledge
605 Third Avenue, New York, NY 10017
4 Park Square, Milton Park, Abingdon, Oxon OX14 4RN

Routledge is an imprint of the Taylor & Francis Group, an informa business

Library of Congress Cataloging in Publication Data
Reid, William H., 1945–
Developing a forensic practice: operations and ethics for experts /
William H. Reid.
p.; cm.
Includes bibliographical references and index.
I. Title.
[DNLM: 1. Forensic Psychiatry—ethics. 2. Forensic Psychiatry—
organization & administration. 3. Expert Testimony—ethics.
4. Expert Testimony—legislation & jurisprudence. 5. Liability,
Legal. 6. Practice Management. W 740]
614'.15068—dc23
2012037423

ISBN: 978-0-415-81705-9 (hbk)
ISBN: 978-0-415-53776-6 (pbk)
ISBN: 978-0-203-11006-5 (ebk)

Typeset in Garamond
by Book Now Ltd, London

To my teachers, friends, and colleagues in the American Academy of Psychiatry and the Law, and to the many fine and ethical attorneys with whom I have worked over the years

CONTENTS

Preface   xi

1 Getting Started   1

2 Vocabulary   16

3 Lawyer–Expert Relationships   24

4 Records and Record Review   30

5 Evaluations   35

6 Reports and Affidavits   47

7 Deposition and Trial Testimony   54

8 Fees and Billing   62

9 Ethics   70

10 Marketing   73

11 Your Office and Office Procedures   81

12 Liability in Forensic Practice   87

13 A Lawyer's Perspective on Forensic Mental Health Experts   90
    SKIP SIMPSON, J.D.

CONTENTS

Appendices: Forms, Letters, Reports, and More   106
Internal Documents, Letters, Communications

A. Initial Attorney Letter   108

B. Fee Sheet   109

C. Settlement Acknowledgment   111

D. Evaluation Appointment Letter   112

E. Evaluee Information Sheet   113

F. Notification of Treatment Need Discovered During Evaluation   114

G. *Subpoena Duces Tecum* Response   116

H. Pre-Testimony Deposit Worksheet   118

I. Pre-Testimony Deposit Letter   119

J. Time Worksheet   121

K. Vendor Confidentiality Agreement   122

L. Employee Confidentiality Agreement   123

Report Examples

R1. Report: Trial Competency (Fitness to Proceed) (Simple)   125

R2. Report: Trial Competency (Fitness to Proceed) (Complex)   127

R3. Report: Criminal Responsibility (Sanity)   134

R4. Report: Criminal Defense, Mitigation of Charge or Sentence   137

R5. Report: NGRI Release, Defense   143

R6. Report: Personal Injury Defense (PTSD)   147

R7. Report: Clinician–Patient Sex, Plaintiff   153

R8.   Report: Malpractice, Plaintiff (Complex, Doctor and Hospital)   163

R9.   Affidavit: Malpractice, Plaintiff Pre-Suit   176

R10. Letter/Report: Malpractice, Plaintiff Pre-Suit, Lack of Causation   179

R11. Report: Malpractice, Plaintiff (Complex)   181

R12. Report: Malpractice, Defense (Complex, Facility)   195

R13. Report: Malpractice, Defense (Facility), Forensic Practice Standards   201

R14. Report: Malpractice, Defense (Clinician) (Alleged Fetal Damage from Medication)   208

R15. Report: Accidental Overdose vs. Suicide   216

R16. Report: Defense, Death in Custody   223

R17. Affidavit: Defense Rebuttal, Death in Custody   227

R18. Report: Workplace Stressors Allegedly Causing Suicide, Expert Report Rebuttal   232

R19. Report: Private Insurance Disability Appeal (Complex)   238

R20. Report: Employee Emotional Injury, Treater–Expert Conflict   249

R21. Report: Professional Licensing Agency Review   262

R22. Report: Professional Licensing Agency Review   264

R23. Opinion Letter: Professional Licensure   268

R24. Report: Civil Capacity, Contracting   270

R25. Report: Capacity, Guardianship (Complex, Contested)   276

R26. Opinion Letter: Capacity, Business, and Testamentary   285

CONTENTS

R27. Report: Auto Accident vs. Suicide   288

R28. Affidavit: Supporting Motion to Strike Expert Testimony
      (Forensic Practice Standards)   292

R29. Letter: Rebuttal of Expert's Report, Forensic Practice
      Standards   297

      Index   300

PREFACE

Nothing in this book should be construed as any form of legal advice. The contents represent the author's opinions and recommendations at the time of writing. Dr. Reid is not an attorney and does not represent that any of these materials meets, or fails to meet, any legal standard.

Once written for psychiatrists, this work has been completely updated for use by any independently licensed mental health clinician who practices—or wants to practice—at the interface of mental health and the law in the United States legal system. The book is written from the viewpoint of a private practitioner or forensic service contractor, one who acts as a forensic consultant or expert in his or her particular clinical field (psychology, psychiatry, social work, mental health nursing, mental health administration, and others.)

I do not provide very much information about basic law or legal cases (such as the "landmark cases" that underlie much of the interface between mental health and the law). This is a *practical* guide that assumes the reader is already well founded in his or her clinical field and wishes guidance about forensic practice matters.

The *nidus* for this work was designed in a workshop format with a qualified discussant available. I have tried to make this new book format stand alone. Most or all of the content should be readily understandable by clinicians with little experience in forensic work, but the very nature of practical books implies that one should often look elsewhere for details, further education, specialized information, and clarifications. One should get relevant (often supervised) training and experience before representing oneself as a subspecialist. Various references and bibliographies should help, but readers should feel free to query and work with experienced, credible forensic specialists and training programs; this, like other professional pursuits, is not a "cookbook" endeavor.

William H. Reid, M.D., M.P.H.
Horseshoe Bay, Texas, 2013

1

GETTING STARTED

Most of this book assumes that the reader has (or is actively seeking) a terminal degree in a clinical mental health specialty (psychology Ph.D./Psy.D./Ed.D., M.D./D.O. with psychiatry residency, M.S.W., R.N./M.S.N./R.N.-P.) and wants to learn about private consultation at the interface of that specialty and the law. (I generally use the terms "forensic professional" or "forensic clinician" for efficiency's sake, including others as applicable.) Many of the principles and procedures also apply to employed clinicians, including those who carry out consultations separate from their employment (such as "moonlighting"), those who perform forensic services through agency or facility contracts, and those who perform forensic services as employees of agencies or facilities.

Much of this book assumes that the reader will be retained most of the time by an attorney in a contested ("adversarial") proceeding. Experts are sometimes retained directly by courts or agencies for other purposes, but it is a common misconception that experts are usually "friends of the court" (a misuse of that phrase as well).

Readers in academic or agency settings may notice differences between the professional viewpoints implied here and those in their own settings, such as (but not limited to) a focus on work done as part of retention by an attorney and one's relationships with retaining attorneys. This should not be construed as suggesting any significant differences in duty or ethics.

My references to lawyers may sound stilted (e.g., repetitive use of "the lawyer who retained you" or "the retaining entity"). That's my inartful way of avoiding any implication that the attorney who retains you is "your" lawyer. Expert witnesses should not be direct advocates for the side on which they work[1] but, rather, advocate articulately for the opinions they legitimately form if asked to do so. Thus it is improper for an expert

---

1 "Consulting" experts who do not anticipate testifying have much more flexibility in this regard.

to refer to "my lawyer" when the lawyer actually represents his or her own client, not the expert.

Similarly, although I sometimes refer to "the opposing lawyer," I actually mean "the lawyer for the party who opposes the client of the lawyer who has retained you." I could have said that every time, but the printer would have run out of ink.

Before we go further, here are five postulates that can guide you to a career that is both successful and rewarding. We'll discuss each of these postulates in various ways throughout this book; keep them in mind:

1. Practice well.
2. Understand the point of the legal exercise.
3. Be serious about ethics.
4. Quality begets quality.
5. Quality begets success.

You will have no trouble competing with forensic professionals who are poorly trained, lazy, sloppy, single-sided, "hired guns," unethical, or just don't get the point of the lawyer's or court's work.

Finally, courts and lawyers need experts with clinical expertise and some understanding of the legal process at hand, not quasi-attorneys or doctors who act like lawyers. Forensic mental health professionals are generally not, and should not act as, attorneys. Simply understand your clinical discipline and how it applies to the forensic arenas in which you work. If you happen to have a law degree in addition to your clinical credentials, note that the material in this book is completely unrelated to legal consultation or representation of legal clients. I strongly recommend that professionals with such dual credentials (M.D./J.D., Ph.D./J.D., R.N./J.D., etc.) refrain from mixing them in the same case.

Training and Credentials

Clinical training, experience, and certification (as relevant to the field of practice) are necessary and expected for every forensic medical/mental health expert. Your usefulness to lawyers, courts, and other entities almost always comes much more from your clinical expertise and experience than from your forensic background. As I have told countless high school, college, medical, and graduate students, one must first be (and want to be) a clinician, then consider working toward forensic goals, not the other way around.

Specifically forensic fellowships, post-docs, and internships can be valuable preparation for a forensic career but are not usually necessary for forensic practice. Many certifying bodies (such as the American Board of Psychiatry and Neurology [ABPN] and the American Psychological Association) require them in order to sit for subspecialty diplomate exams (see below).

Professionally accepted forensic subspecialty certifications include those of the American Psychological Association's American Board of Professional Psychology (ABPP) and the ABPN. In my experience, "forensic" certification is a worthwhile pursuit and useful for practitioners who work in academic or administrative environments, but it is far less important than *clinical* certification when working with attorneys and courts.

There are other "certification" organizations and companies that market their "credentials" to various kinds of mental health professionals. One should investigate their claims and usefulness carefully before applying, since many (but not all) hold no particular influence in either clinical or forensic fields, often giving certificates and titles to those who merely take a simple test and pay a fee (sometimes even waiving the test). Some are outright "diploma mills" that should be avoided. Good lawyers quickly discover which are legitimate and which can be criticized if you list them on your *curriculum vitae.*

Continuing education courses and workshops in forensic practice can be valuable and efficient ways to increase and/or update one's practice skills. Professionally recognized forensic organizations, such as the American Academy of Psychiatry and the Law (AAPL) and the American Academy of Forensic Sciences (AAFS), offer a variety of educational opportunities, usually at their annual or semiannual meetings. One in particular deserves special mention—the comprehensive forensic psychiatry course by Dr. Phillip Resnick and colleagues, sponsored by the AAPL and offered at AAPL and some American Psychiatric Association meetings. Most recognized national (and some state and regional) clinical organizations offer approved continuing education in forensic practice.

Participating in recognized forensic organizations is a good way to stay abreast of important professional information, learn of continuing education opportunities, keep in touch with colleagues, compare your procedures with those of other forensic practitioners, and remain aware of ethical issues and guidelines. Some professions, such as psychiatry and psychology, have active forensic organizations; others have forensic sections or interest groups within their national associations.

Your membership in a recognized professional organization is one sign to clients and courts that you are not some sort of isolated "maverick" practitioner and that you have adopted, at least by your membership, that organization's code of ethics. Conversely, there are poorly recognized organizations that focus more on "guild" issues or superficial titles than professional education or scientific endeavor; in my opinion, many of them should be avoided.

Mentoring by someone you know to have excellent skills, ethics, and reputation is very helpful. *Books and publications* are great sources of information and reference, but are not sufficient for the knowledge and experience you need for practice.

I am often asked whether or not attending *law school* is helpful in forensic practice. I believe law school to be completely unnecessary for forensic practice, and it may be detrimental to some careers. Most M.D./J.D. and Ph.D./J.D. holders practice as either clinicians or lawyers. The combination seems reserved largely for academic settings and a few medical malpractice attorneys. Some R.N./J.D. and M.S.W./J.D. holders find careers in law firms or as legal consultants but not often, in my experience, as forensic experts (the practice discussed in this book). Forensic experts with law degrees need the *imprimatur* and credibility of their clinical professions as they communicate with judges and juries; a law degree may decrease some of that credibility (no offense to our legal brethren). If you decide to go to law school, do it because you want to be a lawyer, not because you think it will make you a better (or more sought-after) forensic clinician.

Reputation and Credibility

Get it. Keep it.

Have the requisite education, training, and experience. Do not misrepresent or "pad" your credentials. First, it's dishonest. Second, lawyers who will question you often check out your background and know the answers to questions before they are asked.

Do quality work. Much of this book is devoted to showing you how to do quality forensic work. Your clinical work should be relevant and free of serious criticism as well.

Do ethical work. Don't get into ethics trouble, and don't do things that are likely to get you into ethics trouble. Be an example of ethical practice in both clinical and forensic work.

Continue to do clinical work. Much, perhaps most, of your forensic work rests on a foundation of current clinical expertise. This is critical for most kinds of malpractice consultation and testimony and important for many other forensic practices as well.

Don't be a "hired gun" (or even look like one). Some of the public, including some lawyers and jurors, get their ideas about forensic experts from television and movies. That means they see dramas about experts who say whatever the lawyer wants, work as "advocates" for the retaining lawyer's case, get paid flat fees to say something, or shade evaluation results to fit the case. Those people are not common, but they do exist. *Do not* be one of them. First, it's dishonest. Second, nothing ruins a career faster than getting a reputation as a hired gun.

Have unblemished licenses and certifications. Your licensing board status and lots of other credentials information is easily available to lawyers and courts.

Guard against hospital or organization censure, such as privilege suspensions, expulsions, or termination for cause.

Avoid malpractice suits, especially if you consult in malpractice cases. No one is perfect, and a malpractice judgment can happen to anyone over a career, but more than one is difficult to explain in the best of circumstances.

Be completely honest in your testimony and reports. Your past testimony is easily available to attorneys, and your honesty and consistency will be scrutinized during trials and depositions.

Your nonprofessional pursuits can affect your forensic credibility. This includes damning items such as arrests and convictions, as well as seemingly less significant things like questionable websites, hobbies, and associates.

A clinician was discussing forensic careers in one of my workshops when the topic of websites arose. She mentioned her nonclinical website dedicated to an interest in witchcraft and the paranormal. She was proud of her reputation in that avocation, said it was quite separate from her mental health practice, and wondered if it might interfere with forensic referrals or credibility. We examined her website with that question in mind.

The website was "dark"—deep red in color, with ominous background music and drawings of satanic-appearing figures and symbols on the main page. It included a forum with comments from visitors, often followed by the clinician's own comments or answers (which focused enthusiastically on wiccan topics, never mentioning that she was also a clinician). She offered a witchcraft-related music CD for sale.

Without knowing more about her clinical practices, I nevertheless suggested that the website and similar pursuits would indeed be a problem, since it could be easily found by lawyers and others and she would have to acknowledge it if asked. I asked her privately to think about what the website and activities might represent about her professional identity and her ability to work objectively with patients and forensic clients. I told her that she should at least disclose the website and related activities to anyone who wanted to retain her, and that it might indeed put off forensic clients and decrease referrals.

The clinician balked at those ideas, choosing to believe that her wiccan pursuits were kept separate from her clinical work and any forensic pursuits, and that they "shouldn't make any difference." Several years later, I learned that she had had both licensure and practice problems as a result of her unusual practices.

5

Lawyers communicate with each other about experts. They ask others for recommendations when they're searching for experts. Once they have your name, they may ask others about you before calling. Those who depose or cross-examine you are likely to have researched your background to a greater or lesser extent.

Duties

Just as a clinician has certain duties to his or her patients or clients, forensic experts have duties that must be fulfilled in order to meet professional practice standards and, in some cases, legal requirements.

You have *duties to the attorney or organization that retains you* (referred to in this book as the "retaining entity"). He/she/it is entitled to know of any issues that may affect your ability to do the work for which you have been hired or which may occur at some future time (such as testifying). Those concerns include, but may not be limited to, conflict of interest (such as relationships with one of the parties, financial conflict, or strong personal feelings about the litigation or the parties), scheduling difficulty, past license problems or relevant lawsuits of your own, and inadequate knowledge, training, or experience. In most cases, you act as the attorney's *agent*, within legal and ethical limits, but almost never as a direct *advocate* for any litigant.

Part of your duty to the retaining entity is to be accurate and objective. You should not offer, nor should ethical lawyers or other clients expect, opinions that lie by either commission or omission. In fact, an attorney's learning things that go against the case can be as valuable to him or her as learning those that support it.

You have *duties of honesty and objectivity to any court or other judicial or arbitrating body* to which your opinions are offered. Your opinions and other comments may reach a judge or court in several ways: in a report, by affidavit or sworn statement, in deposition testimony, or in direct testimony at a hearing or trial. You are expected to articulate your opinions well and defend them convincingly, but you must be honest. Do not allow others, such as a retaining entity, to offer in your name opinions that have not been genuinely and properly rendered.

You have *duties to the retaining entity's client(s)*, including those of adequate qualifications, practice standards, and good faith. However, as already noted, you should not advocate directly for the litigant, nor should the litigant or any interested party be your patient.

You have a *duty of honesty and good faith to the opposing entity.* Being a "hired gun" may be the lawyer's role, but it's not yours.

*Here are some duties you **don't** have.* Forensic consultation or expert witness activity does not, in most instances, create a "doctor–patient" or clinician–patient/client relationship. When you evaluate a person solely for a forensic or administrative purpose (not for direct treatment or contemplating treating the person yourself), you do not, in my opinion, incur the same duties as a treating clinician or clinical consultant. There are times when you cannot place an evaluee's needs before those of others, for example, or maintain his or her confidentiality. It is a good idea to remind evaluees of that fact and to refrain from calling them "patients" or "clients."

Treater vs. Expert Witness or Consultant

One of the most important topics for clinicians doing forensic work is the separation of clinical and forensic roles. A clinical relationship with the subject of a forensic or administrative issue raises very important conflict-of-interest issues and should be avoided in almost all instances. Those who act as both treater and expert without very good reason (such as a genuine emergency) are at best imprudent and at worst knowingly misleading the judicial process.

- With rare exceptions, *a treating clinician should not become an expert witness for his or her past, present, or foreseeable patient.*
- With rare exceptions for emergencies, *an expert witness should not treat a plaintiff, defendant, or evaluee in the same forensic case.*

When these prohibitions are violated, significant conflicts arise for both the patient and the court. Those conflicts are often partially unconscious, and are often irreconcilable.

A psychotherapist treated a man for several years in psychodynamic therapy. When the man was sued over a business transaction, his attorney asked the therapist to become an expert witness in his defense. The therapist agreed, and spent many hours reviewing records, working with the lawyer on her patient's behalf, providing written opinions in the patient's legal defense, and testifying at deposition and trial. In addition to statements about the legal matter, the therapist agreed that she had been paid several thousand dollars over the years for treatment, had received many thousands more as the attorney's expert witness, and planned to continue providing therapy to the defendant in the future.

Although the judge allowed the therapist-"expert" to testify, she was later brought before her professional licensing board for unethical practice and was eventually censured. The licensing case was appealed to civil court, where the therapist did not prevail.

The purpose and goals of a treating clinician are fundamentally different from, and often conflict with, those of a forensic expert. The treater
has "fiduciary" (or near fiduciary; see definition in chapter 2) and ethical
obligations to the patient which demand that the patient's interests be
placed above all else. The forensic consultant's responsibilities, on the
other hand, are to objectivity and the court.

There are at least four reasons that such a dual relationship should be
avoided.

First, a treatment relationship clearly creates a professional and ethical
obligation to act in the best interests of the patient. The patient has a
right to rely on this attitude in the doctor or therapist during (and after)
the treatment relationship. It is a cornerstone of the patient's ability to be
free of concerns about future divulging of confidences, betrayal, or exploitation. Since forensic consultation or testimony, by definition, requires
objective comment regardless of the patient's wishes or needs, an inherent
clinical and ethical conflict is created. This conflict is recognized in the
ethical guidelines of all mental health professions, often expressed as
the patient's right to expect a single, private treatment role from his or
her clinician or therapist.

Second, a treating clinician who testifies regarding a current or past
patient knows (or should know) that he or she is ethically required to act
in the patient's interest. Having spent many hours (perhaps dozens or
hundreds) working with a patient, sometimes quite intimately, clinicians
often feel a personal affinity for that patient's viewpoint. There is thus a
danger of *intentional bias* toward the patient.

Third, separate from the clinician's conscious awareness of a duty or
wish to act in the patient's interest, the obligation to "do no harm" to the
patient is keenly felt by ethical practitioners. Even if they attempt to be
objective in forensic reports or testimony, there is a danger of *unintended
bias* toward the patient.

Fourth, the ethics principles of both the American Psychiatric
Association and the American Psychological Association require that when
a treating clinician believes it may later become necessary to comment to a
third party (such as an employer or insurance company), this is to be discussed fully with the patient as early as is feasible. Awareness of the probability of disclosure affects the patient's conversations and disclosures to
some extent, and this in turn affects the validity of both clinical and forensic participation.

If we look more closely, we can see even more reason for concern. I have
seen examples of each of the following:

1. If the initial referral is forensic and the forensic professional elects to
   treat the person as a patient, the clinical evaluation may intentionally
   be incomplete and/or may not document the evaluation, history,

symptoms, diagnoses, treatment plan, and prognosis as completely or objectively as would a solely treating clinician. That is, the care and documentation may be modified to fit the forensic purpose, thus short-changing patient care.

2. If the initial relationship is clinical but the role later becomes forensic, the diagnosis, treatment, and/or documentation of care may change, to the detriment of the patient's clinical needs.

3. A forensic expert who is treating a litigant may *unconsciously* (i.e., without overt malicious intent) create incomplete or skewed treatment documentation. He or she knows that the notes are likely to be revealed during the litigation. There may be a subtle wish or impulse to support the attorney's case and/or to please the attorney.

4. A forensic expert who is treating a litigant may *unconsciously* diminish or otherwise change his or her treatment or procedures in a way that (a) creates findings that will support the legal case and/or please the attorney, (b) obscures findings that might refute the attorney's case, (c) avoids (or fails to encourage) potentially effective assessment and treatment procedures (e.g., to keep the patient from improving and decreasing damages), and/or (d) prevents timely referral to nonforensic clinicians.

5. A forensic expert who is treating a litigant may *consciously* create incomplete or skewed treatment documentation and/or diminish or change treatment or procedures in the ways described above.

6. A forensic expert who is treating a litigant may *consciously* use a nominal "treatment" relationship to prevent creation of a legitimate factual treatment situation. That is, by controlling the documentation of clinical care, an unscrupulous expert is in a position to control, if he or she chooses to do so, opposing counsel's access to accurate clinical information.

7. A forensic expert who is treating a litigant could *consciously* collude with the litigant to misrepresent symptoms, diagnoses, treatment response, or disability (note that this may occur with nonforensic clinicians as well, often out of a misguided effort to help the patient).

What "treater" situations might be acceptable? The above cautions notwithstanding, some administrative assessments are commonly and reasonably completed by treating clinicians (though a separate evaluator is often a better choice). In the simplest cases, agencies ask treaters to opine from their records about mental disability, fitness for duty, some sort of license or permit, or civil commitment, for example.

Things get a bit more complicated when one is asked for a separate assessment or opinion about a patient's/client's fitness or condition. I do not take a position of forbidding physicians and therapists from filling out disability forms or requests for opinions about, say, eligibility for a driver's license, but there are several inherent sources of conflict. Clinicians know (or should know) that their patients and patient care are affected by what the doctor or therapist says to others, such as employers or agencies. We don't want to upset our patient relationships or make patients/clients uncomfortable. Moreover, we don't want to make ourselves uncomfortable by having to explain a negative opinion. Some of the conflicts are clear; others are hidden and even unconscious.

Some clinicians deal with this by being very open with patients for whom they write letters or complete administrative forms. Others have a rule that the form will not be discussed with the patient at all and will be sent directly to the requesting party. Still others have the patient participate in completing the form or letter, edit drafts, or even write it him- or herself. Although discussion is recommended, *I do not recommend allowing the patient to influence one's wording or opinions and believe that such a process is often dishonest and unethical.*

Career Directions in Private Forensic Practice

"Expert," "Expert witness"   As we will quickly see, the word "expert" has both general and specific definitions and usually includes far more than testifying. Giving testimony is only a small part of most forensic experts' practices.

Litigation consultant   Litigation consulting by itself is a relatively unusual subspecialty. General forensic work may include some litigation consultation, but that is not the primary role of most retained experts, and it may preclude an expert from testifying (because of the advocacy role that it implies). When attorneys hire an expert, they usually want the option of having that expert testify if his or her eventual opinions are helpful to the case. On the other hand, ethical experts who anticipate testifying should be cautious about the extent to which they assist in strategy and advocacy for one side or the other.

Doctor vs. doctor–lawyer   As already mentioned, almost all of the forensic/ expert roles discussed herein stem from a clinical foundation. Clinicians who also have a law degree are considered, in this book, from the standpoint of their psychiatric, not legal, expertise.

Part-time or full time?   I recommend that almost all forensic expert careers be "part-time," in the sense that some aspects of patient consultation and/or care should remain a part of the forensic clinician's practice. Exceptions exist—for example, for a very experienced forensic professional who does not become involved in many matters involving malpractice or clinician competence.

Subspecialization (civil, criminal, child, family, substance abuse, worker's compensation, etc.) I do not recommend subspecialization early in one's forensic career. It is important to gain a breadth of experience in the field as a whole, and limiting oneself to, for example, criminal work reduces the practice "market." On the other hand, it is very important to refrain from accepting cases in which one is not qualified. Some specialty areas, such as child forensic work, require considerable additional clinical training in order to offer true expertise.

Case experience with both plaintiff/prosecution and defense In contested litigation, consulting to one side most or all the time should be avoided by private practitioners, since it may imply (accurately or not) a bias that can be exploited by the lawyer for an opposing side. Some forensic clinicians are employed by court systems or law-enforcement agencies, and thus naturally find themselves working for the prosecution more often than for the defense in criminal matters. Conversely, in cities in which prosecutors employ or commonly use particular experts, it may be difficult to develop local criminal experience except as a defense expert. Note that the proportion of cases in which one testifies for one side or another is not the same statistic as the proportion in which one is retained. If you are retained frequently by both prosecution and defense, or plaintiff and defense in civil matters (in separate cases, of course), but end up almost always testifying for one or the other, be prepared to discuss the reason.

Local vs. broad regional or national practice It is much easier to develop a local practice than a broad geographic one. Local practice has obvious advantages but is vulnerable to local change, such as becoming too familiar to local lawyers and judges, influx of competition in the form of new practitioners, state and local agency and judicial budgets, and changes in state law that may affect one's ability to testify (particularly professionals with less training or certification than, say, a fully trained and certified forensic psychiatrist). Gaining experience in other jurisdictions and states is usually helpful to one's knowledge and career, in spite of geographic inconvenience (but note that, in many cases, almost all forensic work, such as record review or deposition, is done near one's home). Those who have an active forensic practice outside their home communities should consider limiting their clinical work to patients and caseloads that can tolerate unexpected absences.

Kinds of Cases

As noted above, the kinds of cases in which one becomes involved is an individual choice, but one should be sure of actual expertise before representing oneself as qualified in a particular area. This list is not all-inclusive, and the concepts often overlap; most are discussed to some extent later in this book.

Negligence, personal injury   These are broad categories of common civil litigation that include medical/clinical malpractice and standard of care, emotional damage, liability, disability, harassment, and discrimination.

Criminal   This category includes criminal responsibility (sanity, "not guilty by reason of insanity" [NGRI]), trial competency and other criminal-related competencies (e.g., to plead, to represent oneself, to be sentenced, to be executed), and offense mitigation.

Juvenile court matters   These may not strictly be called "criminal" because of the age of the defendant, but include many of the above plus juvenile waiver (related to being tried as an adult) and other topics. Many of these topics suggest that the expert have extensive child or adolescent clinical training.

Competencies and capacities   "Competency" should always be followed by "to . . .." In the civil arena, it may refer to the mental ability to make a will, make a contract, act properly (e.g., drive a car), consent to something, refuse something, marry, parent, or act in light of others' influence. Competencies in criminal matters are noted above. (Note that an assessment of competency to parent is not the same as one for child custody; see below.)

Guardianships, conservatorships   These matters refer to a person's ability to do something independently and, conversely, to a psychiatric or psychological need for outside help or substituted judgment when that ability is compromised. In children, guardianship is often predicated solely on age. In adults, the issues are mental function and capacity (such as the ability to manage one's finances or other affairs). Guardianship and conservatorship are similar concepts which may have specific differences in different jurisdictions.

Child custody or best interest   These matters ordinarily involve comprehensive assessments of both children and adults and thus special expertise in both child psychiatry/psychology and family interaction.

Disability, impairment   The most common tasks in this area are assessments of mental disability or impairment for such things as disability insurance income, allegations of mental damage, and fitness for a particular job or duty. They may also include assessing ability to perform functions for employment or licensure purposes (including professional licensure). Sometimes (often in employment cases) it refers to the interface of mental condition and the Americans with Disabilities Act (ADA).

Worker's compensation   Worker's compensation is a fairly narrow and specialized area of law and forensic endeavor. It has elements of assessment of disability or impairment but is separate from civil liability *per se* (that is, it is related to a form of insurance rather than to the complexities and potential liabilities of civil lawsuits).

Consultations, second opinions   Various kinds of entities (e.g., health-care facilities, businesses, government agencies) sometimes seek forensic clinicians when they encounter mental health issues that may also involve the law (such as potential liability, safety, or civil rights). The clinician may not only address the clinical aspects of such situations but be asked about (or asked to help the entity meet) some legal or liability standard. For example, a company may ask a forensic psychologist to assess the potential dangerousness of an employee; a hospital may ask for a second opinion about suicide risk before discharging a patient; an emergency room or physician may need assessment or certification of a patient being considered for involuntary psychiatric hospitalization; or a school system may retain a mental health expert to assist in writing policies about mental disorders in its students or staff. The clinician is not retained as a lawyer but, by virtue of forensic training and experience, offers something more than clinical expertise alone.

Clinical practice in forensic settings   Although this book is not directed at clinical practice in forensic settings, many "forensic" mental health professionals spend most of their practice time providing patient/client care in jails, prisons, secure hospitals, juvenile residential centers, outpatient forensic clinics, and similar treatment environments.

A Few Practice Principles

Before we get to the nuts and bolts of forensic practice, let's touch upon a few of the basic principles to which those nuts and bolts apply.

Advocacy is the lawyer's job, not yours. When you are working on a case, it's not "your case," and the lawyer isn't "your lawyer." The lawyer's duty is to his or her client; most of your duty, within certain bounds, is to the lawyer or other entity that retained you, not to the litigant. With few exceptions (such as the complex area of being retained by a *pro se* litigant), you should not be retained directly by a litigant if you anticipate testifying as an expert.

*You may (and often should) advocate articulately for your **opinions** (e.g., in reports or testimony), but not for the case or litigant* per se. It should be obvious that the attorney who retains you will not ask you to testify unless he or she believes your opinions are helpful to his or her case, and will attempt to guide your testimony toward those opinions. This can often be done within the expert's ethical bounds, but one should be a bit cautious, particularly if one is asked to gloss over important and relevant information that tends to detract from the lawyer's purpose.

*Don't express an opinion before you have done sufficient objective review and/or evaluation, and be certain you **have** sufficient and representative information before coming to any opinion.* Be sure the retaining lawyer understands that, although you may comment informally to him or her during the course of the case, any "opinion" attributed to you must have an adequate foundation.

If you are retained (or expect to be retained) by an attorney, do not communicate directly with the court, litigant, or opposing lawyer without authorization. Always communicate through the retaining attorney or with his or her approval. This applies to initial case contact (e.g., avoid calls or emails from litigants or potential litigants asking you to become involved), information gathering, obtaining corroborating information, scheduling examinations or interviews, preparing reports, and preparing for deposition.

Don't accept cases in which you aren't really an expert or don't think you can be objective. For example, all psychotherapists know something about psychotherapy and all psychiatrists know something about psychotropic medications, but if the case is likely to involve complex or esoteric knowledge you don't have, refer it elsewhere. With regard to objectivity, if you are particularly opposed to the death penalty, for example, or markedly repulsed by pedophilia, consider not becoming involved as an expert witness in such cases.

Consider not accepting an expert role in cases involving friends or close colleagues, even for malpractice defense, or in those involving your own (past or present) students, residents, supervisees, employees, or employers, for whom there is likely to be a bias or conflict of interest.

It is ethical to offer honest expert opinions against colleagues; however, you may wish to avoid those near whom you practice or whom you know fairly well. I sometimes tell colleagues or students in lectures that, although it is unlikely that I will be involved in a case against them, they might prefer that I were, since they at least would be assured of an honest review.

If you work on a case involving a defendant clinician (e.g., a malpractice action), *resist the temptation to be personally supportive of the physician (or any plaintiff or defendant).* You're not that person's therapist. Your usefulness lies in your independent expertise, not in your personal support. You may suggest (preferably through the attorney who has retained you) someone else to offer counseling or treatment, but you should not be directly involved in either the referral or the clinical case.

What the Heck Does "Do Not Allow the Lawyer to ... " Mean?

From time to time in this text I say something like "Do not allow the attorney to (send you incomplete records, attribute an opinion to you that you haven't genuinely expressed, etc.)." My point is that you should not knowingly participate in whatever shenanigans are being referred to. Sometimes it's an ethics matter; sometimes it's just bad practice or places you on a sort of "slippery slope." You can attempt to educate the attorney about your role and ethics, but your main "power" if that doesn't work is simply to decline to cooperate or, if the matter is serious, to withdraw from the case. Don't do this lightly, and be aware of the possible consequences of abandoning a case after time and money have been spent, but don't be a pushover, either.

The great majority of the attorneys and firms with whom I have consulted over the past 30 years or so are ethical, straightforward, and easy to work with (yes, even plaintiffs' lawyers). They need you for your skill and expertise, not as some kind of mouthpiece for their cases. Most will not ask you to do anything illegal or unethical (and will often help you to better understand legal and judicial propriety).

There are, however, a few real schmucks (like the one who once told a colleague: "Having an unbiased expert in your case is like having a pacifist in your foxhole"). Try to spot them early (there are often premonitory signs in the first phone call); get away from them as quickly as you can; don't go back to them in the future; and don't do anything your mother wouldn't approve of.

2

VOCABULARY

Yep, a whole chapter on vocabulary. Much of your role involves translating clinical information into the language of lawyers and courts, so much of your success is related to familiarity with legal terms. I'm not trying to make you an attorney, but understanding and communicating with lawyers means that "vocabulary" is too important to relegate to an "appendix." I suggest you read this entire chapter *now* rather than simply referring to it when you think you need it.

By the way, don't rely solely on my definitions; *get an inexpensive dictionary of legal terms.*

Ad litem (**Guardian *ad litem***)   Literally, a guardian "for the purpose of legal action." A guardian *ad litem* is a person (often a lawyer, occasionally a program or agency) appointed by a court to represent, in a legal proceeding, the interests of a child or incapacitated/incompetent person. It is not the same as a conservator or guardian of the person; the duty and responsibility are limited to the legal process.

Amicus (***Amicus curiae***)   In the context of this book, literally a "friend of the court." A person or group that communicates facts and/or opinions (via an "*amicus* brief," in a complex format that is never very "brief") to an appellate court regarding a case that it is scheduled to hear or is deciding whether or not to consider. The *amicus* is not a party to the litigation but has an interest in the outcome (for example, the American Psychological Association may file a brief supporting one side of an appeal involving the rights of mentally disordered offenders). The term does *not* refer to the work of forensic mental health professionals unless they happen to be assisting someone who is preparing an *amicus* brief.

Appeal, Appellate   In the context of this book, the rehearing of some aspect of a case that has already been adjudicated in a trial court. Appeals are almost always appeals of matters of *law*, not matters of fact (for example, procedural matters such as whether or not a judge ruled properly on a motion or whether or not a case was heard in the proper jurisdiction). Thus a trial court finding of guilt or innocence, or whether a plaintiff or civil defendant prevails, is not *per se* a matter for appeal (since these are matters of fact and decided by the "trier of fact"; see below).

When an error in law is found by the appellate court (which may be, but isn't limited to, a state supreme court or the U.S. Supreme Court), that court may or may not overturn the trial court's ultimate finding, depending on the importance of the error. An error important enough to justify overturning a trial court verdict is called a "reversible error."

Appeals are generally allowed for any verdict except one that finds a criminal defendant "not guilty." The judgments of appeals courts (except the U.S. Supreme Court in federal matters or a state supreme court in purely state matters) may themselves be appealed to a higher appeals court.

Appreciate, Appreciation   Something more than the simple concept of "knowing" or verbalizing. Legal criteria for competence and responsibility often separate "knowing" from "appreciating" or "understanding." It is important that definitions be clear when using the term in some contexts (for example, one's knowing she is buying a car vs. appreciating whether or not the purchase is reasonable, or knowing that firing a gun may harm someone vs. appreciating wrongfulness and forming criminal intent).

Capacity   A condition of being able to do something. It may be the same as "competence" in some matters but is often slightly different. See "Competence, Competency," below.

***Certiorari* (Writ of *Certiorari*)**   Certain appellate proceedings to re-examine the actions of a trial court. Today this usually refers to a petition to the U.S. Supreme Court, which may be accepted for hearing or denied (the latter letting the next highest appellate decision stand).

Client (Business Client, Forensic Client)   In this context, the person or entity with whom you have a consultative or expert witness relationship. This relationship is different from, and should not be confused with, either a clinician–patient or a lawyer–client relationship.

Client (Legal Client)   A person or entity who has a fiduciary (q.v.) relationship with an attorney or law firm in which certain services and privileges are expected. This relationship is different from, and should not be confused with, a clinician–patient relationship or the relationship a forensic clinician has with a retaining entity. Note that you *do not* have a lawyer–client relationship with any person involved in your forensic cases; that's just for lawyers.

Client (Psychotherapy or Mental Health Client)   See "Patient," below. I often use the term "patient" rather than "client" or "patient/client" when speaking of someone who is being treated by a clinician. I do not use either term when describing a forensic professional's relationship with a litigant, defendant, or other evaluee (and neither should you).

Competence, Competency A condition of being able to do something. The elements of competence and the level of proof required to establish its presence or absence vary from topic to topic (e.g., competence to consent (q.v.), refuse consent, make a will, change a beneficiary, stand trial, plead, manage one's financial affairs, contract, parent, be sentenced, be executed). It may be the same as "capacity" in some matters but is often slightly different. *Note that competence is an **ability** to do some specified thing, separate from whether or not one **chooses** to do it.*

Consent A condition of allowing something. Valid consent requires adequate *knowledge*, *competence*, and *voluntariness* for the particular activity. Note that the concept of requiring "informed consent" is incomplete without the other two elements (competence and voluntariness). The criteria for competence to consent vary with both the complexity and the anticipated consequences of the proposed action, and thus *the criteria for competence to **consent** to something (such as hospital admission or a medical procedure) should be viewed differently from the criteria for competence to **refuse** it.*

Contingency Fee As used herein, a fee that is either based upon the hiring entity's (e.g., lawyer's) winning or settling the case or levied only if the case is won or settled. Plaintiffs' lawyers routinely work on contingency (at least in part). *Contingency fees are unethical for forensic clinicians and expert witnesses* and may be illegal in some jurisdictions. (Almost all forensic clinicians charge by the hour or day only; a few charge a flat rate for certain activities.)

Defendant In civil matters, a person or entity against whom a lawsuit or other complaint or allegation is brought. In criminal matters, a person accused of a crime or juvenile infraction.

Deposition (Discovery Deposition) A formal process of testimony, usually in civil cases, in which the deponent (usually an expert witness or a fact witness [the same as "lay witness; see below]) is asked by the opposing side's lawyer(s) about his or her background, observations, and (in the case of an expert witness) opinions with regard to a case. This allows the other side to assess the strengths and weaknesses of the case and to "discover" what a witness is likely to say at trial. Depositions also allow the deposing attorney to "lock in" the deponent's opinions and other testimony for trial, so that, if he or she later testifies differently, apparent contradictions can be addressed. Deposition testimony is taken under oath, is recorded, and may be used at trial. (See "Deposition (Trial Deposition)" below.)

Deposition (Trial Deposition) Essentially similar to the above, but used in *lieu* of trial testimony if, for example, the deponent knows that he or she cannot be present at trial.

18

Discovery   A process through which each side in a litigation is allowed access to information possessed by the other side. This increases the fairness of the litigation process, prevents last-minute surprises, and provides time to prepare rebuttals. When your work becomes part of the discovery process, it opens your files, notes, and memory to the other side. *You must respond honestly when asked.*

Duces tecum   See "Subpoena."

Evaluee, Examinee   In our context, a person who is evaluated for some forensic or administrative purpose in the absence of any clinician–patient relationship ("plaintiff" or "defendant" may also be correct). *It is important to refer to such a person as an "evaluee" or "examinee" (or "plaintiff" or "defendant" as appropriate) rather than as a "patient" or "client"* (which would imply a relationship with the evaluator, which should not exist).

Expert Deposition   A discovery deposition of an expert witness, in which his or her opinions may be elicited.

Expert Witness   A type of witness who is allowed to give opinions and who is allowed to consider things not directly observed (including "hearsay" evidence), as well as to testify to "facts" (observations). Expert witnesses are qualified by the court before their testimony is allowed. Expert witnesses need not be outstanding in their fields but should have special and reliable knowledge about a matter before the court. Qualifications considered include training and experience relevant to the case at hand, relevance of proposed testimony, and other criteria. (Contrast with "Fact Witness," below.)

Fact   Often merely a statement made by one side or the other which is relevant to that particular side of a case. "Facts" in legal matters are not necessarily "true" unless a judge says they are true, and then they are true (as a "matter of law") whether they are accurate or not.

Fact Witness ("Lay Witness")   The most common type of witness, and one who is allowed to testify only to what he or she knows from actual observation (e.g., things seen or heard firsthand). Fact witnesses generally are not allowed to give expert opinions (although they slip in from time to time, and certain opinions are permitted when they don't require special knowledge; see chapter 13).

Factfinder   The person or persons who determine whether or not a litigant has met his/her/its burden. This may be a jury or, if there is no jury, a judge. See "Trier" (trier of fact) below.

Fiduciary, Fiduciary Duty   An adjective or a noun which refers to a legal requirement to place another person's interests above virtually any others, including one's own. Banks have a fiduciary duty to their depositors. Doctors have a fiduciary (or near-fiduciary, depending on jurisdiction) duty to their patients. As already noted, that duty to patients or therapy clients generally precludes forensic expert

19

objectivity and credibility, because of the conflict between one's duty to a patient and his or her duty to the court.

Foreseeable, Foreseeability   The reasonable expectation, by a prudent person, that something may occur. The term generally refers to *risk*. *Foreseeability is not the same as predictability*, does not "predict" specific events, and usually need not anticipate specific events. Think of a business with a big, unprotected hole in its sidewalk: a prudent person would expect that someone would eventually be injured, even if most patrons avoided the hole. Applied to mental health topics, it may be foreseeable, for example (that is, there is substantial risk), that a patient who has just tried to kill himself will try again if something doesn't change for the better.

Friend of the Court   See "*Amicus.*"

Guardian *ad litem*   See "*Ad litem.*"

Independent Medical Examination (IME) ("Independent Psychological Examination")   Detailed, in-person examination of a litigant, complainant, or other party to a legal or administrative claim, undertaken by a clinician who may be retained by one side of a case but who has no clinician–patient relationship with the evaluee/examinee. Some jurisdictions reserve the word "independent" for examiners engaged by a judge or other disinterested party; others use the term when the examiner is retained by one side or the other (sometimes with the court's approval).

Know, Knowing   May refer to simple, rote knowledge (such as knowing that one is signing a check or firing a gun); however, "know" may also refer to the broader concepts of understanding and/or "appreciation" (q.v.). It is important that definitions be clear when using the term in some contexts (for example, one's knowing she is buying a car vs. appreciating whether or not the purchase is reasonable, or understanding that firing a gun may harm someone vs. forming criminal intent).

Lay Witness   As used herein, a fact witness (q.v.).

Negligence   As primarily used herein (and called "ordinary" negligence), generally a failure to exercise reasonable care under the circumstances, particularly (e.g., in malpractice actions) when one owes a special "duty of care" (such as that created by a clinician–patient relationship).

There are many kinds of negligence, among them *gross negligence* (sometimes called something like "reckless indifference" or "wanton disregard"), which is a failure to exercise even slight care (definitions vary by jurisdiction).

Opine   To offer an opinion.

Patient (or Psychotherapy or Mental Health "Client" [but not a Lawyer's Client])   As used herein, a person who has a doctor–patient (or clinician–client) relationship with a physician or other clinical professional. Such a relationship creates a number of duties of the clinician to the patient/client. A clinician–patient relationship is different from, and should not be confused with, either an evaluator–evaluee relationship or a lawyer–client relationship.

Plaintiff A person or entity who pursues a civil lawsuit against a defendant. May be called a "complainant" under some circumstances ("complainant" has other meanings as well).

Pro se In our context, referring to a litigant who represents himself. Litigants may be allowed to proceed *pro se* in both civil and criminal matters provided they are competent to do so. Sometimes the court appoints an attorney to assist *pro se* litigants or gives them a bit of latitude with regard to legal technicalities. Being retained by, or acting as an expert for, a *pro se* litigant raises a number of practical and ethical issues for forensic practitioners.

Prosecutor A government attorney who pursues criminal charges against a defendant. The pursuit of charges is called "prosecution."

Reasonable A concept dearly loved by the law but rarely defined in statute. Such concepts as "reasonable" actions and a "reasonable" clinician are not informal, but are often used in statute and case law and carefully considered by judges and juries. "Reasonable" is commonly associated with "prudent." *Do not use these terms lightly*, as they often have special meaning in legal settings.

Reasonable Medical Certainty/Probability (Psychiatric or Psychological Certainty or Probability) A legal phrase with no comparable clinical definition, which translates in almost all jurisdictions to "more likely than not." Reasonable certainty or probability *is not* the same as "beyond reasonable doubt" and *does not* refer to any clinical concept (for example, it does not refer to the level of certainty used to diagnose or treat patients). Different jurisdictions use different terms ("certainty," "probability," etc.).

Retain, Retainer, Retention A *retainer* is an advance fee intended to establish a relationship—for example, a payment to an attorney to establish a lawyer–client relationship or a payment to a forensic consultant or expert from a lawyer or other entity who wishes to hire (*retain*) him or her. One may be retained (hired, contracted) without any retainer fee. It is similar to a deposit against future expenses or hours of work, but a broader concept, and it may or may not be refundable. In forensic practice, retainers are optional but often a very good idea.

Retainers help to establish the business agreement before work is started, prevent some income loss if the attorney or other hiring entity refuses to (or cannot) pay the bill, and can provide important "leverage" in disagreements about billing. With the last item in mind, it is very important that forensic practitioners deal fairly with those who retain them and promptly refund any money to which the expert is not entitled.

Retainers should not be confused with contingency fees (q.v.), which are *per se* unethical for expert witnesses.

Spoliation (of Evidence) Destroying evidence—in forensic work, most commonly the inappropriate destruction of records, including one's professional or forensic notes. "Spoliation" itself refers to injury beyond repair.

Standard of Care (SOC) In most jurisdictions, referring to negligence allegations, for example, "that level of care expected from reasonable clinicians of similar training and experience in a similar circumstance." The definition is similar for hospitals and other treatment/care/custody facilities.

The standard of care is generally *national*, rarely local or regional. It usually applies regardless of the sophistication of the clinical setting. Thus a small rural hospital is generally expected to meet the same SOC as a university medical center, given the same clinical situation and its accepting the patient. Similarly, community clinicians are generally expected to meet the same standards for adequate care (see below) as cosmopolitan or academic practitioners, assuming the same situations.

The SOC is a standard of *adequacy*, not of excellence, and is not necessarily what any particular expert would have done. There is often more than one way to meet the standard of care.

Regarding "reasonable clinicians of similar training . . .," controversial care advocated by a relatively small group of practitioners *may* be within the SOC, so long as the practitioners are "reasonable" in their work. On the other hand, if lots of clinicians or facilities practice poorly or inadequately, their numbers alone do not establish the poor or inadequate care as "standard" (or protect negligent practice from malpractice allegations). For example, even though many clinicians and hospitals may allow financial issues (such as insurance policies or managed care plans) to dictate care, that practice often leads to care which is below the SOC.

Subpoena A demand to appear (e.g., in court) or to produce (provide) something (e.g., *subpoena duces tecum*, a demand to produce one's records).

A subpoena may come from a lawyer rather than a judge, the former having less weight of demand. You may or may not be obligated to respond, or respond completely, unless it is signed by a judge, but *never ignore a subpoena. Check with the lawyer who retained you, or your own attorney, before failing to accede to the demand.*

You should not destroy anything in your file after receiving a *subpoena duces tecum* unless a judge or the lawyer who retained you says that it is proper to do so.

Trier The person or body that decides things in a trial or hearing. The *trier of law*, who is always a judge (sometimes more than one in appellate cases), decides points of law. The *trier of fact* ("fact finder"), who may be a jury or (*if and only if there is no jury*) the judge, decides which side's case is the more convincing. All trials have both a trier of law and a trier of fact. When there is no jury (called "bench" trials/hearings), the judge is both the trier of law and the trier of fact.

Work Product, Attorney Work Product   Things a lawyer does, or discusses, for or with a client. Attorney work product is extremely confidential, *but it generally does not include things an expert witness does or things an expert receives from the lawyer*. "Work product" almost never applies to *your* work (there are exceptions).

3

LAWYER–EXPERT RELATIONSHIPS

Forensic Practice Relationships

When you are acting as an expert witness, your relationship should be with the lawyer or other retaining entity, not with the litigant him-/her-/itself. If someone other than a lawyer or judge calls or emails you to inquire about a personal (or family) forensic matter, *do not* do anything that might form a clinical or business relationship with that person. Don't discuss the situation, express an opinion, or make any agreement. Simply say politely that you work only through third parties (attorneys, courts, insurance companies, etc.) and that talking with the (potential) litigant directly may harm any involvement you might eventually have. *Do not* suggest that the person might or might not "have a good case," and refrain from recommending specific lawyers.

When contacted by a law firm, you may talk initially with an assistant of some kind. Be sure your eventual business agreement is with a person who is authorized to contract with you and to guarantee payment from that firm or agency. Payment may ultimately come from a third party, such as a litigant or insurance company, but I strongly recommend that you do not *rely* on any litigant for payment, either directly or indirectly. It should be clear that you will bill, and expect payment from, the attorney or other retaining entity (unless, for example, you have contracted with an insurance carrier itself).

Initial Attorney Contact

Don't charge for the initial call. You'd be surprised how many colleagues try to start charging as soon as they pick up the phone. That's a good way to alienate someone who is considering working with you.

Ascertain possible conflicts of interest early, and discuss them with the attorney. Ask the litigant's names, for example, to see whether or not any of them creates a conflict. Sometimes one has worked with an opposing counsel on another forensic matter. This does not usually create a conflict, but it should be disclosed early. If you are *currently* working with the opposing counsel, the new case should probably be declined. Sometimes disclosing identifying information about other retention or cases is improper. It may be helpful to defer details and, if necessary, contact the other lawyer for guidance. (Note also that some law firms are so large that either you may not know that a lawyer with whom you're working is in the same firm or the branches or sections are sufficiently unrelated as not to create a significant conflict. Government agencies and some nongovernmental organizations, such as the U.S. Department of Justice [DOJ] or the American Civil Liberties Union [ACLU] fall into a similar category; disclose the possible conflict and discuss it with the new attorney as appropriate.)

Lawyers from a "state's attorney's" office (the agency that serves as legal counsel for that state) interviewed me about possible retention in a lawsuit. Although I was willing to serve as an expert, they did not follow up or retain me. Several months later, lawyers for the other side of the same matter contacted me about the same case. I disclosed the earlier contact and the facts that I had no agreement with the state in the case and had not done work on it for them. The second group of lawyers retained me and eventually disclosed to the other side, without incident, that I would be one of their experts.

Many months into the litigation, a lawyer from a different section of the same state's attorney's office contacted me about a different matter. I disclosed the fact that I was already working on a case with private lawyers opposing a government position represented by the same state's attorney's office. I suggested that (1) I discuss the possible new retention with the current lawyers and (2) the assistant state's attorney discuss it with her agency colleagues as well. In the end, the assistant state's attorney did not believe there would be a conflict (because her section was quite separate from the other litigation), and the private attorneys had no problem with my being hired by the "opposition" in a separate matter (indeed, they saw some advantage to the fact that the opposing counsel respected their expert in that way).

Don't believe everything the lawyer says about the case. If you're taking notes, indicate that they reflect what the attorney said in a brief conversation and are not necessarily accurate or complete. Some lawyers are more straightforward than others, and many will be trying to "get you on board" with their cases. Get your facts from your own reviews and examinations.

Understand that your all your notes are probably discoverable should you be retained, and anticipate that they will be seen by the other side. Don't be cavalier when writing things down. Incidentally, it is the *information* you receive or exchange that is discoverable, not merely your notes, recordings, or physical things the lawyer sends to you. You probably will not be able to remember the content of a conversation months or years later, but, if you do, you must disclose it if asked to do so during testimony.

Try to avoid discussing so much before being retained that you can't ethically work with the other side if the first caller doesn't retain you (see example above). It is fairly unusual to be called by both sides of a case, but it can happen under at least three circumstances, two of which are innocent and the other a real pain in the neck. If you practice locally, both sides' lawyers may have you in their Rolodexes (Rolodices?). If you are somewhat well known, both sides in cases outside your locale may call coincidentally. Finally, lawyers for one side or the other may contact you in an attempt to preclude your being retained by the other side (or, occasionally, to intimidate the other side), with no real intention of using you. Sometimes they just call; sometimes they actually hire you; and sometimes they don't bother to hire you but list you as their expert anyway. This is known as a "phantom expert" situation (see below).

Don't offer opinions based on an initial call or even represent that your participation will support the lawyer's side. Remember, (1) you have heard only one side of the story, (2) in brief summary form, (3) usually early in the discovery phase of the case. (4) You probably haven't received any written records, and (5) you haven't put much thought into it.

If you are not a good expert for the case, cannot participate for some reason, or simply don't wish to become involved, consider referring the attorney to another expert. Be polite and helpful, not just self-serving, even if you are not retained.

What You Need from the Lawyer before Proceeding

You will require the following from the lawyer:

- an accurate case description, with the official "styling" (name) of the case if it has been filed;
- a clear understanding of your role (sometimes *you* define it, so be sure it's clear and ethical);
- a clear and binding agreement for your fees;
- an expectation that you will receive all available relevant records (not just summaries or "chronologies");
- time and freedom to review the records completely;
- the general schedule of the case, deadlines, etc., with timely updates (be certain you are prepared to meet the relevant deadlines);
- the attorney's understanding of your work procedure and ethics (e.g., how you review, how you will communicate, and your statement that

you will be honest and objective and will not render opinions that are not justified).

Are you a "phantom expert"? That means being listed or declared without your knowledge—for example, when an attorney lists you as his or her expert after contacting you, but without an agreement, declares that you hold opinions that you've never formally rendered, or even lists you as his or her expert without *any* contact. When this occurs, it's a big problem.

- It misrepresents you and your opinions.
- It limits your ability to contract with an opposing attorney.
- It keeps opposing lawyers from considering contacting you.
- It often cheats you out of legitimate fees.

Using "phantom experts" may not be as unethical for lawyers as one would think. Forensic clinicians who have been used in this way often complain about dishonest practices or listing without compensation (*if* they somehow discover the dastardly behavior), and one can contact a judge or consider legal action for using one's likeness or name without consent (or for "restraint of trade"), but it's tough to get satisfaction. Judges rarely side with experts in such circumstances unless a law or court rule has been broken. (See Appendix A for the wording in my initial letter to attorneys, which may prevent some of these problems.)

A Typical Case Review Process

Initial call from a lawyer or other potential retaining entity Spend 15 to 30 minutes learning about the case or other legal matter, getting to know the attorney, answering his or her questions, deciding whether or not you want to participate and can be useful, and agreeing on the process. Take notes and get relevant identifying information. Do not charge for this call. At this point, you have not been "retained" (see below) and probably owe no duty to the caller.

I do not recommend that this step be completed by email. One can learn far more, and make far better decisions about being retained, in a telephone or in-person meeting than by email or letter. When I get an email offering to retain me, to send records, or asking for detailed information, I always suggest that we speak by telephone and rarely, if ever, answer in detail about the case.[1]

---

1 Note that this email suggestion is different from dealing with an email that simply asks for information without anticipating being hired as an expert. It is fine (and often rewarding) occasionally to answer brief, general questions from students, lawyers, or others. *Your answers should be generic, and should not imply forensic or clinical "opinions" or that you agree to be retained in any matter.*

Establish a written agreement/contract² If you are willing to participate, send some sort of a letter of understanding indicating your willingness and requirements (such as fees, procedures, and schedule). I use real stationery; others may use email. Real stationery looks and feels better (see "Initial Letter" example, Appendix A). If you are presented with a contract that you didn't create, be sure you understand what you are signing and that it covers your requirements as well as those of the client.

Receive records Request, and expect, *all* the available and relevant records. "Records" often include clinical, school, employment, legal, corrections, etc., records, legal materials or citations (as relevant to a forensic clinician), others' forensic or clinical reports, and/or depositions and statements by litigants or other parties.

Complete an initial review You may or may not choose to review only selected records at this point (see below). Take notes as needed, understanding that these are probably discoverable if you are officially "listed" or declared an expert in the case (especially if it is a civil case). *Do not offer opinions without adequate review of the relevant records.* Don't be bullied into expressing opinions in a report or affidavit, or in testimony, if you don't have all the information you believe is important.

It is reasonable to perform an initial, limited review for the purpose of preliminary discussion with the attorney. Talking with the lawyer after a preliminary review helps the attorney, may focus your role in the case, or may even suggest to the lawyer that your work is not likely to be helpful to his or her case (don't take it personally). If you do express opinions at this early point, include disclaimers when they seem necessary. For example,

> *. . . Although I have reviewed detailed records of past hospitalizations and clinic visits, I have not examined the plaintiff. Such an examination could provide information which would change the opinions below.*

or

> *. . . My review to date has necessarily been limited to the clinical record; vocational records are not available to me at this writing. Although some inferences may be drawn based upon his diagnosis and the clinicians'*

---

2 Cases often have multiple litigants, which sometimes creates separate legal cases (such as when more than one person is injured in an accident). When the cases are separate, create separate cases in your own office as well, even though the matters may be tried together. That usually means separate retainers, separate files, separate evaluations, separate billings, etc.

> *progress notes, specific opinions concerning Mr. _____'s actual work performance cannot be rendered without credible information about his workplace functioning and behavior.*

or

> *... It should be noted that the comments and opinions in this preliminary report are based upon the assumption that the events in question happened essentially as Ms. _____ described them to her psychiatrist and in her deposition. I reserve the right to change or withdraw any opinion should additional, credible information suggest otherwise.*

Communicate with the lawyer or retaining entity   Communicate orally with the lawyer or retaining entity about your preliminary review, any need for further records, and/or next steps (such as client examination, report, or testimony). In general, do not communicate opinions in writing, or create any written report, unless the retaining entity requests it. Sometimes, talking with the lawyer after a preliminary review helps focus your role in the case or even suggests that you should stop your participation, particularly if the findings appear to be heading in an unexpected direction.

Many cases – especially civil ones – end here. (See following chapters for later processes and procedures.) The great majority of cases never get to trial (some, of course, are not even filed at the time you become involved); many are resolved one way or another before reports are written or expert depositions taken.

Examinations, interviews, and/or testing   Did I forget about examining the litigant or other party(parties)? No; there's a reason those aren't usually priorities at this point (but we'll discuss them soon).

Lawyers often call saying they just want to schedule an "independent medical examination" ("IME"), *but scheduling IMEs before adequate review and discussion often leads to unnecessary, premature, or inadequate evaluations* (and not a few scheduling headaches). With the exception of insurance company disability reviews, I rarely schedule in-person evaluations without at least some record review and discussion with the attorney.

4

RECORDS AND RECORD REVIEW

First, a point that I used to think was obvious until a forensic supervisee told me he was retrieving an evaluee's past clinical records himself: *Providing the records is the lawyer's (or retaining entity's) job, not yours.*

Obtaining records for forensic review is a big deal. It requires a lot of time and some specific legal procedures in order to be certain the request (often actually a demand) is taken seriously and the materials are complete and unaltered. It's not just a matter of obtaining authorization and asking for them, or of having the evaluee bring them.

Records for forensic review (e.g., of health care, psychotherapy, employment, education, arrest and conviction) are usually obtained by subpoena. The subpoena wording makes sure that the person who complies is a responsible records custodian (such as a hospital records clerk) and demands "true," complete, and unaltered copies.

The level of completeness a lawyer attains is far better than that obtained by most forensic practitioners (and you don't have subpoena power). The lawyer (or legal assistant) already knows where to get various kinds of records (such as schools, archives, law-enforcement agencies, corrections agencies) that are usually unfamiliar to clinicians. Finally, it is handy to be able to hold the retaining lawyer responsible for getting you everything relevant that is available.

The Retaining Entity Must Send You *All* Relevant and Reasonably Available Records

Overkill is better than inadequate records. You are the main person who decides what is relevant for your review. Skim virtually everything to make that decision (but be fair; don't spend the lawyer's money on the details of superfluous materials). Being "blind-sided" by the opposing lawyer with additional, relevant records during testimony is bad for the case and often embarrassing.

You may suggest that the records be organized in some way that is easy to review, perhaps with tabs, a table of contents, or (in some cases) even an index (but not altered or "filtered"). You will receive copies of the lawyer's copies, so they will often have been organized or digitized already, so that it's easy to put them into convenient order. It is very tedious (and expensive for the retaining entity) for you to slog through one or more file boxes of generic, identical-appearing copier pages.

Lawyers often offer to send records electronically or on a DVD. Some people prefer reviewing on a computer or electronic reader; I don't, in most cases (but it's great to have a searchable version handy). They'll usually send you paper if you request it, especially if you tell them your office will have to charge a printing fee after the first 20 or so pages (be fair; don't overcharge).

Do not allow the lawyer to send records piecemeal until you come to an opinion that he or she likes. On the other hand, in matters with voluminous records, I sometimes suggest that a lawyer send me *representative* records for preliminary review (or mark certain records as ones he believes are most relevant) in order to provide some early discussion about the merits of my part of a case. I am careful not to construe this as sufficient to form opinions.

Writing a final report without seeing all available records is at best iffy and at worst unethical and dishonest. Provide disclaimers when relevant records are missing.

With regard to taking notes, it's okay to write on any record *copies* you receive, but those pages may have to be recopied later for the discovery process.

Record Review Is Not as Private as it Seems

Once you are declared as an expert in a case, everything you create is (probably) discoverable. (See "Discovery" in chapter 2.)

Don't be snide or cavalier in notes, letters, or emails. Do take notes (your memory isn't good enough to remember everything important), but write them as if someone on the other side will be reading them in the future (which is often the case). The following doesn't refer to an expert witness's notes, but it makes the point and the example is too good to pass up.

A psychotherapist was sued by the family of a former patient who had committed suicide. The therapist initially refused to turn over his notes to the plaintiff's lawyer, citing a mistaken impression that "process notes" were somehow different from ordinary clinical records and could be withheld from scrutiny.[1] When they were

---

1 That's another lesson of this example: Although one may store psychotherapy notes separately from the rest of the clinical chart, they generally have no special status under the law and must be given up along with the rest of the record when circumstances (such as lawsuits and lawful subpoenas) demand them.

eventually obtained, I saw the reason for his concern. The margins contained a number of embarrassing notations and drawings indicating that he was very bored by the patient; he found her conversations trivial and comical, and he counted the minutes until her sessions were over.

Tell the attorney that you will communicate orally with him or her after your review (not by email) and that you won't write a report without being instructed to do so. Emails, letters, and reports generated during the course of expert review are discoverable and should be carefully composed with the attorney's needs in mind (without doing anything dishonest). If a report is desired, wait for the lawyer to request it, then discuss the format and likely content beforehand (but without allowing the lawyer either to write the report for you or to dictate content which misrepresents your opinions by either omission or commission; see chapter 6). *Lawyers hate surprises.*

Do not destroy your own notes, records, emails, phone messages, report drafts, etc., unless you are certain that doing so is proper. In particular, if you receive a subpoena for your records (a *subpoena duces tecum*, routine when the other side is about to depose you), be certain that you safeguard for the discovery process all the notes and records that you possess.

A somewhat forensically inexperienced clinician was being deposed as a plaintiff's expert in a particularly sensational case involving several defendants. He had been retained as an expert and had not treated any of the parties. Lawyers from several firms were in the room as he began to answer questions in front of the court reporter.

LAWYER: Did you receive my *subpoena duces tecum*, doctor, asking you to bring all of your notes to the deposition?

DEPONENT: Yes.

LAWYER: And may I see those notes, please?

DEPONENT: They aren't available.

LAWYER: Really? May I ask why not?

DEPONENT: I shredded them after I received your subpoena.

LAWYER (SOMEWHAT TAKEN ABACK): May I ask why you shredded your notes in this case after being specifically asked to produce them for this deposition?

DEPONENT: They were my private notes, and I believed they might contain something harmful to [the plaintiffs].

The deposing lawyer spent the next several minutes explaining the concept of "spoliation of evidence" and sarcastically asking, on the record and in front of several lawyers who would likely spread the story to many others, why the doctor should not be charged with a felony for knowingly destroying evidence.

Your work is rarely "work product." That's for lawyers, not experts, even if you happen to be a lawyer yourself. If in doubt about whether or not something in your files is discoverable, consult the attorney who retained you.

Be Objective When Discussing the Case with the Lawyer

Cover the pros and cons of how your findings could affect the case, in terms the attorney can understand. Do not play "shrink" or use a lot of psychobabble; the lawyer wants to know what you think, wants you to be clear and concise, and wants to see that you can convey your findings to others (such as jury members) in an articulate and unambivalent manner when necessary. He or she has probably talked with lots of psychiatrists and psychologists, and is nervous that our stereotypic ambivalence and intellectualization will obscure, not clarify, his or her case in court.

If the findings seem ambiguous or your views are ambivalent, now is the time to talk them out and try to find clarity (if there is clarity to be found). Use this early discussion, going back and forth over the details, to focus your thoughts, so that you can be as concise as the findings allow when writing a report or testifying.

Delegation and Consultation

- In general, *review all records yourself*. If an assistant helps with your review, let the attorney know.
- Be cautious when delegating anything for which you charge *your* fee and/or for which you must take personal responsibility (including anything to which you may testify).
- Don't seek outside consultation without the retaining attorney's agreement, but feel free to suggest it for matters outside your expertise.
- Be sure to "vet" personally those with whom you consult (e.g., have personal knowledge of them or reasonably verify their qualifications). If you do not know them personally, include a *caveat* to that effect.
- Persons with whom you consult about a case usually must be disclosed, and they may be asked by the other side to give their own testimony (e.g., to be deposed).

Giving "Bad" News

What if your early findings don't seem to support the lawyer's case?

Lawyers often benefit from expert findings that go against their clients almost as much as they benefit from findings that support them. They need to know *both* the strengths and the weaknesses of their cases in order to evaluate case merits objectively, save time and money on frivolous litigation, promote reasonable settlements and negotiations, and help their clients accept the truth about their situations. In addition, if you find that there are few merits in the psychological or psychiatric issues of a case, expressing or (if asked) documenting that finding may protect the attorney from later criticism for not pursuing them (e.g., for not pursuing an insanity defense in a criminal matter).

Conversely, however, it is important to realize that *objectivity is not the same as extreme obsessiveness about the pros and cons of a case.* Be able to see the "big picture" and prioritize your findings accordingly, but don't shade your opinions toward what the lawyer seems to *want* you to find.

5

EVALUATIONS

Lawyers or courts sometimes ask experts for "just an IME (independent medical examination), nothing fancy." It may be a "simple" disability or damage assessment or a fitness evaluation, or the attorney may believe he or she has an uncomplicated case. Many of them believe that psychiatrists and psychologists who spend an hour with someone can somehow figure out everything there is to know about that person.

"Simple" evaluations almost always require record review before interview or examination, and they should *always* be treated with the same professional routine as any other case that comes your way. That means the same initial letter, fee agreement, record review, and, usually, discussion with the attorney before proceeding to one's review and examination.[1] Clinicians who do several jail or worker's compensation assessments per week, for example, may argue, and many clinician-employees or contractors for repeated assessments have an acceptable office routine, but I strongly advise a complete administrative procedure for anyone who does IMEs on a private practice basis.

Dr. X, a well-qualified clinician, did "routine" trial competency evaluations at a large city-county jail. He had a court contract to do assessments whenever ordered and to provide reports to both the prosecution and defense counsel, all at a flat rate per evaluee.

Every Monday his assistant would give Dr. X a list of several defendants/evaluees for whom his report was due the following Monday. His contract provided for identical payment for each defendant, about equal

1 The only exceptions I can think of right now are for acute dangerousness and examination of a criminal defendant as soon as feasible after the alleged offense. Assessment of criminal responsibility (associated with a defense of not guilty by reason of insanity {NGRI, NRRI}) is greatly aided by seeing the defendant within hours or days of the incident (provided defense counsel has been appointed and authorizes the examination). If it has already been a couple of weeks since the event, there's probably no rush.

to his fee for five hours of (non-forensic) private practice time. That amount was to cover all necessary review, discussion with counsel, seeking of corroborating information, travel, waiting time, examination, report preparation, and (when necessary) court testimony. Thinking that his usual patient evaluations took far less than five hours, he had calculated that the compensation would be sufficient "on average," and that the money and time charged would "work out in the end."

Dr. X tried hard to meet the court's demands (and his own high expectations) for each case, but what began as a regular schedule soon became crowded and chaotic, and he found himself working late at night and on weekends to meet his deadlines. He often spent more hours than anticipated to do an adequate evaluation.

Then another problem arose. Some of the judges made unusual, burdensome, or even forensically inappropriate requests in their evaluation orders. Many ordered "evaluation of the defendant's competency to stand trial and legal sanity" (adding a criminal responsibility assessment). Some asked for "recommendations for sentencing." Dr. X was reluctant to complain, cite the provisions of his contract, or suggest renegotiation, believing that competition for his job was fierce. On the one hand, he liked the regular income; on the other, life was pretty miserable for him and his family.

When Dr. X consulted me about his dilemma, my recommendations were pretty simple.

1. Terminate the court contract and deal with each case individually rather than "in bulk" (albeit with individual court contracts, a simple process).
2. Use roughly the same administrative and practice procedure for each court-referred case as for his other forensic clients.
3. Demand clear and written expectations in each assessment order (that is, competency vs. criminal responsibility vs. other things) and clarify them with the court as necessary.
4. Consider charging according to time spent rather than trying to "average" the fee per defendant.[2]

I also suggested that Dr. X meet, over time, with the parties usually involved in his cases—the judges, prosecutors, some defense lawyers, and even court clerks—to help them understand his processes and to discuss how he could best meet their needs while dealing reasonably with his own.

---

2 Why do I recommend against most "package pricing" for forensic work? See chapter 8.

Know Your Stuff

- Don't exceed your clinical abilities.
- Know your stuff *forensically*. Forensic work is a subspecialty. Reading this book will help, but don't represent yourself as a forensic psychiatrist or psychologist (or bill as one) unless you have the requisite knowledge and experience.
- Know the clinical subspecialty involved in the evaluation, if there is one (such as child psychology or psychiatry, substance abuse, clinical nuances such as suicidology).
- When relevant, know the language of the person being assessed. Forensic evaluations should almost never be done through an interpreter; refer the case to someone who is fully capable of doing the evaluation in the appropriate language. If the evaluation absolutely must be done through an interpreter, be certain that he or she is properly qualified and that you understand the nuances of using one.
- Avoid, or be able to deal effectively with, significant countertransference and personal conflict (e.g., disgust, titillation, political views).

What if the Evaluee Fails to Appear or Doesn't Cooperate?

Opposing attorney refusal (usually a plaintiff's lawyer in civil matters or a defense lawyer in criminal cases)   The opposing attorney may believe an evaluation would jeopardize his or her case or may not wish to expose it to additional scrutiny. He may allege that the evaluee would be traumatized by the examination. Opposing lawyers may place unreasonable restrictions on one's evaluation (see below).

These are usually matters for the lawyers to work out, not issues for the expert. Tell the lawyer or judge who retained you (a) the extent to which not doing an evaluation may affect your ability to form opinions, (b) the extent to which not doing an evaluation may affect your credibility, (c) the disclaimer you will add to any report or opinions that lack an appropriate examination, and (d) that psychological/psychiatric evaluations are almost never "traumatic" for evaluees.

Evaluee refusal   If an evaluee calls to cancel, or doesn't keep the appointment, contact the entity or lawyer who retained you. Do not reschedule or "negotiate" directly with the evaluee unless it is simply a matter of scheduling a more convenient time (and then notify the retaining entity).

If an evaluee balks after arriving or demands to leave after the interview has begun, be polite, generally encourage him or her to stay, and briefly try to address any concerns that may be making him or her uncomfortable.

Don't "negotiate" extensively or do things that may be construed as manipulation or "extortion" in return for completing the examination. If the evaluee actually ends the interview prematurely, politely tell him or her that you will need to note that in the evaluation record. Keep the lawyer who retained you informed about whatever happens.

Outside Consultation

If you believe outside consultation (such as psychological testing, general medical examination, laboratory tests, or neuroimaging) is needed in order to do a good evaluation, talk with your retaining entity before arranging it. Explain that you believe that the evaluation requires additional procedures or expertise. That discussion should include

- whether the additional person will be "your" consultant or hired separately by the lawyer, court, agency, or other retaining entity (and thus a separately retained expert);
- how the additional consultant will be paid (be cautious about extending payment from your own office);
- telling the consultant that he or she will probably be vulnerable to discovery and deposition by the other side of the case; and
- the knowledge that, so far as you know, any consultant you personally recommend is well qualified, has no prior relationship to the evaluee, and understands his or her forensic role in the case.

Scheduling

In general, *don't schedule examinations before reviewing background information*. If a lawyer asks you to see a client immediately, *slow down* and go through your routine case/evaluation procedures (but note that some evaluations for criminal responsibility or dangerousness should take place as soon as feasible).

Give the retaining attorney or agency your interview specifications and explain *why* they are your specifications (but try not to be a *prima donna*). Make sure everyone understands your role, the procedures you expect to use (including pre-examination review and post-examination communications), what results may reasonably be expected (not a prediction of assessment findings, but the *kinds* of information one can anticipate from whatever type of examination you are contemplating), the likely number and durations of interviews and/or testing (sometimes examination involves more than one session), the location and environment, recording procedures, and approximate cost (which should usually be predicated on time and expenses).

Except for simple things like verifying times or giving directions, *communicate through the retaining attorney or agency, not directly with the evaluee or his or her attorney* (unless the attorney is also the person who retained you).

Be very cautious when someone requests an evaluation for himself or a relative. I do not accept such requests or discuss the matter with the caller. I politely let him or her know that I cannot deal directly with potential evaluees or litigants and would be happy to talk with his or her attorney or the requesting agency.

Avoid evaluations or referral sources that curtail your ability to do a complete workup. If the referring lawyer or agency wants a "quickie," or otherwise unreasonably limits what you may do or to whom you may speak, run like the wind.

The Evaluation Setting

Use a professional office when feasible, either yours or that of a colleague (for example, when evaluating someone in a distant community). Avoid personal settings such as a home office, a hotel room, or the evaluee's home. (An evaluee's home is sometimes appropriate, for example, for some child or family evaluations or civil capacity assessments.) Avoid doing assessments in lawyers' offices.

The furnishings should be compatible with good interview technique. You already know what that is.

See below for law-enforcement, jail, and prison settings and for the interview procedure itself.

Jail/Prison Settings

Have a "contact" visit whenever feasible. That means trying very hard not to have to talk through a security screen or a hole in a plexiglass barrier or on one of those little visitor phones. Interviewing through glass via "telephone" is the worst. Don't accept either unless security needs force them. A face-to-face interview using shackles, or even through bars, is better than one through glass or detail-obscuring screen. "Anchored" shackles are safer but may be prohibited.

A private room that can be monitored visually (e.g., through a window) is ideal. *Ask for the kind of room in which lawyers talk with their clients.* Have the evaluee face away from the monitoring window if feasible.

Have the retaining lawyer or agency arrange the visit in advance, understanding your requirements and preferences. Custody staff are very security conscious (and don't want to put their jobs in jeopardy); carry something in writing that clarifies the conditions that have been authorized.

- *Attend to your safety* (see below).
- *Privacy is second only to security and safety.* Ask the evaluee if he or she thinks the setting is private enough.
- *Do not conduct individual assessments around other inmates* (although you may wish to observe a defendant with other inmates).

- Except in extreme circumstances, *do not interview inmates within earshot of security staff.* You may have to leave a door slightly open for security, but custody officers should not be in the room.
- *Be nice to the officers and security staff,* and they will often try to provide what you need and advise you about your safety (see below).
- *Lawyers should almost never be present* (see "Lawyer Presence," below).

Your Safety

Listen up; this is important. It applies to all evaluation and clinical settings, not just to correctional facilities.

- *First,* **never knowingly put yourself in danger.** Inattention to—*or overconfidence about*—assault by evaluees and patients has gotten several evaluators killed. Your gender and size are relevant to a point, but even large men can be seriously hurt or killed by relatively small, unpredictable evaluees.
- *Do not believe that you can predict, "sense," or "talk down" assaultive behavior in enraged, desperate, frightened, psychotic, or confused evaluees.* If you do sense danger, act on your intuition, but *do not rely on sensing danger to keep you safe.*
- *Do not let anyone put you in danger, or accept a setting you believe is dangerous.* If a correctional officer, nurse, or other person assigns you to a setting that you believe may not be safe, ask for a safer one, a monitor, and/or a chaperone as needed. *Don't be shy about this.*
- "Panic buttons" and advice such as "don't sit between the evaluee and the door" are woefully overrated (especially when the door is locked).
- Security staff can often keep you safe while staying out of earshot (e.g., by monitoring through a window).
- Consider asking the security staff for suggestions about the evaluee and your safety.

Feeling safe helps you (and often the evaluee) complete a better assessment. Noting your own feelings and perceptions during the interview can add to the overall evaluation, but being significantly concerned about your safety, and/or feeling intimidated by the evaluee, is likely to alter the findings to some extent.

Who May Be Present During the Assessment?

I'm referring here to persons actually in the interview/examination room, not those merely monitoring from outside or by video.

Alone is best, if it can be accomplished safely. Security/corrections staff should almost never be within earshot. (See safety considerations and jail/prison notes, above.)

Lawyers should not be present, though they sometimes demand it and may have a legal right to be there (to protect their clients' rights, for example). It's almost always a bad idea from the standpoint of evaluation quality. Discuss your concerns, evaluation requirements, and recording procedures with the retaining attorney; he or she should convey them to the opposing lawyer if necessary. (See "Lawyer Presence," below.)

Videographers are often part of litigant interviews. Experienced ones know how to be unobtrusive, but I prefer an unattended camera. Don't use a "hidden" camera; that's unprofessional and may be unethical (you're not filming a reality TV show).

If you need *a translator or an interpreter*[3], you may not have read the argument (above) against interviewing evaluees without a very good understanding of their language and culture. Be that as it may, be sure you know how to use them properly (many interviewers don't). Use a good one. Avoid those who aren't professionals and experienced in the relevant field. Family members *may* occasionally be acceptable, within confidentiality and credibility limits, but they (a) are not usually forensic or mental health professionals, (b) often don't understand the terms, (c) often misinterpret or misreport evaluees' answers, and (d) are routinely biased.

Sometimes an *attendant, nurse, or chaperone* is required for evaluee safety, examiner safety, or liability concerns. They should be unobtrusive (usually out of earshot), avoid interfering unnecessarily with the interview/examination, and afford as much privacy as feasible.

Family or co-plaintiffs/co-defendants should not be present without good reason. A parent or guardian may be recommended or required for children's interviews/examinations. Sometimes there is a procedural reason or forensic purpose in group interviews (such as for some parts of child custody evaluations or as a preliminary to individual interviews when several people have been involved in a traumatic situation). If you believe that a child evaluee should be seen alone but the family or lawyer demands that a relative be present, assess the extent to which his or her presence might interfere, document your recommendation, and either proceed (with the retaining attorney's knowledge) or postpone the examination until the procedure can be clarified.

Lawyer Presence

I've already said that having a lawyer in the room is not advisable for an accurate evaluation, though the evaluee may be entitled to it. Do not accept a lawyer's presence without careful consideration by you and the lawyer/entity who retained you. An audio or video recording of the

---

3 Vocabularian purists differentiate the two; I won't in this book. They probably don't like being called "vocabularians" either.

assessment, particularly with an unattended recorder or camera (see above), is often a good idea and may decrease the attorney's concerns.

If an attorney is present, he or she must be out of evaluee's vision and be silent. Don't tolerate lawyer interference. If it occurs, document it carefully and consider terminating the assessment.

Even considering the above, be polite and professional, not defensive. It's the lawyer's case and client, not yours.

Recording (Audio or Video)

I recommend recording most IMEs and other evaluations. The benefits usually outweigh the drawbacks. Video, when feasible, is usually preferred over audio.

- Recording provides accurate, usually unimpeachable, documentation.
- It decreases some evaluator liability (e.g., for alleged inappropriate behavior).
- It renders detailed note-taking unnecessary.
- It helps with report writing.
- It may increase the evaluator's credibility (e.g., by showing willingness to subject one's process to scrutiny).
- It may defuse attorney requests to be present in the interview.
- It may reassure the evaluee that the evaluator will be honest and objective.

Drawbacks (or purported drawbacks) include lawyers' concerns that recording everything will reveal things they don't wish to highlight (remember, lawyers hate surprises). This is insufficient reason to decide not to record, but one may have to abide by the attorney's wishes. If you are asked during testimony why you did not record the interview, simply tell the truth.

Concerns that recording will alter the accuracy and atmosphere of the interview are overblown. Properly done, the process is usually innocuous. Employing a videographer, however, *is* often intrusive. When using a videographer, try to have him or her start the video, then leave the room, and later verify that the camera was running continuously.

Professional videographers are often preferred, particularly when the record must be certified. Use forensically experienced ones when feasible.

Do not record interviews or examinations surreptitiously.

If the equipment malfunctions or you make a mistake in the recording process (formerly known as leaving the lens cap on), simply document the problem promptly and carefully.

Sometimes evaluees bring their own recorders (which they are probably entitled to do). Don't make a big deal of it, but *do* record the interview yourself.

If you make your own recording, *keep the original in a safe place. Do not* alter or destroy the original. It is probably discoverable. If you later use parts of the recording for testimony or demonstration (for example), be sure to work from a copy to avoid altering or deleting the original.

Evaluation Format and Behavior

Evaluation format and content vary with the purpose of the evaluation and other factors. It isn't feasible to become too specific in this practical guide, but the following are some principles.

- Forensic interviews are a bit different from ordinary clinical evaluations (see examples in the appendices). Do not think of them merely as extensions of the things we do with patients. You should know the purpose and context of the evaluation and modify the format and style accordingly.
- Do not limit your evaluation to the common time constraints of routine clinical exams. Many kinds of forensic evaluations should take several hours, not including psychological testing and other special procedures. It is often useful to schedule two or more interviews (e.g., morning and afternoon of the same day). All of this makes forensic assessments expensive, but getting to the truth is paramount, and the findings affect case outcome, which in turn may affect the evaluee's life, his or her liberty, and/or significant amounts of someone's money.
- Be professional and as friendly as is reasonable and compatible with the circumstances. Explain the process and format to the evaluee (see "Consents and Notifications," below). Be aware of evaluee fatigue or discomfort and offer breaks as appropriate.
- Be respectful, but be don't be "sandbagged" by the evaluee. Be persistent; follow up your queries. Watch for conscious or unconscious evasiveness and be very thorough. Although the forensic question may seem very focused (such as the person's condition at some specific point in time, or whether or not the person has been injured by some event), a broader complete assessment (with focus on the relevant item) is usually indicated.
- Be honest (just as you expect of the evaluee). Avoid "tricks" (e.g., making a sudden loud noise to assess startle effect). "Honesty" does not suggest that you should answer all an evaluee's questions, however (see below).
- Consider (through the retaining lawyer and with his or her permission) inviting the evaluee to bring one or two other people to the interview in order to provide corroboration, expansion, support, and/or contradiction of the evaluee's statements. At least part of such interviews should be in the evaluee's absence and without giving an opportunity for the evaluee and corroborating person to compare notes.

Forensic vs. "Patient" Interview Styles

A forensic evaluee almost always has a non-clinical interest in the outcome of the evaluation and the case. Sometimes the person is a criminal defendant, sometimes a civil plaintiff. Sometimes the interest is capacity or permission to do something (such as practice a profession, manage one's affairs, or gain custody of a child).

A forensic evaluee usually has good reason to try to fool or mislead you, and most can probably do so to some extent. Do *not* assume that you can discern whether or not the evaluee is telling the truth, or whether or not an answer is accurate (in addition, accuracy is not the same thing as veracity). Thus, *forensic evaluations often require extensive corroboration.* Review the records in advance. Ask about other information sources, and use them.

A forensic evaluator generally has no duty of "patient" confidentiality or clinical care to an evaluee and fewer other duties than he or she would have to a patient (but see "Consents and Notifications," below).

Questions from evaluees during or after the examination may or may not be answered directly. You have no obligation to answer every question (and often should not), but queries and concerns should generally be handled with openness and sensitivity.

Evaluees often ask for a copy of the evaluator's report. Although they may be entitled to a copy, it should not come from you. Refer the evaluee to his or her attorney or other party (insurance company, employer, etc.) as relevant.

A few experts are willing to give evaluees feedback about to the evaluator's impression or the case itself (particularly if they have been retained by the evaluee's attorney). *I strongly recommend against this* for a number of reasons (one of which is the evaluator's lack of an overall view of the case or any real knowledge of the probable outcome). Simply acknowledge that the question is reasonable, but refer the evaluee to his or her attorney or other relevant party for case-related questions.

Consents and Notifications

I'm not a lawyer, and jurisdictions may differ, but I believe it is rarely necessary to obtain written consent from forensic or administrative evaluees. Some professions recommend it.

- The evaluee is not your "patient."
- The evaluee has probably already agreed, (a) through his or her lawyer, (b) by virtue of his or her pursuing a claim or action, (c) as part of an employer or agency requirement (such as in employment or "fitness for duty" evaluations), and/or (d) in following an attorney's instructions, to be evaluated for the purpose contemplated.

- Many evaluations are pursuant to (i.e., done because of) a court order. The evaluee may have little or no choice in the matter unless he or she simply refuses to participate.
- The evaluee has usually arrived at the evaluation site in anticipation of the evaluation and can usually be assumed to have chosen to participate in it.
- The evaluee is free to stop the evaluation at any time (although the consequences of stopping may be detrimental to his or her case).
- Minor (underaged) evaluees, or those who are or may be incompetent in some relevant way, should already have been through a proper avenue of substituted consent (e.g., through a parent, guardian, judge, or appropriately empowered attorney).

The above do not mean that the evaluator should proceed without respect and regard for the evaluee's need for information. The evaluator should provide simple but clear information about the following (I summarize it in an information sheet—see example, Appendix E—giving a copy to the evaluee and keeping a copy for my file):

- the evaluator's name and profession (and explanations about others in the room, including trainees or videographer, if present);
- the purpose of the evaluation;
- the evaluator's role in the case and who retained him or her;
- the fact that the evaluation is being recorded (in writing, by video, etc.);
- the uses to which the information obtained may be put;
- some idea of who will have access to the information obtained;
- the general format to be followed;
- the fact that the evaluation is not intended to be stressful and breaks may be taken at any time;
- the fact that the interviewer is not interested in the legal strategies of the case and will not ask about them except as relevant to the evaluation task;
- an invitation to ask questions about the format and other topics as appropriate;
- the need for honesty and frankness from the evaluee.

This introductory process should not be overly formal or sterile and will often set a tone of comfortable professionalism with a minimum of adversarial stance.

Evaluees with Clinical Needs

Absent a crisis or emergency, *do not* treat or give specific clinical advice or referral names to an evaluee. Simple, generic encouragement is often nice (e.g., "I hope you feel better soon"), but, if you believe care is necessary, recommend it through the attorney who retained you. If the evaluee is a client of the lawyer who retained you, or in the case of disability or competency evaluations, it may be appropriate to discuss treatment needs with the evaluee's treating clinician.

Special Note Regarding Criminal Defendants

Do not forensically interview an arrestee before defense counsel is appointed and notified. When criminal responsibility (the mental ability to form criminal intent) is an issue, it is very important to interview the arrestee/defendant as soon as possible after the alleged crime. Nevertheless, if you are asked by an officer or prosecutor to see a person soon after he or she is arrested, *ask* if defense counsel has been appointed, *document* the answer, and *decline* if you believe the arrestee has not yet had benefit of defense counsel.

It is ethical to evaluate and treat an unrepresented arrestee or defendant for *clinical* purposes, but you must not do any "forensic" evaluation or assume any expert role. If such a person blurts something out, you may record it, as well as your impression of the person's state of mind at the time (e.g., delirious, intoxicated, psychotic, or not). Do not pursue the topic with the person unless it is *clinically* necessary.

If you treat an arrestee/defendant, avoid becoming an expert witness in the same case (you may be a fact witness, and have to testify to what you saw or heard).

6

REPORTS AND AFFIDAVITS

If someone had told me when I was in college that I would make much of my living writing "term papers" and having to get an "A" on every one, I'd have laughed him into the next county.

Reports and affidavits are lasting representations of your opinions, abilities, expertise, and effectiveness. Once submitted, you can't take back the words (though you can often amend them). *Take your time and do them right.*

Forensic reports are different in format and intent from clinical reports. Don't assume that your clinical report style is appropriate for forensic reports.

Don't write a report unless the retaining entity requests it.

What do reports and affidavits accomplish?

- They formally *convey your opinions* and/or other information to others, often including the trier (a jury or judge).
- They *organize and clarify* your opinions for the lawyers on both sides, the court, and yourself.
- They're *a tool for resolving cases* (settlement in civil cases, plea negotiation in criminal ones).
- They establish how (or whether or not) your expertise will be used in the litigation process.
- They help focus your study before testimony.
- They may be required before a lawsuit can be filed or proceed (cf. presuit affidavits or reports that are required in many jurisdictions).

Who asks for reports? Reports are usually requested by the retaining attorney, not a court, even when they are required by court rules.[1] Thus you're usually writing them for a lawyer. Always remember, though, that your report will probably be read by the other side's lawyer and perhaps a

---

1 There are exceptions. Sometimes one is retained by a court rather than a lawyer or other entity; reports prepared by agency professionals (such as state hospital or correctional facility clinicians) often go directly to a court.

judge and/or jury. It may become part of a public record, and it will be in someone's files for a very long time.

Some states require a preliminary expert report or affidavit before a malpractice suit can be filed. These may be in the form of a letter, with format dictated by the statute or jurisdiction (but the *content* must be your own). The retaining lawyer may help with the formatting and framing of the report, but be sure the opinions are your own. Although lawyers often say they "just need a letter so I can file the lawsuit," treat such requests seriously and write them only after adequate record review.

*Who **doesn't** ask for reports?* It's simple: lawyers for whom your opinions don't support their cases or for whom a report is not required to pursue or defend the case. Many cases for which you will be retained won't generate "favorable" opinions (that is, ones that support the attorney's case). In those matters, the lawyer is unlikely to ask you to write a report (and probably won't need your further services). It's nothing personal; that's to be expected. If you end up writing reports in every case you accept, then you are either tailoring your opinions to what you think the lawyer wants (a bad thing), or the attorneys who contact you have infallible judgment about the cases they accept (an unlikely thing).

The only situations I can think of right now in which a lawyer may want a report with your non-supporting opinions are criminal cases in which the attorney wants to protect him- or herself from being accused of not exploring every possible defense, and cases in which the lawyer is trying to convince a persistent litigant that his or her case has no merit. I've encountered both. The former is more common, especially in capital cases when the defense lawyer needs reassurance that there is no chance of an insanity plea or sentencing mitigation due to a mental disorder.

Resist requests to produce a "quickie" report. Lawyers often ask for "nothing fancy; just a couple of pages with your opinions." Things done in a hurry are often sloppy or incomplete, rarely show you at your best, and are often embarrassing later in the case. (I once saw a report addendum written in pencil on lined paper—necessary perhaps, but not a very good reflection on the expert.) *Take the time to follow your usual routine.*

Lawyer Participation in Reports/Affidavits

Do not let a lawyer (or anyone else) write your report or your opinions without your guidance or attribute opinions to you that you have not genuinely rendered. You may accept the lawyer's predetermined *format* or a request to limit your report to specific topics (unless you believe that would make your report dishonest). You may also talk with the attorney about helpful ways to frame your opinions once they have been formed. Remember that part of your goal is to provide opinion and comment in a way that is consistent with the *court's* language and purpose. It is acceptable (and ethical) for a lawyer to attribute opinions to you in legal documents (such as "answers" or discovery documents), provided you have discussed those opinions beforehand and the wording accurately reflects them.

It is not acceptable to our profession (though it may be legal for lawyers) for an attorney to publish detailed opinions attributed to you without your knowledge. This sometimes occurs, and you may first hear of it when you are deposed or testify at trial. I tell lawyers that this kind of "surprise" during testimony is very irritating to experts and suggests that the lawyer has been shifty or dishonest with them. No lawyer wants an irritated expert testifying in his or her case.

Various rules often require that you divulge, if asked, how you discussed the report with the lawyer, what was in report drafts, etc. Keeping most attorney communications oral is one approach to keeping them private, but be aware that (a) many things *should* be documented in your records (don't play "hide the ball") and (b) oral communication is as discoverable as written communication, provided you remember it at the time you are asked.

Report Format

Format and style vary with case, jurisdiction, and expert. The examples in the appendices are not the last word, but they illustrate what I believe are useful styles and contents. The following reflect what I tend to do, not a mandate.

Short is usually better than long. I usually suggest to lawyers that my report answer specific questions rather their giving me *carte blanche* to write whatever I wish. No one wants to read volumes (I've seen them over 100 pages), and the more free the prose, the more likely the report will contain a lot of extraneous material (perhaps harmful to the case). Short reports, whose content and format has been discussed with the attorney beforehand, mean fewer "surprises," and (all together now) lawyers hate surprises.

Short "telegraphs" less to the other side than long. I'm not suggesting that you omit important opinions or information, just that you stick to the point (as usually best defined by the person requesting the report).

Short often takes longer to compose. You may want to let the requester know that well-written brief reports generally take extra thought and care. Certain things have to be included, and winnowing the important points from everything you've done and reviewed over many hours of work is time-consuming. That means that *short is rarely less expensive than long.*

"Short" is relative. Sometimes it means three pages, and sometimes 10 to 20.[2] In my practice, which includes some very complex matters, I rarely

2 In high school, that's a thesis, and it's longer than most clinical reports.

write more than 15 pages, and the opinions themselves are almost always conveyed in fewer than five.

Many good forensic reports do not contain detailed case information, long discussions of findings, extended recitations of psychodynamic or medical issues, or pseudo-legalistic prose. You may be prepared to comment on those when you testify (except the legalistic stuff), but even then the questions and answers should be short. In your report,

- include all required topics (see below);
- answer the questions asked;
- don't answer questions that have *not* been asked (unless not to do so would be misleading or dishonest by omission);
- write for a lay audience rather than a professional one; and
- don't try to sound like a lawyer.

Be clear for the reader. As a rule, state your opinions early in the report. Report formats require lots of things besides opinions (such as lists of records reviewed, statements about your qualifications, etc.), so make your opinions easy to find.

Be aware of (and ask the lawyer about) legal requirements for format and content in the particular report. In malpractice cases, for example, reports regarding the standard of care may require that you state that standard for each behavior you question, whether or how the standard was breached, and, if breached, what the damage was and how the breach caused it. *Cases have been dismissed because an expert report did not obsessively address the required elements.*

Be complete (but not overly wordy). In some jurisdictions (especially federal ones), your future testimony will be limited to the opinions and issues enumerated in your report (thus reports in federal matters may be longer and more detailed than those for state courts).

In almost all cases, each of your opinions must be accompanied by a reasonable explanation. One cannot simply write, "It's true because I said it's true." I generally recommend that the explanations be limited to a few paragraphs apiece (at most). Courts have rules about the credibility of expert opinions (look up *Daubert* v. *Merrell Dow Pharmaceuticals* or *duPont* v. *Robinson*).

If in doubt, ask the person who requested the report how much explanation is required, whether or not you should cite specific references from the record or examination, and whether or not you should include references from the professional literature.

Use relevant legal terms correctly. See chapter 2[3] for definitions of important words and phrases such as the following:

---

3 Don't always take my word for it; get your own legal dictionary, and don't be afraid to ask the lawyer whether or not you are using a term correctly.

- reasonable medical certainty/probability (psychiatric, psychological "certainty," depending on jurisdiction);
- standard of care;
- foreseeability;
- cause (causation);
- competence (competency);
- responsibility;
- know;
- appreciate;
- negligent (negligence);
- gross negligence.

Include relevant disclaimers and caveats. One of the most common and important *caveats* is that your report may be preliminary and that you reserve the right to amend or add to it should additional information be obtained. *Most reports are "preliminary" in this sense.* You should usually mention that your report

- is "preliminary";
- may be amended or expanded at some future time;
- assumes that the records received and reviewed were reasonably complete; and
- assumes that the records received were reasonably representative of the overall facts (in case those facts are later discovered to be wrong or incomplete).

In addition, you should disclose whether or not you actually examined relevant persons (e.g., a criminal defendant or allegedly injured civil plaintiff) and, if they were not examined, whether or not adequate examination might change your opinions.

I often add that my opinions were formed "using information and procedures generally relied upon by forensic psychiatrists in such work."

Drafts, Discovery

You are not generally required to keep report drafts in computer files if you type over them in the usual course of your work. However, if you do keep any drafts or notes (in hard copy or computer files), most jurisdictions require you to produce them when they are subpoenaed. *Do not* destroy copies of anything you have sent to the attorney (including drafts, letters, and emails), and *do not* destroy anything related to the case once your records have been subpoenaed.

If you or the attorney believe(s) something is not discoverable, or need not be provided to the other side when subpoenaed, discuss that with the lawyer who retained you.[4] If you were retained by someone other than a lawyer or judge, don't rely on his or her word for a legal opinion about what you must produce.

Grammar, Spelling, and Vocabulary

Write as if your report were going to be graded by an English teacher and you're hoping for an A-plus. People who use poor grammar and spelling usually never realize it. They remain unaware that they are embarrassing themselves in front of people who matter (i.e., those who will use your words in a legal forum and who are in a position to affect your future practice).

Sometimes the mistakes are glaring (such as misusing "your" for "you're," using plural pronouns such as "them" and "their" in place of a singular "him or her" and "his or her," or inserting erroneous apostrophes). Sometimes they're little things that only a lawyer or the opposing expert might notice, such as saying that one is a "diplomat" of the American Board of Psychiatry and Neurology (the proper word is "diplomate") or referring to one's "*curriculum vita*" (*curriculum vitae* is correct; if you have two, they are *curricula vitae*).[5]

Poor or erroneous vocabulary is not just embarrassing; it can get you or the case into trouble. The language of the legal arena is often very specific, and its definitions sometimes differ from ordinary usage (cf. "fact," "reasonable certainty"). Read chapter 2.

Unless you minored in English composition, buy a good grammar guide such as the slim W. Strunk and E. B. White: *The Elements of Style* (4th ed., Boston: Allyn & Bacon, 1999). You'll be glad you did.

How it Looks

How your report appears to the reader is important, not only for its evidence value but as a representative of you and your work. Most of your future referrals will probably come from lawyers and others based on their impressions of the quality of your work.

First, be competent, accurate, and honest, then be sure the report

- is properly formatted;
- is clearly organized;
- contains everything required;
- is carefully and clearly worded (see above and examples in the appendices);

---

4 In some cases, I give everything requested to the lawyer who retained me and let him or her decide what is proper to produce.
5 If you're translating old Latin texts, it might be *curricula vitorum*.

- contains excellent grammar and spelling;
- is very neat;
- is printed on quality letterhead and paper (not computer-printed letterhead); and
- is mailed flat (don't just fax or email the original; if time is short, fax it and follow up with the original).

7

DEPOSITION AND TRIAL
TESTIMONY

If someone had told me when I was in college that I would make much of my living taking oral exams, and having to get an "A" on every one, I'd have laughed *him* into the next county, too (see the opening of chapter 6).

General Notes on Testimony

Depositions can usually meet your schedule. *Trials* are less flexible, but scheduling is not generally onerous.

The lawyer is the litigation scheduling boss. In trials, he or she is orchestrating a very complex and important process controlled by the judge. Be reasonable about meeting scheduling needs; don't be a *prima donna*.

Don't assume that court dates are set in stone. Once you have agreed to a date, you must be available for it, but you may be able to schedule some flexible activity at the same time. In civil cases particularly, over 90 percent of even "certain" trial dates will be changed or the case will be resolved before trial.

Have a pre-testimony conference with the retaining attorney. Do *not* simply show up to testify. At that conference, the retaining attorney should bring you up to date about the case, go over likely questions and what he or she thinks is important, and maybe tell you about the opposing lawyer. He or she may also give good advice, such as:

- "Listen carefully to the question."
- "Don't let the other lawyer mislead you."
- "Don't answer too quickly. Think first."
- "It's not a memory test."
- "Don't speculate" (that is, don't make statements that are not based on credible information).
- "Give short, direct answers."
- "Don't answer more than you're asked."
- "Don't be misled by the informal setting" (depositions only).

Many years ago, I had a pre-deposition meeting with a "country law-yer" who had a heavy southern drawl. After I had dazzled him with my sophistication for a few minutes, he finally said, "Doctor, if you'll be quiet and listen to me for about 30 minutes, the deposition will go a lot better for both of us."

I did, and it did.

Be clear and firm with your answers. (Your testimony will usually consist of answering questions, not giving lectures.)

Don't argue (but *do* correct misunderstandings). Being argumentative usually weakens testimony.

Don't be flippant, cavalier, or arrogant. Your usually good sense of humor can be misconstrued (and may be purposely misconstrued), weakening your credibility. Show that you take the case and your opinions seriously. Don't be disrespectful to anyone (you need not be a *milquetoast*, either). Most mental health professionals aren't arrogant, but if you begin to feel superior to the opposing lawyer, think again: He or she probably already knows the answers to most of the questions you'll be asked.

Don't say anything you can't support. Testimony, the court's way of getting to the truth, is a stepwise process. If you can't support each of your state-ments and opinions, your conclusions are unlikely to stand (or to be allowed to stand).

Stick to forensic opinions, not philosophy, unless asked. Opposing lawyers will listen as long as you want to talk and sometimes ask open-ended ques-tions to invite you to talk. Most of the time, they are less interested in your verbose presentation than they are in finding some statement within it that they can turn to their advantage. Answer the question; tell the truth concisely; remember the context and environment of your testimony; and *answer only the question that has been asked* (i.e., be cautious about volunteer-ing answers to questions that *haven't* been asked). Don't over-explain your answers; off-the-cuff explanations often weaken the response and give undeserved information to the other side.

Lawyers sometimes demand that you answer "yes" or "no." *Ignore that demand if the question can't reasonably be answered by yes or no (or if a strict yes or no would misconstrue your meaning)* and politely explain why. You are entitled to explain your answer if you wish. One way to think of this often false dichotomy of "yes" or "no" is automatically to add at least four more choices to it: "I don't know"; "I can't accurately answer the question 'yes' or 'no' as you've phrased it"; "answering 'yes' or 'no' would misconstrue my opinion for the jury (or judge)"; and "I don't understand your question."

If the *judge* says you must answer "yes" or "no," try to explain, but you may not succeed. The retaining lawyer will have a chance to clarify. "I don't know" or "I can't answer the question as asked" are quite acceptable.

Try to answer questions only once. Lawyers sometimes ask the same question several times, then choose the most advantageous answer. Don't let them talk you out of what you believe are accurate, appropriate answers. If you don't know an answer, say so.

Consider answers to standard questions in advance. You will almost certainly be asked about your background, and some other common questions crop up in many depositions and trials.[1]

"What is forensic psychology?"
"Is psychiatry an art or a science?"
"What's the standard of care?"

Some questions are potentially insulting.

"How many tries did it take you to pass your Boards?"

Politely set limits on irrelevant personal questions, but note that whether or not something is relevant is the judge's decision, not yours. Before declining to answer, wait for the lawyer for whom you are testifying to object. "How much have you charged in this case?" is fair. "How much did you make last year in your forensic practice?" may or may not be fair. "What was your gross income last year?" is out of bounds unless the judge tells you to answer.

Be able to tolerate criticism. This is neither a collegial process nor a scientific one. It is not quite "inquisitory," but it is *adversarial.* You should not be an adversary yourself, but you must tolerate questioning from lawyers who vigorously oppose the side for which you are testifying and who may be very good at turning your words, opinions, and even behaviors to their own advantage.

Do not be alarmed if the opposing lawyer appears frustrated or irritated. Keep your cool and be polite. The lawyer for whom you are testifying will intervene if necessary. Don't take it personally, and do not offer rejoinders or verbose explanations.

Don't give your social security number, home address, or home phone number. Most testimony is public information.

Be prepared to have your credibility questioned, especially if the other side cannot refute your opinions. Past trial and deposition testimony, licensing and hospital privilege status, references to you on the Internet, and much of your writing (including nonprofessional pursuits) are easily available to lawyers and may be highlighted by the other side.

---

1 Some come from a three-volume self-published book, called *Coping with Psychiatric and Psychological Expert Testimony*, that a particular psychologist used to sell to attorneys. Don't try to cover all of them.

Don't try to bluff or get outside your expertise. Assume the opposing lawyer knows the answer to every question he or she asks (especially at trial).

Listen carefully to each question. Avoid the "primrose path" phenomenon of rapid-fire easy questions with a surprise kicker at the end. *Don't try to figure out the opposing lawyer's strategy or to "outsmart" him or her.*

Objections by the attorney who retained you may be his or her attempt to telegraph "be careful." Don't answer too quickly, and give the attorney time to object to questions before you answer them.

When questions from the opposing lawyer are vague or unanswerable (e.g., "Tell me every opinion you have in this case, Doctor"), ask for a more specific question. Note that some ("compound") queries include more than one question. This is often on purpose and can either be confusing or lead you to answer poorly. If you notice a compound question, say so, and ask something like "Which question would you like for me to answer?"

It is quite acceptable to disagree with experts for the other side and, if you know they are outside the standard of practice for forensic psychiatry or psychology, respectfully to criticize their methods. However, avoid *ad hominem* (personal) criticisms.

Depositions

All of the above is relevant for both depositions and trials. Read it. And, in addition . . .

Your depositions will almost always be "discovery" depositions, a chance for the other side to learn what you will say in court (and thus very important for positioning cases for settlement or eventual trial). Discovery depositions (as contrasted with "trial depositions") are usually in civil, not criminal, cases.

The attorneys will arrange the deposition to fit your schedule. The opposing attorney may be responsible for this portion of your fee, but I suggest you bill the *retaining* lawyer, since that's the person with whom you have a billing agreement. He or she will collect it (sometimes you'll get a check from the opposing lawyer/entity).

Deposition testimony has the same weight as trial testimony, even though it may or may not eventually be heard by the trier (jury, or a judge in a bench trial).

If you have never been deposed before, consider arranging to sit in on a couple of expert depositions. It's worth the time.

The deposition setting is relatively informal, perhaps an office (*preferably not yours*) or a hotel conference room, but the rules are strict. Several people may be present:

- the retaining lawyer (always);
- the opposing lawyer (always);
- a court reporter (always);
- other consultants or co-counsel;

- lawyers for other involved parties;
- litigant(s) (occasionally);
- the other side's expert (occasionally);
- forensic trainees (occasionally, with each party's permission).

Once everything is scheduled, you will probably receive a *subpoena duces tecum* from the opposing lawyer (a demand to show up and bring your records, files, billing materials, etc.). It comes from an attorney, not a judge. You may question, or even decline, its requests (e.g., for highly personal items or onerous demands such as "every article you have ever read that's relevant to the case at hand"), but be sure to do so through the retaining lawyer.

When you are asked to produce your notes and records, consider giving them to the retaining attorney for transmittal to the opposing attorney. He or she can then determine whether or not the other side is entitled to everything. Do not remove items from your file unless you are sure it is legal and ethical.

Consider supplying *copies* of your notes and reports rather than the originals (but bring the originals as well). That usually prevents the court reporter from taking your original files for a couple of weeks in order to have them copied.

Dress appropriately (see below). Many depositions are videotaped[2] and may be shown to the jury, and you should show professionalism and respect for the process in any event.

If your deposition is being videotaped, behave (and dress) as if you were actually in court, and direct most of your answers to the camera. Parts of the deposition may be played at trial, and the judge and jury will be watching it on a monitor.

"Is that all your opinions, Doctor?" is a common question. Simply say that you aren't sure what you'll be asked at trial, so you don't know what your answers will be, and you'll be happy to answer any questions the opposing lawyer wishes to ask now. Reserve the possibility of forming new opinions if additional information becomes available.

Trials

Everything in the generic section on testimony at the beginning of this chapter is relevant. Read it. In addition . . .

When testifying, *speak to the factfinder* (the trier of fact, usually a jury but sometimes the judge). It is tempting to focus on the person asking the questions, but jurors are the important listeners.

---

2 O.K.; I know "videotape" is obsolete, but I don't know how to spell "video-ed."

Communicate to/with the jury. Observe some of their reactions to your testimony if you can.

Speak clearly and simply. Make the issues less complicated if possible, with concise points of importance. Jurors usually like doctors, but they hate arrogance and being "talked down to." And their eyes tend to glaze over when listening to "fuzzy-headed shrinks."

Be respectful to everyone.

A small thing: Many experts choose not to carry anything to the witness stand except perhaps copies of their reports and/or depositions. Prepare well enough to testify primarily from memory, but ask to refer to notes or records if necessary. *Testimony is not a memory test.*

If you do take your notes or file to the stand, consider making an extra copy in advance to give it to the opposing lawyer if he or she asks to see what you're referring to during testimony. Taking the expert's notes is an old lawyer trick; you don't want to beg to get them back in order to consult them.

If you are experienced, don't hesitate to suggest questions to the retaining lawyer before you testify at trial. In trials, that is the lawyer who will ask you questions first, then the other side will have a chance to "cross-examine" you. (In discovery depositions, the other side's lawyer questions you first, and the retaining attorney may not ask anything.) *Both you and the lawyer who retained you should know the strengths and weaknesses of your opinions, background, etc., before you testify.*

Appearance and Dress

Some of you won't like this section. Think about your role and purpose in court, and consider the following objectively. (See also chapter 13, "A Lawyer's Perspective . . . ".)

Look professional and credible, not flamboyant, wealthy, or effete. Be aware of the jury's background, but don't "dress down" to try to "identify with them." Jurors expect you to be an expert, not "one of the guys" (see below).[3] Try not to have to "act" the part, since jurors easily spot experts who are "acting"; be comfortable with the way you present.

Got hair? Keep the cut and color conservative. Very long hair in men is not usually associated with expertise and credibility. Spikey doesn't work for either gender, in my view. Pencil-thin moustache? Only if you want credibility similar to that of a used-car salesman. And those beards that some of us like so much often make jurors suspicious or give the impression of a fuzzy-headed (rather than clear-thinking) shrink.

---

3 If you have doubts about whether or not this section applies to you, check with the retaining lawyer or read John T. Molloy's *New Dress for Success* (New York: Warner Books, 1988). You'll hate it, but it works.

Styles are changing, but I still recommend that men have no body jewelry (including an earring) or visible tattoos. Women are allowed, in my view, up to two tasteful earrings per ear but no other visible piercings (and no tattoos) before credibility starts to deteriorate.

Non-traditional dress (*burqas*, Sikh turbans, *dashikis*, etc.) is often off-putting to jurors and, in any event, distracts from one's testimony. Studies indicate a negative effect (see below).

The "audience" to whom you are speaking matters. Style may be a little more flexible in some settings and parts of the country and less so in others (such as courts martial or rural settings).

Sometimes I'm asked whether or not an expert witness should look and act in some way that makes the jury "identify" with him or her (such as dressing down for rural or uneducated juries or lawyers' choosing a black or Hispanic expert for a particular case). My answer is generally no, and I believe most (though not all) lawyers who try cases agree. There are a few notable exceptions but not as many as one might think (e.g., female experts in certain child-related matters or sexual harassment cases, black or Hispanic experts—with little accent—in a few geographic regions, Caucasian experts in a few regions; see below).

Juries and judges respect, and *believe*, people whom they associate with credible professional status. That means looking, speaking, and acting like the *jurors'* image (not necessarily yours) of a qualified professional, whatever that may be, not like their neighbor or friend.

"Foreign"-appearing experts   Like it or not, surveys indicate significant differences in credibility and jury acceptance among expert witnesses who have different physical appearances and accents. It's getting better, but the expert's race (separate from being "foreign") is still an issue in some U.S. courts (not just southern ones). Gender is less important *per se*, unless associated with such things as youth, flamboyant dress, or accent.

Setting aside other physical characteristics which may be relevant to superficial credibility—or at least distracting—for some U.S. juries (e.g., speech impediment, marked obesity, some beards or very long hair in men, youth [ouch]), there is no question that "foreign" appearance affects juries. Experts with thick accents appear uniformly to have a credibility, distraction, or communication disadvantage (from the jury's and perhaps the judge's standpoint). Those with slight accents have fewer issues, but some are more acceptable than others. British (including Australian and South African) and German accents seem acceptable, or even preferred; Middle Eastern ones are negatively perceived; Hispanic or East Indian ones seem in between unless the person is hard to understand or has difficulty with American idiom.

Appearance that differs from the expected U.S. professional look can be important. The surveys that exist indicate that swarthy or hirsute experts are, on average, perceived as less credible and more distracting. Unfamiliar dress (such as *burqas* or *dashikis*) adds to distraction and should be avoided.

The lawyer's choice of expert in this regard is not usually based on the attorney's biases but on the very practical matter of how best to win the case. He or she knows the "audience" that will consider the case. Distracting that audience before they even start to listen can't be good.[4]

Don't shoot the messenger.

---

4 This information may also apply to initial interactions with lawyers who are deciding whether or not to retain you. In important cases, lawyers may travel long distances to meet personally with potential experts before hiring them, perhaps in part to assess their appearance and interpersonal skills.

8

FEES AND BILLING

Fees, billing, and collection procedures in forensic practice are quite different from those in general psychiatry and psychology. Most forensic practices have far fewer clients, and the individual bills are usually larger. Collections are usually better (and less frequently discounted) in forensic practice, and resolving billing disputes is far more straightforward. Medicare, Medicaid, other insurance coverage, provider networks and agreements, procedure codes, and diagnosis-related groups (DRGs) are all largely irrelevant in forensic work (although sometimes important to direct clinical services in correctional psychiatry or forensic treatment clinics). Understanding the practicalities and ethics of charging and billing for forensic services greatly simplifies practice management. You will probably get "stiffed" (more than once), but this chapter should reduce the odds of that happening.

Many years ago, a nice lawyer with whom I was working asked to meet over lunch to discuss her ongoing case and her overdue bill. Her office would supply the sandwiches, and I'd bill for my time.

The discussion began with a request for a supplemental report. New facts had surfaced and, she said, the other side was making her job very difficult. The supplemental report was due in a week (she had known of that deadline for several months). She knew my schedule was tight, and that I usually require payment before releasing reports. She balked at bringing her account up to date and providing the usual deposit, and said this was *really* important and "Don't worry; I always pay my experts."

I can be a pushover, but I'd been stung before. And as I'd passed through the parking garage I noticed a very expensive car in the lawyer's parking space.

By the end of the meeting, we had discussed the new situation and the deadline had been relaxed. I had agreed to review the new materials, discuss them with her, and write a report about my findings if warranted. And I had a check that covered past billings and an appropriate deposit toward the time to be spent on the upcoming review.

This vignette is not a criticism of the attorney, nor is it about some sort of gamesmanship between forensic consultants and lawyers. It's an example of common issues facing forensic clinicians (and many other self-employed professionals) as they try to do their jobs and manage their practices at the same time. Expert fees represent only a small part of overall litigation costs for the attorney or other retaining entity, but they're how we pay our rent.

If the financial aspects of forensic practice were as simple and straightforward as most people think they are, there would be a lot more forensic psychiatrists. This chapter illustrates some practical billing and collection procedures and, perhaps more important, a shift in fee and billing *attitude* associated with moving from general to forensic practice.

The Basics

Be clear about your rates and fees, responsibility for payment, expectation of payment, and schedule and method of payment. Remember, *lawyers understand hourly fees and the value of professional time and expertise* (and they are far less neurotic about fees than most mental health professionals). Talk about fees early and whenever indicated for clarity, especially in your initial lawyer contact.

Realize, but don't overestimate, your value. Be reasonable. Consider your experience, your expertise, fees charged by comparable colleagues, etc. Forensic professionals usually charge more per hour for forensic services than for clinical ones (but not for forensic *treatment* services such as correctional psychiatry, psychotherapy, or work in a secure hospital). Forensic psychiatrists generally charge more than forensic psychologists (but less than some other forensic specialists). Actual rates vary with training, experience, reputation, geography, and personal preference.

Your charges should almost always be time-based. "Package" pricing is not usually a good idea, and "contingency" fees (those based on case outcome or lawyer recovery) are unethical. Your hourly fee should be consistent. Discounting (or forgiving) fees is up to you, but increasing them for a big case or wealthy client may be unethical.

Require a retainer or deposit against billings[1] in most cases (especially for new clients, reports, and testimony; see below). Lawyers are accustomed to working with retainers. Promptly refund any portion of a retainer or

---

1 Properly worded government or agency contracts can be an exception; see below.

deposit to which you're not entitled (for example, when a case is resolved before you do much work or are listed as an expert, or when the deposit exceeds your charges).

Watch for early portents of fee and collection problems (and other problems as well). Be cautious if the attorney does not agree to a retainer (see below), is late with payments, wants a "quickie" review or assessment, or does not send you all the materials you need to do a proper review or evaluation. Run the other way if the lawyer wants you to do the work free or at a discount because "I have a lot of other cases that I could send for you." *That's a red flag for both business and ethics.* Your fee may be a factor, but it's rarely the primary one, in whether or not you are chosen as an expert. It's fine to discount fees or work *pro bono* (without payment), but do it because you want to, not because you think it will bring big bucks in the future.

In general, *bill the person or entity that retained you.* Your financial agreement *should not* be directly with a litigant or other client of a lawyer who retains you, even though that may be the source of the lawyer's own reimbursement. (The above obviously does not apply when an insurance company or other non-attorney has engaged you, such as for an insurance review or disability evaluation.)

Fees or fee agreements may have to be approved by the lawyer's client or court before the lawyer can accept your fee agreement, or before payment is authorized, but your routine should be to deal with the retaining entity (e.g., lawyer) and to hold that entity responsible. *This makes billing, fee discussions, and collections much easier in most situations.*

Bill regularly, and don't let client debt get out of hand. Do not wait for the case to be decided, and try not to surprise the contractee with a huge bill.

My very first forensic case involved consulting to a rural New Mexico court in a serious criminal matter. The judge who retained me (a fishing buddy of a lawyer-uncle at the time) was cordial and everything seemed to go smoothly. I reviewed the records, traveled a long distance to evaluate the defendant, communicated with the attorneys as directed by the judge, wrote a report, and returned for two days of testimony a few months later.

Not having read this chapter, I wasn't very careful in my agreement with the court. I didn't prepare the bill until the case was over. It came to $3,600. The time and charges were scrupulously documented, but it looked like a lot of money, so I arbitrarily cut the amount in half[2] and mailed the statement.

---

2 I told you we can be neurotic.

I didn't hear from the court for months. After a few queries, a small check arrived along with a letter from the formerly pleasant judge. He said that (1) the "large" bill had come as a surprise; (2) no expert is worth $1,800; (3) his county maximum for expert witness payments was $375; and (4) I could take it or leave it.

I took it.

A court order or government contract for payment does not guarantee you'll be paid what you bill, or that you'll be paid at all. This may be particularly problematic in small or rural communities with whom you have not worked in the past. To minimize problems, be sure the court order or agency contract specifies your hourly rate, any maximum or restrictions that apply, and who actually pays your bill.

When payment is late, do not accept the excuse that the litigant hasn't paid the lawyer yet (with some exceptions for insurance companies, government agencies, etc.). Be reasonable and polite, but your agreement should be with the attorney, not the litigant (after all, the power company doesn't wait for its utility payments).

Be able to explain your fees to a jury. You will be asked about your fees during testimony. Simply be straightforward and don't apologize (unless you're gouging or doing something unethical). Remember, the lawyer who asks the question probably has an expert who is charging about the same.

Put it into Writing

I recommend that your client agreement contain a standard, written summary of your fees, billing procedures, and any special considerations for the case at hand. Your "fee sheet" should cover a wide variety of topics and circumstances (see examples in Appendix B). Follow that information to the letter; when you go outside your standard procedures, the probability of something bad happening, such as collection problems, increases.

Your fee sheet should contain:

- *the person or entity responsible for the charges.* Be specific.
- *the services to be charged.* Review time, interviews, conferences, report preparation, and testimony are obvious, but what about time spent waiting, unkept appointments, and travel (including time spent in hotels or waiting for planes)? Some experts charge different rates for different services and may or may not charge for travel and waiting. I charge all time-based activity at the same rate (since an hour spent reading records is just as long as an hour spent testifying). I also

charge that rate for interim time, such as waiting, unless I fill it with some other income-producing or recreational activity.

- *your hourly and daily rates.* A time-and-expenses fee schedule is the foundation of your compensation. I use a "day rate" (in my practice, 10 hours) as a maximum so that clients know they won't be unreasonably charged when I travel.
- *standard additional charges,* such as travel expenses, courier charges, large amounts of copying or printing, or exhibit preparation. Don't abuse your expense rates; it's nice to establish a reasonable maximum for hotels and food, for example, or to ask the lawyer for lodging suggestions in his or her city.
- *what's **not** charged.* Reassure the retaining entity that you don't "nickel and dime" your clients. Let him or her know that you don't charge for time spent working on other cases while traveling for the current one or for time engaged in recreation (though I do charge for other "down" time spent away from home or office, up to the daily maximum). I don't charge for alcoholic beverages and have a reasonable maximum for meals and hotels. If you wish to charge for business- or first-class travel, make that clear in the fee sheet; otherwise note that you bill only for "coach."[3]
- *the expected payment schedule.* Your fee sheet should specify your billing and collection practices, including any consequences of nonpayment (see below).

In addition to the above, consider one or more of the following:

- *requiring a partially or fully refundable retainer before beginning work.* I find this very important for guaranteeing billings and stabilizing office revenues. In my practice, the retainer is refundable unless I have been listed as an expert in court papers or represented as an expert to the other side (at which point I consider my name to have been "used" in the case, for which I want to be compensated). Sometimes, a case is resolved after a few hours of review or my services are no longer wanted. In such cases, as long as I have not been "listed" (and sometimes when I have), I promptly refund the unused portion of the retainer.[4] *I keep retainers and deposits in a separate account until they have been earned,* in order to avoid inadvertently spending the money.
- *requiring a deposit against billings for testimony, travel, and/or reports.* This is important as well, and not quite the same as a retainer. Some

3 You need not bill the lowest available fares, since business travel often cannot be scheduled well in advance, and many trips are canceled at the last minute. Just be fair and charge what it costs, no more and no less.
4 It's fair, and it builds goodwill. You'd be surprised how many lawyers are amazed to get money back from an expert.

attorneys, especially ones with whom you have not previously worked, who are on tight budgets, and/or who live in other states are riskier than others with respect to paying their bills, particularly once they have gotten what they need from the expert. Many cases are resolved soon after reports are received or depositions completed. With no disrespect intended to the many reputable retaining entities with whom I work, I like to hold the money myself.

Many experts travel for cases. Travel expenses are not inconsequential; you can't afford to "float" them for very long, much less do without reimbursement altogether. I often tell lawyers that I can't leave the office until an appropriate deposit has been received (see "deposit letter" example, Appendix I).

There's also the matter of "testifying under a bag of money" (see below). If a lawyer owes an expert a substantial amount of money, there is at least an *appearance* of possible coercion (that is, if the testimony doesn't please the lawyer, or the case is lost, one may not get paid). Appearance or not, if the expert's bill has been paid and a deposit received against the time and expenses of testifying, then he or she has no financial incentive to testify inappropriately. I like that, and most lawyers do as well.

- *the consequences of nonpayment.* Note on the fee sheet that you may cease work if bills are substantially in arrears or deposits are not received. This can include not releasing reports, not being available for deposition, or not being present for trial (experts can generally do that, since they are entitled to be paid for their time; subpoenaed fact witnesses cannot). Be reasonable and polite (but firm) in your communications. Try to prevent problems with clear communication and early action rather than letting payment problems go until the last minute.
- *minimum hours for testimony.* Some experts charge for a minimum number of testimony hours (often half a day) regardless of the actual time spent. I don't. As I've already noted, time is time. Once prepared, if I can get to the testimony site, testify, and get home in a couple of hours, that's fine with me.

Avoid (or strongly consider avoiding) the following.

Contingency fees and fee splitting[5] Don't just avoid them; never use them. They are categorically unethical for experts and may be illegal.

"Letters of protection" A letter of protection is a guarantee from a lawyer that a clinician or other vendor will be paid for treating a client if the

---

5 Yes, lawyers can engage in both, but you can't.

client's legal case is successful.[6] If the client (patient) loses, the clinician must seek payment from the patient. Used mostly in worker's compensation and personal injury cases, a letter of protection generally promises a physician, therapist, chiropractor, etc., who has treated a client for an allegedly compensable injury or condition that the first dollars of any judgment or settlement will go to the clinician (even before the lawyer or client is paid). Such promises create a conflict of interest and are often tantamount to a contingency arrangement, since the clinician knows that his or her records, and often testimony as well, will influence the legal case (and thus the clinician's compensation).

Those who wish to draw a distinction between letters of protection and contingency fees sometimes note that, if the case is lost, the clinician can seek compensation from the client him- or herself (or an insurance company). That's bullpucky, in my opinion. The clinicians who do it generally know exactly what they're doing, and I believe it's unethical, especially when combined with offering opinion testimony.

Agreeing to wait for a settlement or verdict before getting paid   I never accept such arrangements; they are arguably unethical if entered into beforehand (cf. contingency fees) and are poor business in any event.

Charging interest on overdue bills   I don't do it, and I don't recommend it. Do keep track of your accounts receivable and collections, but charging interest for overdue bills is a real hassle (and involves some legal rules). Almost all collection problems are solved by clear communication, understanding the above, choosing clients wisely, and not allowing clients to run up large bills.

"Package pricing"   Some forensic professionals have fixed-price arrangements for frequently repeated services such as disability or jail competency evaluations. Although this is understandable, one should be careful that the "per-evaluation" rate doesn't create an ethics or credibility problem (for example, a temptation to shorten fixed-price services in order to make them more profitable). I strongly suggest that more complex cases, at least (such as those that may involve future follow-up, testimony of some kind, appeals, etc.), be done on an hourly basis. This is particularly applicable to professionals in private practice, as contrasted with those who receive a salary from an agency or other employer who negotiates a third-party service contract.

---

6 Of course, you shouldn't be the expert witness if you're treating the patient; I'm generally referring to treating clinicians who end up being fact witnesses and whose records and/or testimony can have substantial impact on case outcome.

Working without a retainer or properly worded agency contract   If you haven't been stiffed yet, you haven't been in practice for very long. This applies particularly to lawyers and firms with whom you are not familiar, but I strongly recommend treating everyone alike (lawyers understand this, and it prevents you from promoting an appearance of biased relationships with some law firms).

Allowing debt to mount   There are both practical and ethical problems associated with allowing the lawyer's or contracting entity's bill to get out of hand. *This is probably the second most common source of not being paid.*

Testifying with a large bill outstanding   There are substantial ethical, practical, and credibility problems associated with "testifying while the lawyer holds a bag of money over your head." Remove the money issue by requiring that the outstanding bill be paid and a reasonable deposit be received before you leave for a deposition or trial. Having said that, be scrupulously honest (and prompt) in returning any portion of the deposit that is not used. (See the appendices for discussions and examples of charging—or not charging—when trials or depositions are canceled.)

(See chapter 11 for information about collections.)

9

ETHICS

Ethics principles and ethical practices are illustrated throughout this book and in the forms, letters, and report examples in the appendices. Take them seriously.

Many clinical duties and issues do not apply in the absence of a doctor–patient relationship (which is the case for most forensic work). But many clinical *ethics* issues *do* apply, and there are additional guidelines to consider as well.

"Official" ethics guidelines are a professional matter. They generally have no "legal" standing unless they have been incorporated into a statute (cf. many states' laws against clinicians having sex with patients).

Almost all ethics enforcement is done by professional organizations, such as the American Psychiatric Association or the American Psychological Association. Smaller professional organizations with ethics codes and guidelines may have no enforcement ability, but they often require that their members belong to a larger organization to which ethics violations can be reported and where they can be enforced. The worst punishment is banishment from the organization, which may then become an issue for credentialing or even licensure.

There are many reasons to belong to accepted professional organizations. One is the ability to say that you are expected to adhere to their ethics guidelines and (one hopes) that you have never been censured by them.

There are ethics "slippery slopes" in forensic work as well as in clinical work.

Common Ethics Issues

- Litigant advocacy
- Bias (vs. objectivity)
- Double agentry (including treater-expert)
- Disclosures, explanations, disclaimers
- Dishonesty (by commission or omission)
- Misrepresenting experience and credentials to attorneys and triers
- Pre-attorney interviews of criminal defendants

Being a forensic expert for a person who is also your patient, or who becomes your patient in the future, is usually imprudent and often unethical. Clinician–patient relationships can form in many ways, sometimes inadvertently. Be cautious about forming relationships with litigants or evaluees, and be sure everyone understands that your role is agent of the attorney or other retaining entity, not of the individual. Make it clear to the evaluee or litigant that you are not his or her clinician.

If you are treating a patient/client, be cautious when a lawyer wants to talk with you about that person, and more cautious if you are deposed about him or her. Understand the difference between a "fact" witness and one who offers "opinion testimony" (an expert witness).

You can choose whether or not you become involved as an expert in a forensic matter. If you discover something intolerable about a case after you have been retained, and you cannot resolve it with the attorney, you may resign or not participate.

Experts are sometimes tempted to disclose serious case problems (such as improper demands from the retaining lawyer) to the judge or court. It is often improper or unethical to discuss such things with the court or (especially) the other side (there are exceptions, such as when the expert is being threatened or extorted).

If you believe there is a significant danger to someone or some other serious problem that you have been unsuccessful resolving with the retaining attorney, you may consult an experienced colleague (who may discuss the practice or ethics issue but should not give "legal advice") or discuss it with your own lawyer.

*You may or may not **generally** be obligated to report clinicians for impairment (e.g., substance abuse or dementia) or improper behavior (e.g., patient exploitation) when you discover (or confirm) their problems in the course of being an expert in a forensic case.* Nevertheless, I recommend contacting your state licensing agency for guidance and/or discussing reporting duties with the retaining lawyer.

*You may or may not **generally** be obligated to report persons, hospitals, or other entities for abuse, neglect, or exploitation when you discover (or confirm) their problems in the course of being an expert in a forensic case.* Note that "reportable" conditions are often not limited to known or proved ones but include reasonable or good-faith suspicion as well. In many instances, discussion with the retaining attorney or entity, along with an expectation that "reportable" behavior will be reported appropriately, will resolve the issue. Determine for yourself whether or not the law requires that you report such "reportable" conditions if you discover them in a "forensic" rather than a general clinical context.

It may or may not be ethical to form opinions about someone without examining him or her. It is often impossible to examine the person about whose care or condition one may opine (e.g., a person who has committed suicide). It is acceptable to offer opinions without direct examination if one has sufficient reliable information and, in many cases, offers a disclaimer that no examination has been done, often with a comment about whether or how an examination might reasonably affect the opinion.

10

MARKETING

Marketing refers to the entire process of bringing a product or service to the public and creating a demand for it. It is not simply advertising. If it were, I wouldn't consider it for this book. *Your most important and effective marketing is the quality of your work and reputation.*

Quality is great marketing.

The job you do and the credibility you develop are your most important marketing tools.

You will be asked about your marketing methods at deposition and trial.

Your Target Market

Most successful forensic clinicians do little or no direct marketing. If you decide to market directly, remember, *your target is potential forensic contractees and referral sources.* Don't waste marketing efforts elsewhere.

Attorneys Attorneys are the most common clients for the majority of private forensic professionals. It's logical, then, that lawyers who specialize in criminal matters, malpractice, personal injury, insurance defense, worker's compensation, and family law use mental health experts more often than, say, real-estate specialists or corporate attorneys.

Courts Courts themselves (that is, judges or local judicial systems) may refer cases to experts who meet some criterion (such as being on a referral panel). Most experts don't (and shouldn't) depend on a local court system to support their practices.

Other clinicians and forensic specialists These are nice folks (just as you are) and interesting to be around (ditto), but rarely important forensic referral sources. Your *reputation* among them is important, however (which *is* a marketing issue).

Litigants (or potential litigants) and patients are not part of your "market." Leave the back cover of the phone book to lawyers. In fact, leave the entire Yellow Pages to them.

Recommendations

Reputation and word of mouth are your best marketing tools Lawyers remember good experts and often find new experts by talking with other lawyers.

The Internet Web searches are probably the second most common method used by lawyers to find new experts (after word of mouth), especially attorneys in smaller cities and rural areas. Unfortunately, it is difficult to attain prominent search-engine placement (largely because one of the most important search-engine placement criteria is time on the Web, and many other experts' sites have been online for over a decade—mine started in 1998). Ask your webmaster about things such as keywords and metatags in order to make yourself easier to find.

Don't pay anyone big bucks to create your website. There are lots of folks out there who will happily charge unsuspecting clinicians thousands of dollars for a pretty vanilla site and a domain name such as experts.com/mental/psychologists/eastcoast/newark/drfredsmith.com (which doesn't exactly stick in a potential client's memory). On the other hand, a new and much better domain name costs under $25 per year (you'll need to search a little, but I'll bet fredsmithpsychology.com is available). Reliable hosting is easy to find yourself, and very reasonable, and setting up a simple website should be inexpensive (a few hundred dollars at most; less if it is done by you or your spouse).

If you work with a professional website designer (not a bad idea), remember that, although they are very good at bells and whistles, "gee whiz," and designing for advertising or sales, *that's not what you want*. Your purpose and needs—quiet credibility, information, and professionalism—are different from those of their other Web customers. Spend those dollars on such things as host reliability, site flexibility, and setting up a site that you can easily update yourself.

I believe lawyers and other potential forensic clients respond most positively to websites that are straightforward, professional, and *not* full of "advertising" or self-aggrandizement. Educational material targeted to the kinds of cases with which you work seems logical and helps increase your search-engine placement (as does a high ratio of text to photos in the content). Some information about your qualifications and background is important, but don't list past legal cases or post a detailed *curriculum vitae*. Your name and contact information shouldn't be in a flashing 36-point font; once at the site, if your qualifications are interesting to the reader, he or she will find it.

Don't fall for the many scams that promise to improve your search-engine placement. Even honest consultants probably can't do it much better than you can (with a little research), and no one can do it very well without paying for the placement—usually a mistake, in my opinion.

You will receive emails from strangers asking to "exchange links" or place links on your site (and maybe an ad or two). Resist them. First, you don't know these people and you have no control over their content. Second, link exchange, while it may have a tiny effect on search-engine positioning, doesn't help you much. Do it with a colleague or friend if you wish (I do), but keep it professional.

Update *and test* your website and search-engine placement regularly (at least once a month). Google and other search-engine companies keep their ranking formulas secret, but frequent updates seem to be important and "stale" sites seem to disappear from top search rankings. Changing a few commas won't cut it; add something substantial (such as a new article or fresh blog). Test search-engine placement using key words a lawyer might use when looking for an expert in your field (e.g., a grouping of "psychologist" and "testamentary capacity" or "psychiatrist," "suicide," and "standard of care"). Don't forget that quotation marks around search words create a search for that specific phrase, not its component words. *Be sure your site's keywords and metatags reflect the words and phrases that you believe potential clients will use in their searches.*

Follow your website traffic with a monitoring program (usually free). Ask your Web host what statistics package they provide and use it every few weeks to gauge number of visitors, movement patterns within your site, and the like.

As far as social media marketing is concerned, Facebook is great for attracting restaurant customers or promoting your kid's rock band, but refrain from using it for forensic marketing. LinkedIn may work for entrepreneurial networking, but I'd be cautious about using it for forensic practice marketing.

Finally, feel free to visit www.reidpsychiatry.com for suggestions (but don't just copy it). It's primarily educational, with lots of student/trainee visitors, but it has also been a significant source of referrals (in part because its search-engine placement, for searches in my areas of interest, is excellent).

Certifications Professionally accepted certifications may be helpful in separating you from those in the field who are not certified. General and child psychiatry certification by the American Board of Psychiatry and

Neurology (ABPN)[1] is important for psychiatrists in those fields, and subspecialty ABPN certification (such as psychopharmacology, substance abuse, or geriatrics) may be relevant for particular kinds of practice. Specific ABPN forensic psychiatry certification is often irrelevant to lawyers (who are more interested in your clinical and scientific knowledge about their cases), though it establishes a certain level of formal training and understanding of the legal exercise. Psychologists' certification by the American Board of Professional Psychology (ABPP) is a good thing, and certification in neuropsychology is quite valuable in that subspecialty (e.g., for cases involving brain injury or damage).

Don't bother with the many pseudo-certifications offered online (anything you can get with just a degree, a questionnaire, and a credit card); they often do more harm than good.

An excellent interface between your office and new referrals   Your success is a combination of the number of potential clients who call and the number who actually become clients after contacting you. Be easily reachable and easy to work with (but not "easy to manipulate" or a "hired gun"). Lawyers and their staff people will remember courtesy, competence, intelligent discussion, and generosity with your time.

Less Useful but Often Worth the Trouble

Tasteful announcements to attorneys are acceptable and sometimes helpful. Don't include a *curriculum vitae* or list of cases or lawyers with whom you've worked. What kind of announcement might *you* seek that professional rather than ask a colleague for a referral?

Teaching mental health-related courses or seminars in law schools, legal or judicial continuing education settings, law-enforcement training sessions, or risk management symposia is a fine contribution (and you'll learn a lot as well). You're not the first expert to think of it, so opportunities may not be immediately available.

Media interviews are often a public service, but be sure the topic is newsworthy and not self-serving fluff. Be conservative, not sensational. The contacts you will receive from media exposure are less likely to be from attorneys than from potential litigants (whom you'll want politely to avoid, and some of whom have been turned down by lawyers). Many attorneys prefer an expert who is not a television personality.

Nonprofessional service organizations (Rotary, Kiwanis, Lion's Club, etc.) are a traditional networking tool and good for your community. Join

---

1 Recognition by equivalent bodies, such as the British or Canadian Royal College of Psychiatrists, is usually fine. Osteopathic Board certification is unusual but equivalent.

them because they do good works, not because the members will refer you business.

Not Recommended

The following are not recommended (but are usually ethical):

- marketing brochures;
- legal directories, Yellow Pages, other ads;
- self-serving media interviews;
- flashy Internet pages, website banners;
- Internet expert directories, referral brokers, paid referral services.

Don't believe anyone who says he or she can increase your referrals through some "expert listing" or "expert finder" website. Be cautious about expert "brokers" who have a stable of forensic practitioners to whom they refer cases. Many (not all) use procedures that are ethically acceptable, but the fine print in their contracts can limit your flexibility and practice style. I never pay for such services, and I believe that sounds good to lawyers and juries.

The following are not recommended and are often unethical:

- marketing to patients or litigants;
- advising people to sue or referring them to lawyers for personal gain;
- offering to become be an expert for your own patients or former patients.

Access and Availability

Make it easy for the lawyer or other retaining entity.

Be very available to callers. New attorney calls are among your highest priorities. Return missed calls immediately. You are probably not the only expert the attorney is considering; if you aren't available, most of them will simply go to the next person on their lists.

Consider a toll-free phone line or a permanent, very reliable cell phone number (the toll-free number can "roll" to your local number). Although the cost of long distance is largely irrelevant these days, a toll-free number still highlights convenience for the caller. Even more important, if you move across country, the number can move with you. *Lawyers may have your number on file for years before dialing it*, and it is very common to receive repeat referrals several years after an earlier case. If you use a cell phone number in your practice, *always carry that phone*. If the other golfers complain when it rings, tell them you're on call.[2]

---

2 I used to say, "Tell them your wife is having a baby," but that's 'way too sexist.

*Have your office phone answered by an intelligent, professional **person**,* not an answering machine, voicemail, or twit.

Have at least two business phone lines (one of which rolls automatically to the unused line) and a separate fax line, and don't use cheap or unreliable telephone or email services.

Test *your office telephone and email procedures occasionally* to be sure they're professional and responsive to callers.

Don't miss referrals because your phone number, address, or email address has changed. Use a post office box for U.S. mail rather than a physical address, and maintain your box, email address, and phone number indefinitely, no matter where you move. Use a toll-free number, a permanent cell number, and a national Internet service provider (not a local one that will change if you move) for email. As already noted, referrals may come months or years after someone gets your name; cases may be quiescent for months or years; months may elapse from initial call to retainer or agreement, and lawyers who liked your work in earlier cases may call years later with new ones.

Remember, contrary to ordinary clinical practice, *each new forensic client provides a significant portion of your office income.* It's simply a business fact that forensic work is a low-volume, high-revenue-per-client profession. A missed call, or one that is returned late, can be very expensive; if the potential client reaches someone else before you call back, or if reaching you is inconvenient, you'll never know what you missed.

Make Every Public Interface Very High Quality

Some of the items below may seem trivial. They're not. Forensic clients, such as attorneys, may never see your office (particularly if your work is regional or national), so make sure the other interfaces you have with them reflect professional quality, whether you work from a fancy office or review records in your spare bedroom.

Many of the people who matter to your success understand the difference between engraved letterhead and computer letterhead, engraved parchment business cards and "thermo" fakes, minimum-wage staff and sophisticated assistants. Every interaction you have with the professional public should be consistent with an impression of competence, solid reliability, top quality, and customer service.

By the way, you'll like the way the items below make *you* feel, too.

- *Staff* Hire intelligent, helpful, polite, reliable, professional staff. Don't be penny wise and pound foolish when hiring (or in any of the items in this section).
- *Stationery and business cards* Consider engraved letterhead, on excellent stock (few commercial printers offer true engraving). Engraved business cards (on parchment) are worth every penny. Design letterhead

and cards tastefully; don't fill cards with extraneous information (or your photo). Avoid bargain printers (and for goodness' sake don't print your own letterhead or business cards). Many people won't notice these touches, *but those who do can contribute a lot to your success.*

- *Telephones and telephone answering*   See above.
- *Fax machines and copiers*   Make them fast, reliable, and fairly high capacity. Avoid "all-in-one" printer/fax/copiers.
- *Have absolutely reliable, high-speed Internet service*   You will often receive large attachments, do online research, and exchange time-sensitive emails.
- *Deliver what you promise, on time, every time*   No . . . deliver it *early.*
- *Dress and groom professionally when meeting with attorneys or other clients and when examining evaluees*   That doesn't mean "fancy" or "rich," but never take a "casual Friday" if you're meeting with a lawyer or examining an evaluee. If you're a male, wear a tie unless you know the uniform of the day is "business casual." If you're not sure how to do this, ask a successful, court-savvy lawyer for sartorial advice (don't ask one who is not very successful).
- *Have excellent manners and diction*   Your manners and dress communicate volumes about you and imply a lot about your social and forensic competence. If it doesn't come naturally, or if you believe your cultural background may interfere with getting along in professional situations, don't be afraid to get some friendly consultation or a simple book on etiquette. It matters to your career.
- *Be easy to work with*   Once you've been engaged by a lawyer or other client, the quality of your service is judged in part by the ease with which he or she can work with you. This doesn't mean bending to unreasonable or unethical expectations; it means *understanding the client's needs, being available and attentive, knowing your stuff, and caring about your work.*

Referral Courtesy

One day I got a call from a lawyer who practices only a few miles from my office. It was a bit of a surprise, since forensic cases rarely come up in my community. He was defending a client in a murder case and had called a prominent forensic colleague in a faraway state. The colleague told him, in essence, "I'd be happy to work with you, but did you know that there is another qualified forensic psychiatrist just down the road from you?"

I thanked my colleague, and years later had an opportunity to do the same with a lawyer in his city.

Offer to refer attorneys to other forensic colleagues when you can't, shouldn't, or don't want to accept a referral, or simply when you know there's a colleague who might be more convenient for the attorney (e.g., in his or her geographic area). This starts the relationship off on a good note by illustrating your willingness to help the caller get what he or she needs. It's nice for your colleagues, too. And send a brief heads-up email to the person/people to whom you're referring the caller, perhaps with the lawyer's name (but without case details).

Don't refer lawyers to colleagues unless you have reason to believe they are competent and ethical. You probably have a directory of forensic professionals and can help attorneys find one, but don't do it blindly (any more than you would unqualifiedly refer a patient to a clinician without knowing something about him or her). I always tell the caller whether or not I have actually observed the work or skill of the person whose name I give out, or am giving the name merely because the person belongs to an organization and is certified in his or her field. I quietly avoid sending referrals to people I believe may not meet standards of practice quality and ethics.

Express appreciation. Send thank-you notes and annual holiday cards. Follow up after cases are resolved, not to "keep score" but to see if there was anything you might have done differently, or just to congratulate the attorney on settling. Send good clients small holiday gifts (it's not a "bribe," it's a *courtesy*).

11

YOUR OFFICE AND OFFICE PROCEDURES

A successful forensic practice does not need a very large administrative operation, but it must have a very *good* administrative operation.

Staff

People, even if it's just one assistant, are the backbone of your practice and the arbiters of your success. *Employ the very best staff you can.*

- They often have more contact with your clients than you do.
- They are usually the first people your potential clients encounter.
- They are the public face of your practice and the interface between you and your clients.

Choose them carefully; train them well; treat them right; and, if you have to skimp, skimp on something else.

Keep Your Files and Practice Secure

- It's your duty to the attorney-client.
- Do background checks on new staff.
- Train staff in basic security procedures.
- If you don't do your own cleaning, lock everything daily (cleaning people can be very curious).
- Be aware of, and deal with, the substantial security risks associated with email.
- Don't be too dramatic; you're not the CIA.

Telephone Coverage

Best: A real person, in the office
Second best: A real person, in the office
Fall-back: A real person, in the office

The telephone is your main interface with clients and potential clients. (Your written material is second.) Carry your cell phone everywhere you go (see chapter 10).

Email is convenient, but it does not replace telephone contact. New attorney-clients often contact me first by email, but I uniformly suggest that we speak by phone (at no charge) and not discuss the case by email. You learn more in a direct conversation, and so does the caller.

Records and Logs

Log everything that comes into and goes out of your office, including phone calls, letters, records, deliveries, and visitors. Make file notes of telephone conversations, scheduling agreements, billing changes, etc. You will list what you reviewed when deposed or writing reports; referring to a log of records received (and pasting it into a report, for example) is much easier than shuffling through boxes of paper.

Keep track. Have a procedure for keeping track of current and past cases, case types, past testimony, referral sources, etc. These seeming "details" are very handy for analyzing your practice patterns, keeping track of referral sources, adhering to jurisdiction rules for testimony lists, and verifying your practice makeup when asked during testimony.

Have a system for keeping track of case expectations and deadlines as well (e.g., a simple spreadsheet). It's also useful for quick review for conflicts in new referrals.

Client Files and Records

Keep them secure and keep them accessible. You'll often have to locate records after several months, even years.

Consider creating a very accessible *summary file* for each case, with copies of your notes, reports, and other frequently addressed information (including everything you created personally). I call this our "main file." Keep a separate *financial file* with time sheets, bills, invoices, payment records, etc.

You'll need lots of on-site, accessible storage for *bulk records* and a good system for filing and locating them, as cases move from active to quiescent and back over months or years. Scanning and DVDs may help, but those who think they can create some sort of "paperless office" . . . let me know how that works out for you. *Do not* store client records in the "cloud" without the client's permission and a very reliable system.

Old case archives should be kept until the client says they may be destroyed. I strongly recommend keeping your "main" or summary files, and perhaps case financial files, forever. I've been called for information over a decade after case resolution (in one case many years after the defendant in question was executed). If you use off-site storage, be sure that it is secure.

Many offices log and track access to all of the above. I recommend it . . . see what I mean about needing good staff?

Opposing lawyers often ask for copies of your old depositions. I rarely keep mine. If you have yours, you may have to produce them unless you can reasonably establish that doing so would create an onerous task (e.g., searching through piles of off-site storage). Lawyers can get most old depositions themselves using search services; if you do the search yourself, charge a reasonable fee.

Get a good shredder for disposing of obsolete records. Don't just send them to a landfill. If you use a shredding service or commercial recycler, be sure the records are rendered unreadable.

Billing and Collections

Try hard to prevent collection problems beforehand (see chapter 8). Most lawyers pay promptly. A few make it very hard to collect. Have a specific billing procedure which is understood *in writing* before agreeing to provide services. Just a few deadbeats can lead to substantial loss of income.

- Require retainers against billings.
- Consider requiring replenishment of retainers.
- Consider requiring payment before releasing reports.
- Settle outstanding bills before testifying.
- Require deposits for estimated testimony or report preparation time and expenses.

Expect an adequate retainer and prompt payments. Strongly consider not testifying, and perhaps refraining from releasing reports or opinions, when the outstanding bill is large (and warn the client well in advance). Note the ethics and credibility issues of offering opinions while owed lots of money; some juries and judges reasonably suspect that would affect your testimony. You need not hold lawyers "hostage," but have a clear understanding with the retaining entity that payment must be current before testimony (or release of a report).

On average, you are likely to have more problems with lawyers who are new to your practice, those who represent civil plaintiffs or criminal defendants (and thus rely on individual clients, or on winning the case, for their own income), plaintiffs' and criminal defense lawyers who lose their cases, and those outside your geographic area. Attorneys who are paid by insurance companies or government agencies may be slow in paying, but they tend to have better track records.

Plaintiffs' attorneys who have invested large amounts of their own money in a case and lost (perhaps in a faraway state) have little motivation other than their own sense of fairness to pay you after your usefulness has passed. A few may try to tell you that your testimony hurt their cases and refuse to pay on those grounds. This is obviously an unfair and unethical stance, regardless of your testimony, since you work by the hour and winning the case is not, and should never be, your responsibility (it's their job to use your opinions wisely).

When bills are overdue, don't waste time with the firm's or agency's accounts payable clerk. He or she is not the decision-maker. You or your staff person should talk to the person who can write the check.

Once again,

- be fair;
- bill regularly;
- itemize statements;
- make your time sheets and billing records available;
- don't "nickel and dime" clients with charges for very brief services, routine office procedures, short phone calls, curbstone advice, etc. (I like to enter a "no charge" for such things on the bill; it just looks nice);
- *do not* cheat or pad billings;
- charging interest on overdue bills is subject to legal procedures and rarely worth it.

Serious Collection Problems

When you know you've done your job and deserve to be paid, try not to be bullied by lawyers who threaten to sue you, say they'll besmirch your reputation, etc. (often saying you screwed up when you didn't). I know I've said your reputation is critical and lawyers are your best referral source but, in this case, ignore the threats. After all, whether or not such a lawyer pays you is unlikely to affect what he or she says to colleagues or puts on his or her Facebook page, and you'll feel better if you don't knuckle under. And it's amazing how often other lawyers know that the one who is stiffing you is a schmuck.

If you find that a lawyer or other influential person is saying or writing bad (and untrue) things about you (e.g., on Facebook, LinkedIn, or an attorney forum or list-serv), consider pursuing the matter vigorously. *It's slander or libel*, and damage to your reputation is damage to your livelihood.

A couple of years ago, I Googled a very reputable forensic colleague's name and came across a terrible post about her on a prosecutors' online forum. I notified her at once. She contacted the forum administrator, who removed the offensive message, posted an apology, and offered other ways to correct the forum record. No one knows how the post may have affected her reputation or referrals during the years it was there, but the problem was eliminated.

Don't forgive a large overdue bill in the hope of mollifying the lawyer. I've actually seen experts do this, and it's stupid.

Some years ago, before I knew better, a well-known attorney retained two other experts and me for a civil matter that involved a great deal of money. He and his firm paid the bills promptly for the first several months, then the "tab" began to mount as he requested a lot of time-consuming record review, travel to attorney meetings, etc. The case went to trial and the lawyer's side lost. I had not been paid before the trial, and was owed over $40,000.

I billed the attorney for over a year with essentially no response. Finally, I contacted the other two experts, who lived in the same city as the attorney, and discovered that they were owed similar amounts. I suggested that we take legal action as a group, but both said, in effect, that they did not want to irritate the attorney for fear of not getting future cases from him!

I retained a lawyer, who wrote a letter threatening to sue for breach of contract, citing our original fee agreement, my detailed time sheets, and earlier bills. Within a couple of weeks, I accepted a settlement check for about 75 percent of the bill.

How many of the business and billing principles mentioned in this chapter does the above vignette illustrate? I suspect the other two experts didn't get more cases from that lawyer anyway (and why would they accept them?).

Prevention is much better than cure, but, for the rare times when things get nasty, you should know how to find a lawyer who sues other lawyers. Lawsuits for nonpayment (generally a contract issue and thus fairly simple) are usually successful but not worth the trouble for just a few hundred bucks. I've done it only once in over 30 years of practice. Most collection processes begin with a letter from your lawyer and are resolved once the deadbeat knows you're not going to take it lying down. (Do not threaten to sue if you have no intention of doing so.)

State bar associations have complaint processes (sometimes specifically for clinician-lawyer issues) which are *occasionally* helpful in billing disputes. They are almost never helpful if the lawyer is in another state.

Budgeting

Learn to budget. Compensation in private forensic practice usually comes in fairly large amounts, but infrequently. Sometimes the pipeline is full;

often it is dry (especially in small practices). Unlike salaried positions or clinical practices in which one may have dozens of paying patients/clients each week, slack periods and long payment delays are routine.

Don't take that tempting $5,000 retainer and make a down payment on a new car.[1] The retainer isn't yours until you've earned it (you are merely holding the money, which is better than letting the client hold the money, but you must be honest with it). Besides, you're responsible for income-tax deposits, tax withholding, employee salaries and benefits, prompt client refunds, insurance, etc., in addition to your family expenses.

It is very helpful to keep a separate account for retainers and client deposits, to remind you that the money is not yet yours and to make it easy to send refunds promptly when necessary. More than one of my forensic clients has told me that the promptness of the refund—and the fact that an expert actually sent money back—was a much appreciated surprise.

---

1 I recommend that you pay cash for cars anyway, and for other depreciating assets.

1 2

LIABILITY IN FORENSIC PRACTICE

Even more disclaimer: I'm not a lawyer, and this isn't legal advice! It's merely my non-lawyer thoughts.

*Liability arises from a **duty** that one person or entity has to another.* You have duties to the person (e.g., lawyer) who retains you. For example, you must be reasonably diligent in your work, avoid misrepresentation, provide adequate quality of work, and not abandon the retaining person without an acceptable reason.

You *may* have duties to that lawyer's or entity's client or litigant—for example, to provide such diligence and quality of work that you do not unreasonably endanger the case through failure to perform (*not* the same as failure to support the client's side, to advocate for the litigant, or to do everything the lawyer may demand).

You may have duties to other people—for example, those whom you evaluate (such as refraining from acting in bad faith, being dishonest, or negligently causing a loss or damage).

You have a strong duty of truthfulness to the court, and you probably have some duty to be reasonably objective.

Negligent breach of a duty may cause damage, for which the negligent person (you, in this case) may be found liable. Other problems that could apply (but are rarely seen among qualified experts), some of which can involve criminal charges, include perjury, contempt of court, and spoliation of evidence. You are more likely to be accused of a breach of duty if the lawyer or litigant with whom you are associated loses his or her case. (Duh.)

Be sure you are insured. In my experience, most forensic work incurs far fewer malpractice allegations than clinical work, but be sure your insurance policy covers your forensic work, including being sued for damages outside the usual "malpractice" realms. Some malpractice policies cover forensic work without an additional rider; others don't. *Ask your carrier!*

Working in States in Which You Aren't Licensed to Practice Medicine, Psychology, etc.

Note that I didn't say "practicing" in those states. Most litigation- or administratively related forensic work does not seem to me to be psychology or medical "practice" for licensure purposes, but state Board rules vary about some of the items below.

Consider the various possibilities when

- reviewing materials for an out-of state case while in your home state;
- reviewing materials for a lawyer or agency while in another state (i.e., "on site," in a state in which you are not licensed);
- working with a lawyer or agency while in another state;
- testifying in another state;
- doing a forensic interview in another state;
- performing a broader examination of an evaluee[1] (e.g., an IME) in another state;
- offering a diagnosis or treatment recommendation for a *clinical* purpose (not a forensic or administrative one) in another state.

I have worked with forensic matters in more than 35 states over the years (not always actually testifying in those states, and not usually examining evaluees in them). It seems to me[2] that forensic work of the kind outlined in this book is not done on behalf of one's own "patient" or clinical "client" (see discussions earlier in these pages) or for any direct purpose of treatment (although treatment and its costs may be discussed as part of a damage assessment).

Reviewing records and discussing them with a lawyer or other person for a nonclinical purpose is not similar to activities commonly called the "practice of medicine" (or "psychology"). Almost all review occurs in one's home state anyway.

Examinations or consultations done for forensic or administrative purposes, or done for non-health-care professionals and nonclinical purposes, and which do not contemplate participating in the evaluee's clinical care or making recommendations to treating clinicians regarding that care, are quite different from those done for health-care professionals. I'm speaking here of consultations to attorneys, law-enforcement agencies, correctional systems, or judges, as well as companies, schools, or organizations that are concerned about, for example, an employee's or student's dangerousness to others.

---

1 One more reason to make it clear that the evaluee or interviewee is not one's patient or client.

2 The non-lawyer, remember?

Testifying or reporting about one's opinions, no matter how "clinical" or nonclinical the opinions may be, seems to me a matter of simple freedom of speech (one often exercised by both clinicians and nonclinicians in courts, the media, and other fora). In addition, I believe it is reasonable to assume that, if a judge of proper jurisdiction allows an expert to testify or otherwise participate in a forensic matter (or, especially, *directs* the expert to testify), then the expert's decision to do so should not be constrained by an absence of licensure.

Some persons who are the focus of forensic work are deceased (cf. many malpractice cases). It seems logical that one cannot "practice medicine/psychology" by reviewing their records or testifying about what those records contain or imply.

Some evaluees or litigants cannot reasonably travel to the expert's home state (e.g., those confined to hospitals or correctional institutions). I agree with the common argument that those persons are entitled—as are litigants on the opposing side—to access to expertise which is not available, or not deemed to be optimal, in their own states.

As a practical matter, some experts try to shift this issue to retaining lawyers—for example, by reminding them in writing that they (the experts) have no license in the states in question and giving the attorneys responsibility for notifying them of licensure requirements or otherwise making everything okay. I have often let a retaining entity know that I am not licensed in his or her state and am uniformly told that it will not be a problem. I'm not at all sure that means there *couldn't* be a problem. *The lawyer who retains you is almost certainly not in a position to be "your" lawyer and may not be in a position to give you legal advice.*

Finally, at the time of this writing, a few states (notably Florida) issue a time-limited "expert witness" permit (for physicians at least) that is quickly and easily obtainable for a small fee. While I do not agree that such a permit should be necessary in most cases, I would not recommend challenging the system unnecessarily, and the permit does eliminate any question of propriety or liability for "practicing without a license."

13

A LAWYER'S PERSPECTIVE ON FORENSIC MENTAL HEALTH EXPERTS

Skip Simpson, J.D.[1]

No matter what I say in the following paragraphs, remember that I am writing this chapter to brighten your day and make your decision to become an expert a joy. I'm currently a plaintiff's lawyer who works a lot with mental health malpractice, but I've had lots of other trial roles during my career. I've tried to make these comments apply to many kinds of legal practice.

You've already read that most expert activity does not involve testifying, but my perspective, which includes whether or not I retain you to help in a case, must assume that each case *will* go to trial and that you will be the person who testifies on behalf of my client. Jury impressions and reactions are very important to my work; I consider and retain my experts accordingly.

What is your motivation? Why have you decided to be a forensic mental health expert? To help others? To improve society? To serve as a watchdog for your profession? For professional stimulation? To protect your colleagues from unfair accusations? Did you choose this line of work to be a part of the action and glamour of the courtroom? Or is it for the money?

The jury already "knows" the answer: It's money. They will learn what you are charging for every hour you speak to them. They believe you are in the courtroom because a greedy, money-loving lawyer hired you. They will learn what you charged for every hour you prepared to speak to them. They may learn what percentage of your income comes from expressing

---

1 Skip Simpson, J.D., is a successful trial lawyer in the Dallas–Fort Worth area with experience in criminal and civil matters as a prosecutor, criminal defense attorney, and plaintiffs' lawyer in state, federal, and military courts. His current work and positions include cases across the U.S. in state and federal jurisdictions, speaking before mental health forensic groups on providing care without fear of being sued, research associate in the Harvard Medical School Program in Psychiatry and the Law, national expert on suicide risk and prevention, and Adjunct Associate Professor of Psychiatry at the University of Texas Health Science Center, San Antonio.

opinions for money (the way the other side will ask them to think of your work). Those amounts are much more than jurors themselves earn.

That's not an unfair position for jurors to take, given their limited knowledge and their exposure to television, websites, and lawyers' advertisements. Both the lawyer and the expert should recognize that fact from the outset.

Why am I highlighting money? I start this chapter talking about money because jurors know there is at least *some* level of motivation for experts simply to dance to the tune of the lawyers who hired them. If a jury believes my expert is dancing for money, they will disregard his or her testimony and punish my client. Consequently, I must seek experts not only for their skill and experience but, more important, for their integrity and their attitude: to help the jury reach a correct and reasoned verdict.

Rules

Courts and judges have rules about experts. The trial judge follows various requirements for allowing experts to testify. They are based on longstanding "rules of evidence," as well as the individual judge's interpretation of them. We'll touch on just a few in this chapter.

It is important to know the difference between lay (fact)[2] witness testimony and expert testimony. Lay witnesses are restricted to testifying only about their personal knowledge of the matter at hand.[3] A lay witness can give an opinion only if (a) it is rationally based on the witness's perception; (b) it helps the court to understand the witness's testimony or to determine a fact in issue; and (c) it is not based on knowledge that requires an expert.[4] For example, a lay witness can say someone *seemed* to be drunk, depressed, or anxious, or acted weird.

In contrast, an expert (once "qualified" by the judge; see below) may express opinions on facts and evidence about which he or she possesses special knowledge beyond that of most lay individuals. The legal basis of expert testimony is provided in federal and state rules of evidence.[5] The expert must possess scientific, technical, or other specialized knowledge or skill that will aid the trier of fact (the jury or, in a "bench trial" [which has no jury], the judge) in understanding the evidence or will help to establish a fact in issue. The witness must be qualified as an expert—by showing the court that he or she possesses requisite special skills, knowledge, experience, training, or education—before being allowed to offer an opinion.

The rest of this chapter is largely about *my* rules in expert selection and use. (Yes, I "use" you.) My rules were handed down to me initially by my

---

2 For our purpose, a "lay" witness is the same as a "fact" witness, as defined in chapter 2 on vocabulary.

3 Federal Rules of Evidence (FRE) 602.

4 FRE 701.

5 E.g., FRE 702–705.

parents and later by my teachers, the military, mentors, colleagues, and my church. Jurors have had similar influences in life. That helps.

I use you to help assess my case, teach me about some of its elements, assist in framing its presentation, and increase my chances of winning (or settling wisely). Although you aren't a direct advocate for my client, you and I must become a team. We participate in an "adversarial" system of justice whose advantages have proved themselves countless times over many centuries.

My first rule is the rule of *integrity*.

> My first rule is *integrity*.

You're probably saying "How dare a lawyer talk to me about integrity."

In my 36 years of being a trial lawyer, the majority of the attorneys that I have worked with and against have been honest men and women. Many lawyers are truly honorable; a few much less so. As a former state, military, and federal prosecutor, I put several bad-actor lawyers into prison (as well as a few doctors, ministers, and politicians).

Integrity means, in part, that you're not interested primarily in yourself but in others. If my potential expert is focused on him- or herself, he or she doesn't make the cut. For my clients (largely civil plaintiffs who have suffered tragic losses), I need experts who want to make the community a better, safer place. But, regardless of a lawyer's "side" (plaintiff, prosecutor, civil or criminal defense), most of us look for a sense that the expert believes our cases occupy the moral high ground.[6]

Since I carefully choose and research my cases before filing them, I expect my expert, after appropriate review and contemplation, to conclude that my client deserves to win, that he or she (the expert) is on the "right" side of the case. (I'm not talking here about technical nuances or individual facts, although those must fall into place as well.) If that doesn't happen, then either there is something wrong with my case or I have chosen the wrong expert. I consider both possibilities. *Believing that one is on the right side is a big deal* and adds greatly to one's credibility.

Of course, attorneys don't always know whether or not they have good cases. Some rely more than others on the expert's review and opinions in order to decide whether or not to proceed, figure out how to frame the case, or support a poorly conceived (by the lawyer) case impression. Sometimes

---

6 Some cases involve more "moral high ground" than others, of course, and some (often inexperienced) lawyers try to convince experts that their causes are just. Mental health cases often involve human tragedy and real suffering. Juries are guardians of the community. At the end of the day, the jury wants its verdict to protect the community.

you end up disagreeing significantly with the attorney; good lawyers will question you about areas of both agreement and disagreement. Don't adjust your views and opinions just to fit a bad case or to please an erroneous or inexperienced lawyer. That's bad for all concerned and will hurt your reputation in the long run.[7]

What Can You Teach Me?

Tell me the truth. My experts are told, and understand in my first conversation with them, that what will please me is the unvarnished truth. I am interested only in solid, meritorious cases. They know I would much rather decline a case early than waste months of time and money locked into one that is unworthy.[8] My experts know that I want their opinions to be solid and easily defensible in court and to uphold reasonable clinical standards (safety rules) that the community needs. Lawyers who oppose my clients may want many of the same things, as do those who work in criminal law, family law, and every other legal field. We have to know (at the outset when possible) when to fight, when to compromise, and when to fold up our tents and go home (and, as Dr. Reid says elsewhere in this text, we hate surprises). If, after adequate review, evaluation, and contemplation, an expert doesn't think his or her opinions will withstand detailed scrutiny by a vigorous and educated *opposing* lawyer, that part of the case is probably weak and the expert should let the retaining attorney know as soon possible.

Help me assess my case. It is very useful to have a forensic expert help me value the case. On a scale of 1 to 10 (1 being pathetic and 10 being outstanding), if the case is an 8, I need to learn about clinical factors that might make it a 10. When it's not a 10, an expert can help me decide whether to settle a case or bring it to trial. (If the other side's settlement offer does not compensate my client according to my view of the damages, and recognize the safety violations,[9] I am likely to try the case in any event—I already know it is a strong case, otherwise I would not have pursued it to that point.) I rely on my trial team, including experts, to be frank with me about cases; I try hard to avoid drinking whiskey from my own barrel.[10]

---

7 News travels fast among lawyers. If you want the news about you to be good, you must be highly competent and ethical and understand our needs.

8 One potent safeguard against frivolous malpractice cases is cost to the plaintiff's attorney: hundreds of hours and, ordinarily, $50,000 to $100,000 (often much more) from the lawyer's own pocket. Poor cases are very expensive!

9 Wording is important. "Safety violation" is my non-jargon phrase for violation of the clinical standard of care (SOC). I view SOC breaches as a matter of personal and public safety, and I believe juries understand "safety" better than "standard of care."

10 If this metaphor escapes you, you're just more sophisticated than I. No problem.

I want my expert to be experienced and knowledgeable enough to let me know the strengths and weaknesses of my case, and of the other side's case, and how to phrase the strengths to my client's advantage. If there are flaws in an opposing expert's opinions, I need to know about them and have them explained, so that I can use that information in framing my case. In addition, if there are parts of my case that aren't consistent with my objective (winning) or that appear to contradict each other, an expert may be able to point those out within his or her field of expertise. That doesn't mean my expert is "advocating" in the same way I do, but rather that he or she can articulate important aspects of the case for me to use on behalf of my client.

A consulting expert can suggest deposition questions for me to ask opposing experts and lay witnesses. One purpose of depositions is to discover the strengths and weaknesses of the other side's case. My expert can assist me in that objective and help me get answers that clarify the clinical issues. If my case assessment has been accurate, and the expert's work is accurate and complete, then my case always becomes stronger after the depositions.

In my plaintiffs' practice, expert review of the records can tell me about others who have been negligent, including potential defendants I may have missed, so that I don't weaken the case for my client. If I were a malpractice defense lawyer, I could use that same knowledge to deal with potential additional liability.[11] I also need to know which expert can testify against which allegedly negligent defendant. Can a psychiatrist testify about a nurse's behavior? Sometimes the answer is yes, but each jurisdiction has its own rules. One of my trial team's jobs is to make sure the expert is on solid ground with regard to whom he or she can testify about concerning the standard of care for a given professional discipline. Some psychiatrists are expert in psychiatric hospitals or clinical staffing; many are not. Sometimes a psychologist can opine about a social worker's counseling, and sometimes not.

What Can You Teach the Jury (and How Will You Talk to Them)?

The forensic mental health expert must not stop after cataloguing the case information, digesting it, and interpreting it. He or she must be able to present the information to a trier of fact (usually a jury)[12] in a helpful manner.

---

11 Most examples in this chapter apply to experts on all sides, not just my particular type of practice.
12 Note that, when a judge rather than a jury is the trier of fact, the task usually does not change. Testimony to a judge should entail the same kind of presentation, clarity, credibility, etc., as testimony to a jury.

Framing the issues   The expert helps me—and eventually the jury—to frame the issues. I'm not looking merely for someone who qualifies technically as an expert. I need those who, for example, can point out why it is dangerous not to follow certain practices and standards of care. In my practice—plaintiffs' cases often involving suicide—they must know that standards of care (safety rules) are important and protect people, and must be able to explain that, simply and concisely, to a jury.

Reasonable certainty   In the world of litigation (especially civil litigation), experts must express their opinions to a "reasonable certainty" or "reasonable probability"[13] (cf. reasonable medical, psychological, psychiatric, or professional certainty/probability). *That phrase simply means "more likely than not."* That is, in order to be "certain" in the context of an expert opinion, you need only exceed a 50+ percent threshold.

> "Reasonable probability" or "certainty" of opinions
> means "more likely than not."

A great many experts misunderstand this simple, crucial definition, probably because it differs from the way clinicians usually view "certainty." Don't be one of them.

"Possibilities" and opinions   Expert witnesses must also know the difference between expert opinion and "possibility." It is not sufficient to offer mere "possibility" as an opinion; *probability* is the requisite threshold, and probability is defined as "more likely than not." If your opinions in my favor don't reach probability, then they don't help my case, *and you must tell me that long before any deposition or trial.*

Your Courtroom Presentation

First I must have a case that deserves to win. Then I need to have it presented in such a way that the jury or other trier of fact (judge, panel, licensing board) *listens* to the evidence and to my witnesses. That means you must *(1) change their inherently negative expectations about expert witnesses, (2) instill an assumption of competence and credibility, and (3) help them see your (and my) points in a way that they will remember during their deliberations.*

---

13 Some jurisdictions say "certainty," others "probability." *They mean the same thing in this context* ("more likely than not").

The experts I retain don't use lots of mental health jargon. They talk plainly and to the point. Jurors do not like pretentious experts, and their eyes glaze over when they hear psychobabble. They take it to mean that the expert is hiding something, which immediately translates into a loss of credibility—more on this point later.

The expert's most advantageous courtroom appearance, presentation, and demeanor depend to some extent on the "audience." Is it a jury? A judge? A court-martial panel? An administrative board? Whoever it is, *the audience is initially suspicious of the expert.*

Trust and believability   Trust and believability are key. That's easy to say but not so easy to implement. The main point of what follows is that lawyers don't want experts who *distract* their audiences, whether with appearance, demeanor, speech, or attitude.

> Your *appearance, demeanor, speech,* and *attitude*
> should never be distracting to the jury.

What is presentable in Vermont may be questionable in Alabama and terminally distracting in a military court martial, and vice versa. Trial lawyers want to present experts whom the audience views as caring about doing the right thing, as respected (and respecting the audience in return), and as very competent, honest, and fair. Evolving social mores notwithstanding, most trial audiences *sense* (if not overtly believe), to a greater or lesser degree, that an expert who sports visible tattoos, piercings, or lots of earrings (even one can be "lots" in men), or who is significantly "different" from them in some way they believe is negative, is less than credible.

Appearance   Appearance (including dress) is the first thing the audience sees. Juries start making decisions about an expert's credibility as the expert is walking to the witness stand. They sense, at some level, "believable or not believable" in a second or two. Gender, age, length and style of hair, skin color, and a dozen other factors, some subtle and some not, may be relevant. *Lawyers cannot let social fairness or political correctness guide their decisions about hiring and presenting expert witnesses.*

> Lawyers cannot let social fairness or political
> correctness guide their decisions about hiring
> and presenting expert witnesses.

Trial lawyer Don Keenan tells his friends he has learned his best lessons about courtroom dress from jurors. Like Don, I've been to many seminars where "experts" told us to wear a power suit, a brown suit, a sport coat and slacks, suits with vests, suits without vests, and on and on. One of these fashion experts told Don, "Never dress better than the jury."

Based upon this newly found wisdom, Don went to JCPenney and bought three suits and a sports jacket for the price of a single good suit (or half a custom-tailored one). He says the polyester fabric made the shoulders peak up and the bottom of the jacket looked sort of like a ski jump, but he was convinced that juries would give him great verdicts.

One day early in his career Don got a pretty good verdict. He'd probably still be wearing JCPenney suits except for the conversation he had with one of the jury members after that trial.

The former juror, an older man, came up to the young "puppy lawyer" and asked him whether he was satisfied with the verdict. Don said yes, and thanked him for it. The juror then said, "Kid, can I give you some advice?" The juror continued, "You may be a good lawyer one day, but you've got to dress a little better." He went on to say, in a lowered voice, "Don't tell your client, but we actually put a little more in that verdict so that you could go out and buy some new suits."

Bottom line: Be who you are. Don believes the lesson is one of authenticity. Jurors can smell a phony from a hundred miles away. They may not know *why* a person's a phony, they just know. Don't pay too much attention to all the noise about dress. If you prefer JCPenney suits or a particular kind of dress—remembering my *caveats* about arrogance and distracting the audience—stay with your normal attire. My own preference is to dress conservatively, have no facial hair, and say "yes sir" and "no sir," but that's just me (a former military officer).

Clarity   Lawyers want their courtroom audiences to trust their experts. Clarity of demeanor and speech is very important. If an expert is unclear, uncertain, or ambivalent, the jury will not pay attention to what he or she has to say.

Think of the part of the brain that responds instinctively (sort of the "reptilian" brain). The part of the juror's brain that is alert for danger hates experts who seem to be acting or trying to be clever or who just sound slippery. It implies the expert is hiding something, and it telegraphs to the rest of the brain that the witness shouldn't be trusted.[14]

Clear, unambivalent statements are the ones that ring true in the reptilian brain. That's not to say that jurors are primitive but that they form first impressions just like the rest of us, often based on unconscious and nondeductive factors. Many experts feel a need to explain every nuance and possibility of their findings, but if the jury senses that an expert is going to great lengths just to appear fair, they often suspect he or she is being dishonest (or at least not straightforward). If I think one of my experts is doing this, I won't present him or her at trial or even deposition. If I sense it in an opposing expert, that person's testimony will be easy for me to shred.

Attitude Attitude conveys volumes. For example, if an expert is arrogant in court, his or her testimony will be rejected. That means that if you sound arrogant the first time I talk with you, it will be a short call.

Cultural markers (real and stereotypic) Accents and cultural markers (some not controllable, such as skin color, and some more stereotypic than real) fall into the category of potential distracters in some forums. For example, in all candor, one cannot expect a court-martial panel not to be biased against an expert who is dressed in clothing, or has a cultural background or demeanor, that reminds the panel members of folks in the Middle East who have killed their friends. In large cases, it's not uncommon for lawyers to use focus groups to determine whether or not an expert will encounter such problems.

Professional Experience and Training

Qualification of experts and application of opinions State and federal rules require experts to be "qualified" before their opinions can be offered in court. In addition, the opinions offered must be able to be properly applied to the facts in issue. The Federal Rules of Evidence state, in part,

> If scientific, technical, or other specialized knowledge will assist
> the trier of fact to understand the evidence or to determine a fact
> in issue, a witness qualified as an expert by knowledge, skill,
> experience, training, or education, may testify thereto in the form
> of an opinion or otherwise, if (1) the testimony is based upon sufficient facts or data, (2) the testimony is the product of reliable

14 Interestingly, the worst impression that can be gotten about an expert opinion is not so much that it is a lie but that it is *unreasonable*, and that no competent expert in the field would hold that view.

principles and methods, and (3) the witness has applied the principles and methods reliably to the facts of the case.[15]

Experience   Both court rules and juror perception demand adequate real-world experience in the field in which one testifies. Merely having a certain degree and job title is often insufficient.

During an expert deposition in a malpractice case, a medical doctor testified that he based his opinions on his prior experience with radiation-induced cataracts. Upon further questioning, however, the doctor was forced to reveal that he had treated only five patients with radiation-induced cataracts in over 30 years of practice. The court later ruled against admitting his testimony, saying, "We do not believe that this limited exposure to radiation-induced cataracts qualifies as a basis for a scientifically sound opinion."[16]

You should know the general expert qualifications in the jurisdiction in which you may testify. Discuss them with the lawyer who retains you, and perhaps ask counsel to send you the law itself. Each state has different rules regarding who can testify about what issue. For example, the testimony of a registered nurse generally cannot be used to establish the standard of care required of a physician.[17]

If a potential expert has been very recently trained, the facts of the case determine whether or not I will hire him or her. If, for example, a physician defendant in a malpractice case has been practicing for 20 years, the jury will probably question opinions from such a young clinician. If the issue revolves around relatively new knowledge or procedure, however (such as psychopharmacology or a recently validated psychotherapeutic technique), recent training can be a plus.

Reviewing and Testifying About Those in Other Professions

Psychiatrists and other qualified mental health professionals *can* testify about clinical staff issues (e.g., nursing duties and monitoring, unit

---

15   FRE 702.

16   *Accord Porter* v. *Whitehall Labs*, 9 F.3d at 614 n. 6 (stating that seeing disease five times during lengthy career is not sufficient basis for scientific opinion under *Daubert*). *O'Conner* v. *Commonwealth Edison Co.*, 13 F.3d 1090, 1107 (7th Cir. 1994).

17   See, e.g., *Seisinger* v. *Siebel*, 220 Ariz. 85, 94, 203 P.3d 483, 492 (2009).

staffing, importance or adequacy of nursing notes, unit safety, patient abuse, etc.), provided a proper foundation has been laid that illustrates that they have the training and experience required to do so.[18] This applies particularly to experts who are leaders of, or take responsibility for, clinical teams, groups, clinics, facilities, and the like, and to clinicians whose work exposes them, for example, to critical aspects of hospital policy.

Issues occasionally arise about a psychiatrist or psychologist being asked to testify about mental health assessment or care by an emergency room or primary care physician, a psychologist being asked to opine about psychological testing by a psychiatrist who lacks appropriate training in the procedure, or similar cross-discipline topics.

If it can be demonstrated that there is a standard of care for the *activity*, separate from the credentials or specialty of the *actor*, then an expert in the activity (e.g., in psychological testing) is likely to be allowed to testify as to whether or not the standard was met. That is, if a primary care physician, for example, chooses to assess a depressed patient for suicide risk and treat the person with psychiatric medications or psychotherapy, then protection of the patient demands that the physician be expected to meet the same standard as a psychiatrist or psychotherapist. The latter professionals are the logical source for determining the standard of care.

A Colorado appellate court ruled that a trial court did not abuse its discretion by allowing expert physicians with specialties in areas other than orthopedic surgery to testify as to the *general* standard of care applicable to all physicians with respect to the diagnosis and treatment of deep vein thrombosis and pulmonary embolism. The record demonstrated that the specialty experts established that the standard of care for diagnosing and treating blood clots was identical regardless of specialty and was a standard of care common to all physicians and fourth-year medical students.[19]

Having said the above, a few states' courts are quite particular about plaintiffs' experts in malpractice cases having experience very similar to that of the clinician-defendant. In those jurisdictions, a solely outpatient psychiatrist would probably not be allowed to criticize inpatient care. If the issue involves cognitive behavioral therapy, the expert must be

---

18 A football coach knows what his players should be doing even if he has never been a tackle or quarterback. The coach sees the bigger picture; individual players often don't.
19 *Hall* v. *Frankel*, 190 P.3d 852 (Colo. Ct. App. 2008).

experienced in that technique and not simply a generic psychotherapist. If the defendant has a particular certification, the expert must usually hold a comparable one. If the lawyer who is not experienced in medical malpractice doesn't mention this subject of "comparable experience," you should ask about it early in your work (preferably before being retained).

It's a good idea to ask the retaining attorney about his or her experience with the topic at hand (e.g., psychiatric medical malpractice). The answer may provide a clue to how comfortable you—a non-lawyer—can feel working with the attorney in that legal area.

Academic Credentials

Academic credentials can be important. All other things being equal (they rarely are, of course), it may be better for my expert to have been trained at a prestigious university, particularly in the state in which the case is being tried. Your *curriculum vitae* matters, but often not as much as one would think. Juries like clinician-experts who are currently in practice and doing what they are preaching or teaching and experts who are currently in touch with their professions. In matters that involve clinical work (e.g., malpractice lawsuits, emotional damage assessments, predictions of prognosis or cost of care, actions involving professional practice or licensure), if the expert is not currently in private practice, is he or she in an academic setting teaching practitioners? Once the expert is qualified by the judge or other arbiter, the most important thing continues to be the audience's impression of competence, trustworthiness, and credibility.

Professional Blemishes

I will not hire an expert who has a history of significant professional blemishes (licensing board censure, suspensions from medical/clinical staffs or professional organizations, lost malpractice lawsuits [there are exceptions], or beliefs I think are odd or non-credible). You need not have passed your Board exams on the first try, but when the chips are down the other side *will* attack your background as a way to discredit you. (Note that if a recently trained potential expert I'm considering has not passed his or her Board exams, I won't hire that person.)

Please do not lie about these things (or anything else), and don't think you can hide them. Be straightforward. The other side's lawyers and investigators are very good at finding things, including that "humorous" website you created a few years ago and the information you thought was confidential in the National Practitioner Data Bank. In addition, I will vet you myself before taking any chances with my client's case. (I'm a friendly guy, but remember that my duty is to my client, not to you.) Tell me about such issues in the first telephone call, and I'll make the decision I think is best for my client. Nothing personal.

Past Testimony

The number of times you've testified is not nearly as important as the *quality* of that testimony. It must be consistent with the testimony you plan to offer in the current case. If it's not, I can't retain you.

If you have testified only (or primarily) for one side or the other in certain kinds of cases (whether plaintiff, civil defense, criminal defense, or prosecution), I need to know why. If the reason makes sense (e.g., the local prosecutor works only with in-house, contract experts), it may not be an issue. If not, juries may view you as less than trustworthy. You become, to them at least, a "hired gun."[20] That's the kiss of death for a forensic clinician's testimony (and career) and will be mercilessly exploited by lawyers for the other side.

If an expert has testified very often for the same firm or agency, the question again becomes "Why"? Law firms may refer an expert's name to colleagues within their organization, sometimes in different cities or states. The reason may simply be that the expert is highly credible and very good at what he or she does. Any appearance of bias may easily be overcome by the expert's background and other characteristics or by the similarity of the cases and evidence (and sometimes there are only a few highly trained and experienced clinicians available in some narrow field at issue).

A psychiatrist who often testified in death penalty cases became known in some circles as "Doctor Death" because of his testimony in over 70 capital cases that the defendants were dangerous "sociopaths who would kill again," even if imprisoned for the rest of their lives. He was retained over and over by state court prosecutors—in spite of eventually being censured by the American Psychiatric Association for expressing his opinions as "fact" (rather than opinion)—and jurors kept handing down death penalties.[21] Why? Perhaps he struck a chord with jurors who were afraid of alleged sociopathic killers or who wanted a reason to vote for the death penalty.

In one of my malpractice cases, an expert for the other side (the defense) told the jury that he testified as often for malpractice plaintiffs as for defendants. During my cross-examination, it became clear

---

20 There are other, more colorful terms, including one coined by outstanding trial lawyer Don Keenan: "painted ladies."

21 M. Neil Browne and Ronda R. Harrison-Spoerl, *Putting Expert Testimony in its Epistemological Place: What Predictions of Dangerousness in Court Can Teach Us*, 91 Marq. L. Rev. 1119, 1212 (2008).

that the "50 percent" was accurate for only one state and not for his national testimony (which was 95 percent for the defense), and I asked him to explain why he had tried to mislead the jury. When the case was over, I questioned the jurors about their verdict (which was in my client's favor). They told me they were very upset that the other side's expert had tried to mislead them, and, since he had misled them about his prior testimony, his opinions became largely irrelevant.

If a firm has hired you repeatedly, or you always testify for the same side, the jury must be told why. If the answer is sincere and believable, there may be no issue. If the jury gets the impression that you are a liar, a hypocrite, or a "painted lady" (man or woman), the case will likely be lost.

Working with the Expert and His or Her Staff

The expert's *staff response* is important. When a lawyer calls for assistance, he or she often needs an answer quickly, or at least to know that the expert will be given the message as soon as feasible. Sometimes, for example, lawyers encounter unexpectedly short deadlines for things like motions and affidavits. I'm reasonable (to a point) but, if I don't think I can reach you when necessary, I won't hire you. When I am initially seeking an expert, if I don't get to the expert or a relevant staff person (in person, not voicemail or an answering service) within a reasonable amount of time, I go elsewhere. It is imperative that deadlines be met and promises be kept.

Your staff should get to know me and respect my needs. Sometimes I (or my staff) spend as much time talking with your secretary or other assistant as with you. If your office doesn't reflect the style and professionalism I sensed when I made the decision to retain you, it reflects badly on you.

Lawyers communicate among themselves (our livelihood depends on it). Good and bad news about experts travels fast. We consider many things when hiring experts, but, if you want to work with us regularly and be referred to our peers, your professionalism must include accessibility and an understanding of our needs (which are often a bit different from those of patients and clinical colleagues).

Be able to listen to the lawyer. Mental health professionals are supposed to be very good at listening. There are times when I need for you to listen to me, whether about case needs, your testimony style, or something else. A smart and ethical lawyer will not try to bend you to his or her will with regard to your opinions or your ethics. A smart and ethical lawyer *will* want to know how you reached your opinions. Don't confuse the former with the latter. Take some time; an expert should listen to the retaining lawyer without a "rushed" attitude. If I sense you are a "yes man," saying only what you think I want to hear, I will not trust you and will search for a more honest expert.

Understand that the advocate (that's me) wants to win. A good lawyer knows what is required of his or her witnesses to get that done. For example, when a lawyer preparing you for testimony encourages you to listen carefully to the question and answer it briefly, pay attention. We understand that expert witnesses have a hard time with this concept; they usually want to talk and talk—perhaps because they are teachers at heart—but that may be bad for my case.

It is good to remember that *the case is not about you.* You should be able to subordinate "you" in favor of the relevant points of the case. The stakes are high for every litigant, whether my own client, the other side's client, or someone else whose liberty, money, career, or reputation is on the line. The outcome of the case is always important (often to the community and the nation).[22]

Lawyers rarely want you do anything unethical. If you feel your ethics don't allow you to do what the lawyer is asking, discuss it promptly and openly. Like the jurors and other "audiences" mentioned earlier, we want clarity: nothing hidden, no lying, no sloppy work, no ambiguity, and no pandering compliments.

A Word About Expert Depositions

Most cases are settled prior to trial, and experts' depositions sometimes influence settlements. The settlement value corresponds, in part, to how well my expert presents his or her opinions at deposition. That's why I want you to remember these final paragraphs.

Depositions are a discovery device taken to learn what a witness knows, how the witness knows it, and how the witness communicates what he or she knows. They also preserve testimony. The trial lawyer's main purpose for taking a deposition is usually to lock in the testimony of the deponent, and later to impeach the deponent if the deponent says something at trial that differs from his or her deposition.

Depositions usually take place in an office or conference room with attorneys for both sides and a court reporter present. Such an informal setting can put the uninitiated into a dangerously relaxed state. *You are under oath; your words have the same importance as if you were testifying in court.* Some

---

22 This is not just lofty thinking. Think about cases that influence community safety in some way: expert witnesses are almost always involved in civil ones and often in criminal ones as well.

depositions are videotaped, so comport yourself just as if you were addressing the jury (the jury may well see the video).

I advise experts never to be deposed in their own offices. The convenience (and sometimes money saved for whoever is paying the expenses) is not worth the extra advantage for the other side. Just one example: The deposing attorney will note the books and journals on your shelves and ask—either in the deposition or later at trial—whether or not you have read them. If you say no, you'll sound superficial; if you say yes, you'll be asked about their content (and relevance to the case). If you have tried to exaggerate your reading, you'll get caught.

The expert should be prepared for the deposition by the retaining attorney. You are expected to have reviewed all the materials furnished earlier and should understand that your entire case file (including billing records) is open to the opposing lawyer. The attorneys for both sides have usually learned beforehand how you have testified in earlier, similar cases. Anything you have written (such as journal articles or book chapters) or stated in a prior deposition will likely be compared to what you say in this one. Prior inconsistent statements are gold mines for opposing lawyers.

No pressure.

APPENDICES

Forms, Letters, Reports, and More

Purchasers of this book may adapt the following copyrighted examples for their personal use, but they should not be copied verbatim. No other persons may use their format or content. The author makes no representation as to their quality of content or adequacy for any particular purpose. Itemized fees and charges mentioned herein are not intended to encourage others to use the same rates or to influence or "fix" prices in any way.

All examples of reports or case material have been modified to remove reasonably identifying information. While the result is intended to illustrate real-world situations, no similarity to specific persons or cases should be inferred. If you think you recognize someone, think again.

The format has been compressed in many examples. Letterhead, headers, and standard "boilerplate" sections have often been removed, and the actual report appearance may not be exact. Many reports were in the form of a letter, but the greeting has also often been removed.

Internal Documents, Letters, Communications

A.	Initial Attorney Letter	108
B.	Fee Sheet	109
C.	Settlement Acknowledgment	111
D.	Evaluation Appointment Letter	112
E.	Evaluee Information Sheet	113
F.	Notification of Treatment Need Discovered During Evaluation	114
G.	*Subpoena Duces Tecum* Response	116
H.	Pre-Testimony Deposit Worksheet	118
I.	Pre-Testimony Deposit Letter	119
J.	Time Worksheet	121
K.	Vendor Confidentiality Agreement	122
L.	Employee Confidentiality Agreement	123

Report Examples

R1.   Report: Trial Competency (Fitness to Proceed) (Simple)   125
R2.   Report: Trial Competency (Fitness to Proceed) (Complex)   127
R3.   Report: Criminal Responsibility (Sanity)   134
R4.   Report: Criminal Defense, Mitigation of Charge or
Sentence   137
R5.   Report: NGRI Release, Defense   143
R6.   Report: Personal Injury Defense (PTSD)   147
R7.   Report: Clinician–Patient Sex, Plaintiff   153
R8.   Report: Malpractice, Plaintiff (Complex, Doctor and
Hospital)   163
R9.   Affidavit: Malpractice, Plaintiff Pre-Suit   176
R10.   Letter/Report: Malpractice, Plaintiff Pre-Suit, Lack
of Causation   179
R11.   Report: Malpractice, Plaintiff (Complex)   181
R12.   Report: Malpractice, Defense (Complex, Facility)   195
R13.   Report: Malpractice, Defense (Facility), Forensic Practice
Standards   201
R14.   Report: Malpractice, Defense (Clinician) (Alleged Fetal
Damage from Medication)   208
R15.   Report: Accidental Overdose vs. Suicide   216
R16.   Report: Defense, Death in Custody   223
R17.   Affidavit: Defense Rebuttal, Death in Custody   227
R18.   Report: Workplace Stressors Allegedly Causing Suicide,
Expert Report Rebuttal   232
R19.   Report: Private Insurance Disability Appeal (Complex)   238
R20.   Report: Employee Emotional Injury, Treater–Expert
Conflict   249
R21.   Report: Professional Licensing Agency Review   262
R22.   Report: Professional Licensing Agency Review   264
R23.   Opinion Letter: Professional Licensure   268
R24.   Report: Civil Capacity, Contracting   270
R25.   Report: Capacity, Guardianship (Complex, Contested)   276
R26.   Opinion Letter: Capacity, Business, and Testamentary   285
R27.   Report: Auto Accident vs. Suicide   288
R28.   Affidavit: Supporting Motion to Strike Expert Testimony
(Forensic Practice Standards)   292
R29.   Letter: Rebuttal of Expert's Report, Forensic Practice
Standards   297

A

INITIAL ATTORNEY LETTER

(Date)

_____

_____

_____

FAX TO: _____ (Complete *curriculum vitae* to follow by mail)

RE: _____

Dear _____ :

This will follow up our telephone conversation, in which we talked briefly about the above matter. I should be pleased to examine the details and consult with you regarding my findings. As we discussed, my review will be objective, and I have not represented to you that my findings will be helpful to your case.

The next step would be a review of relevant medical/psychological records, _____, _____, and other facts and litigants' contentions. These should be sent to _____.

Enclosed please find a *curriculum vitae* and a statement of fees and charges. My retainer in your matter will be $_____. Any unused portion may be refundable unless a report is prepared or I am listed or declared in the proceedings. Accounts are billed every thirty days, with payment expected as fees are incurred (except in the case of advances against billings for reports or testimony).

Please note that this letter does not constitute an agreement for services until either a retainer is accepted or such an agreement is established in writing. You <u>may not</u> list me as a witness in any action in the absence of such an agreement and, once an agreement is established, you <u>may not</u> represent to others that I hold any opinion which has not been genuinely rendered.

Cordially,

William H. Reid, M.D., M.P.H.

WHR/kp
encl

B

FEE SHEET

Fees and Charges
Please read this document carefully before contracting for services.

Fees and charges for_____, dated _____, for forensic consultation and related activities by William H. Reid, M.D., M.P.H. If you have a question or special request, please contact Dr. Reid.

All fees are assumed to be guaranteed by the retaining attorney or organization at the rates below. Consultation and financial agreements are with the contracting lawyer, firm, jurisdiction, or organization alone, regardless of the ultimate source of payment. I am not expected to bill any litigant, patient, family member, insurance company, or opposing or additional counsel unless arranged in advance, in writing. The retaining party agrees to bear all costs of collecting overdue accounts, unless otherwise agreed in writing by Dr. Reid.

Fees. All work is time-based. Consultations will not be accepted on any "contingency" basis. No fee will be adjusted or "discounted" in any way related to the outcome of a case.

All activities, including travel ("door-to-door") and time spent waiting, are charged by the hour, at a maximum of **$__ per hour, plus expenses,** up to a 10 hours per calendar day.

The day-rate is **$__ per calendar day, plus expenses.** For partial days, the client will be charged the lesser of the hourly rate or day rate. Time will generally be measured from my leaving home or office until my return to home or office, by the fastest reasonable conveyance and reasonable travel schedule. Any time spent working on other professional matters will be subtracted from the total. Should I choose to travel by some means other than the fastest reasonable conveyance (e.g., by car or train rather than by air), the total time and expense required will be compared to those of reasonably scheduled first-class air travel, and the lesser total will be billed.

A **retainer of at least $ __** is required. In government matters, an acceptable contract for services may be used. No obligation or agreement for services exists until a retainer is accepted or my agreement to forego a retainer is established in writing. The retainer is not a "deposit" and may, at my option, be nonrefundable. If the retainer is exhausted, a refundable credit balance may be required.

Unkept appointments not cancelled more than 48 hours in advance may be charged at the regular rate, unless filled with other gainful activity. Time will not be "double-billed."

Deposits. Unless otherwise agreed in advance, no _testimony_ will be scheduled without payment of any outstanding balance and a pre-testimony deposit against reasonably anticipated charges and expenses. _Written reports or affidavits_ usually require payment of any outstanding balance before release, and may require a deposit. Except as noted below ("Reserving Testimony Dates"), the portion of any deposit which exceeds actual charges and expenses is refundable.

Reserving Testimony Dates. Pre-testimony deposits are applied to actual charges unless the testimony is cancelled or postponed, in which case refunds will be made as follows.

Cancellation with at least 5 calendar days' notice: Full refund less outstanding balance.

Cancellation with 3–4 days' notice: At least 50% refund less outstanding balance.

Cancellation with fewer than 3 days' notice: Refund of expense advance, less outstanding balance.

Note that the above is intended to protect our office against loss of blocks of schedulable time; larger refunds may be sent. We try to accommodate reasonable scheduling changes.

Expenses. All expenses other than office routine are additional. Air and rail travel will be first-class/compartment unless prohibited by government rule; all fares will be at a "changeable/refundable" rate. Car rental will be at "full-sized" rates; private automobile travel at $ 0.__ per mile. Accommodations will be in business-class hotels or motels, with a food allowance of $____ per day. Alcoholic beverages and entertainment will not be billed to clients.

Billing. Accounts are billed about every thirty days, net due upon receipt of statement. Time sheets, billing notes, receipts, etc., will be provided upon request. _Overdue accounts may precipitate stopping of work on a case; such action will not be considered abandonment of the client or any litigant._ Work may resume upon payment of the outstanding balance and an appropriate deposit against future billings.

C

SETTLEMENT
ACKNOWLEDGMENT

(Date)

_____
_____
_____

Re:

Dear _____:

Thank you for your communication advising that this matter has been resolved. Settlement is usually a good thing, and I assume the resolution was favorable to your client, _____.

As requested, we will send a final statement for services without delay.

We will retain all files and records for a period of time, and will attempt to contact you before destroying them. Our "main file" and financial files in the matter will be retained indefinitely.

Again, I appreciate the courtesy of your communication, and hope we have a chance to work together again in the future.

Cordially,

William H. Reid, M.D., M.P.H.

WHR/mm

D

EVALUATION
APPOINTMENT LETTER
(Sent through Retaining Attorney/Agency)

(*date*)

TO: _____

RE: Your upcoming psychiatric evaluation

Dear _____:

Your evaluation is scheduled for:
    (*Date* and *Time*)—Dr. _____ (psychological testing)
    (*Date* and *Time*)—Dr. Reid (interview)
Dr. _____ is a clinical psychologist. He will interview you briefly and perform one or more psychological tests. Dr. Reid is a psychiatrist. He will interview you at greater length and confer with Dr. _____.

Both sessions will take place at _____, _____. Directions to the office are enclosed. If you can't find it, please call (___) ___-___.

There will be ample time for breaks and lunch. The evaluation is not particularly stressful, and will not include a general physical examination or laboratory work.

You are encouraged to bring anyone you believe might have additional information or be helpful to Dr. Reid's understanding of your situation (such as a spouse, relative, or friend).

Please notify our office immediately at (___) ___-___ if you are unable to keep the above appointments.

Sincerely,

Kathy Pomeroy

Administrative Assistant

/kp, encl:

112

E

EVALUEE INFORMATION SHEET

(Given to Evaluee)

Understanding Your Forensic Psychiatry Evaluation

I, _____, understand that I am seeing Dr. Reid for psychiatric evaluation. The purpose of my evaluation is legal or administrative, not treatment or treatment-related diagnosis. This means, in part, that Dr. Reid is not "my doctor"; I do not have a "doctor–patient" relationship with Dr. Reid, and this evaluation does not create one. I understand that Dr. Reid may discuss my evaluation with, or write a report for, a court, an attorney, or other person or organization who is entitled to information about my evaluation, and that Dr. Reid may be asked to testify in court or at deposition about the things I discuss during the evaluation.

If any portion of my evaluation is being recorded (audio or video), I have been informed of that fact.

If any other person is present during the evaluation, such as a trainee, chaperone, or security person, I am aware of that fact.

If I am involved in litigation, I understand that, although psychiatric topics related to the litigation will be discussed, this evaluation is not intended to explore my legal strategy and will not include detailed questions about it unless they are necessary for the evaluation purpose.

This statement has been explained to my satisfaction, and a copy will be given to me to keep. I may ask questions of Dr. Reid at any time during the evaluation. If I have questions after the evaluation, they should be referred to my attorney.

_____ Date _____

_____ Date _____
Witness

F

NOTIFICATION OF TREATMENT NEED DISCOVERED DURING EVALUATION

(Sent to the Retaining Attorney or Entity)

FAX TO: (____) ____-____

RE: Evaluee A.B.: CONFIDENTIAL: Observations and recommendations for clinical referral

Dear _____:

As you requested, this communication is intended to convey my observations about Mr. B.'s condition and to provide Dr. C. (or whoever assumes his care) with relevant clinical information. There is also information regarding other matters, such as his care in the jail. You and I generally discussed the material below by telephone.

Mr. B. is mentally ill and needs psychiatric care. Since my role is a forensic one, as your consultant rather than Mr. B.'s physician or agent, and since I see no emergency that would require me to step outside that role, I have avoided providing any direct medical care. **I recommend that you consider the following and convey the clinical information below verbatim to Dr. C. or whatever psychiatrist assumes Mr. B.'s care after his release from jail. I also recommend that you convey the recommendations in items 2 and 3, below, to jail medical personnel.**

1. Mr. B. is currently ([*date*]) suffering from acute psychosis, a severe psychiatric condition, with poor contact with reality, unstable mood, very poor judgment, and no insight into his condition. He needs psychiatric care and further evaluation in a closely monitored, inpatient setting as soon as feasible. I do not believe that he can receive adequate medical/psychiatric care in _____ jail.

    S.C., M.D., is a well-qualified psychiatrist with whom I spoke earlier today. He will be "on call" for his psychiatric group through (*date*). Another member of the group, also highly qualified, will be on call after that (K.J., M.D.; same telephone numbers below).

114

Regardless of who is on call when you contact the group, Dr. C. is willing to assume Mr. B.'s care, and has the advantage of having already treated him. He is awaiting your call at _____ or _____. Dr. C. recommends that you contact him as soon as you have information about Mr. B.'s release, so that he and the hospital can be prepared to receive him.

The following summary of clinical factors should be helpful to Dr. C. or other treating clinicians:

(Clinical summary deleted in example)

2. Mr. B. should be carefully monitored until he can be hospitalized. Although he was not known to be acutely suicidal when I saw him, his mental state can fluctuate rapidly and unpredictably. He is at some risk of self-harm and is not capable of caring for himself in some ways. You have conveyed this to the jail personnel, who say they have placed him on suicide watch.

If Mr. B. will accept it (and assuming he remains psychotic), antipsychotic treatment should begin as soon as feasible, optimally in the jail itself. My examination and review indicate that appropriate medication could be started by the jail physician, Dr. F., with necessary monitoring and safeguards. If there is a psychiatric consultant for the jail, that person is probably quite competent to begin treatment in anticipation of transfer to a hospital. If there is no psychiatrist, Dr. F. may wish to call Dr. C. directly for consultation. If Mr. B. refuses medication, that further suggests the need to pursue care outside the jail.

3. As we discussed, I am concerned that in his current condition Mr. B. may harm himself or others if released directly to his home. In addition to the above, his interest in and collection of guns is a concern. Driving his car or motorcycle would be dangerous in his present condition.

I will try to call next week, and will contact you within a few days. Please feel free to keep in touch as necessary.

Sincerely,

William H. Reid, M.D., M.P.H.

WHR/kp

115

G

SUBPOENA DUCES TECUM
RESPONSE

(Sent to the Retaining Attorney)

NOTE: Concerns about subpoenas should usually be handled through the retaining entity, not directly with the sender of the subpoena.

TO: (Retaining entity)
RE: (*case*); Recently received Notice of Deposition and *Subpoena Duces Tecum*

I have just received a Notice of Deposition with *Subpoena Duces Tecum* from _____. With all due respect to the other attorneys, parts of their request are onerous, unreasonable, subject to privilege, and/or overly time consuming. Please convey my response (below) as you believe appropriate; if this is insufficient, please let me know without delay.

Item 4. A copy of each *curriculum vitae* Dr. Reid has prepared in the last five years.
Only the most recent *curriculum vitae* is available.

Item 5. Any and all scientific, technical, or medical publications authored by Dr. Reid which he claims have relevance or relates to this matter or subject matter at issue;
This request is onerous and unreasonable. I am happy to discuss the contents of my *curriculum vitae* at the deposition.

Item 8. Any and all scientific, technical, or medical publications claimed by Dr. Reid to be reliable and/or authoritative in connection with this matter:
To the extent that it refers to materials not reviewed specifically for this case, this request is onerous and unreasonable.

Item 10. Any record or list of any and all lawsuits, including the style and cause number of each, in which Dr. Reid has given testimony, whether by deposition or live at trial, and transcripts of such testimony;

116

I will bring a list going back about four years, as required for federal cases. We do not keep further records and it would be onerous to create such a list. I do not keep transcripts of my testimony.

Item 13. All billing statements, including computer disks, computer records, hard copy printouts, time sheets or any other document indicating time expended in review of this matter, amounts paid to date and billing rates;
We do not provide computer disks. The complete financial file will be provided.

Item 14. One page from each and every other legal matter currently being reviewed by Dr. Reid which identifies the style of the case or the names of the parties involved:
This request is unreasonable and, further, much of the information requested is private and/or privileged; it will not be provided. Reasonable questions which do not involve breach of privilege will be answered at deposition.

Item 15. Any and all documents from 2005 to the present which in any way demonstrate, record, or otherwise show the percentage of money or amounts billed by Dr. Reid for reviewing records, consulting in medico-legal cases, giving depositions or testifying at trial;
This request is unreasonable and onerous, and/or the information is private and/or privileged; it will not be provided. Reasonable questions will be answered at the deposition.

Item 16. Any and all documents from 2005 to the present which in any way demonstrate, record or otherwise show the percentage of money or amounts billed by Dr. Reid for reviewing records, consulting in medico-legal cases, giving depositions or testifying at trial as a total percentage of income;
This request is unreasonable and onerous, and the information is private and/or privileged; it will not be provided. Reasonable questions will be answered at the deposition.

Item 17. A copy of any advertisements offering Dr. Reid's services as an expert witness;
I do not "advertise" in the sense apparently contemplated by this request. Notification of services is occasionally sent by letter, but no copies are easily available. I maintain a website with educational and referral information, among other things, which may be viewed at www.reidpsychiatry.com.

H

PRE-TESTIMONY DEPOSIT WORKSHEET

(Internal Form)

Pre-Testimony Balance/Deposit Form

Case	_____ v. _____
Attorney	_____
Firm	_____
Dates available	Trial—(month, days)
Location	_____
Current outstanding charges	$ _____
Pre-travel hours anticipated (includes reviewing records, conference, preparation, etc.) (hours @ $__/hr.)	$ _____
Time anticipated for travel/testimony/ other (days @ $___/day)	$ _____
Expenses anticipated	$ _____
TOTAL required to schedule testimony, as of _____ (date)	$ _____

cc:_____, Business Manager

118

I

PRE-TESTIMONY DEPOSIT LETTER

(To Retaining Attorney/Entity)

RE:_____

Dear _____:

This information is important to your scheduling of Dr. Reid's testimony in the above matter.

Dr. Reid will be available for testimony, in (city), with the conditions noted below.

(1) Your office should advise us of the specific date(s) to reserve and the exact location.

(2) All current accumulated charges must be paid in full. ($ _____ as of _____).

(3) We will need to receive advance payment for time expected to be spent traveling to and from _____, reviewing materials, meeting with you before testimony, and testifying, as well as reasonable expenses. Dr. Reid estimates a maximum of ___ hours of pre-travel review (at $_____/hour); _____ days total for travel, meeting, testimony, etc. (at $_____/day); and a maximum of $ _____ expenses.

Thus a deposit of $ _____ will be needed in order to reserve the above dates.

If there is an overpayment, the balance will be promptly refunded. If we reserve a date which is later cancelled, the advance payment for unused hours or days will be refunded according to the following schedule.

Cancellation with at least 5 calendar days' notice: full refund.
Cancellation with 3–4 day' notice: at least 1/2 refund, less outstanding balance.
Cancellation with fewer than 3 days' notice: no refund except as noted below.

NOTE: If cancelled time is filled with other billable hours, we will not keep that portion of the advance payment; that is, we will not "double bill" for such hours. Unused advances against expenses are always refunded. This refund schedule is meant to protect Dr. Reid from significant loss, and does not preclude our working around ordinary scheduling problems.

Cordially,

Kathy Pomeroy

Administrative Assistant

/kp

J

TIME WORKSHEET
Forensic Time and Charges

Att'y/Contractee: _____ Case/Ident: _____ Date(s): _____

PROFESSIONAL SERVICES	SvcDate	Hours	Rate	Who/Comment	NOTES
Record Review	____	____	____	_____	
Conference/Interview	____	____	____	_____	
Report Preparation	____	____	____	_____	
(may include review and research)	____	____	____	_____	
Testimony Preparation	____	____	____	_____	
(may include review and research)	____	____	____	_____	
Testimony	____	____	____	_____	
(may reflect min. hours and travel)	____	____	____	_____	
Travel Time	____	____	____	_____	
(not included elsewhere)	____	____	____	_____	
Research	____	____	____	_____	
(not included elsewhere)	____	____	____	_____	
Other Hourly Service	____	____	____	_____	
Day-Rate Charges	____	_Days	DayRate_____		
(may include any of above)	____	_Days	DayRate_____		

Additional Description _____

EXPENSES

Contracted Outside Services	Amt._____		Descr. _____
(see itemization)	____	____	_____
Secretarial/Abstracting	Amt._____		_____
(outside office)	____	____	_____
Copies @ 0.20 ea.	Pages_____		_____
Express/Courier/Shipping	____	Amt.__	_____

Travel-Related Expenses (see itemization and/or receipts)

Transportation	____	Amt.__ Descr. _____
Lodging	____	____ ____ _____
Food	____	____ ____ _____
Car rental, taxis, etc.	____	____ ____ _____
Parking/tolls	____	____ ____ _____
Other	____	____ ____ _____
	____	____ ____ _____
Other Billable Expense	____	Amt.__ Descr. _____
	____	____ ____ _____

K

VENDOR CONFIDENTIALITY AGREEMENT

(Used with Copy Services, Cleaning Services, Computer/Information Technology Services, Records Disposal and Recycling Companies, etc.)

Vendor Confidentiality Agreement

I _____, representing myself and _____, understand and agree that neither I nor any person under my aegis or control will discuss or divulge to any person, organization, or other entity any information, data, or other material of any kind which I may discover in the course of performing services for Dr. William H. Reid, his office, and/or his practice.

This agreement includes, but is not limited to, written or graphic materials, client/patient files, records of any kind, any computer or other electronically stored records or materials, the contents and information within such files or records, conversations which may be overheard, and identities of clients/patients or other persons.

No files, records, materials, or equipment is/are to be removed from the premises without Dr. Reid's knowledge and permission. Any material or equipment removed from the premises is subject to certification before and after its return.

No person is authorized to perform work which allows access to any files, records, information, etc., unless he or she has signed this agreement and agreed to its provisions. This requirement applies particularly, but not exclusively, to off-site secretarial services, filing, storage, document disposal, and work on computers and other storage media.

_____   _____date

_____ witness

L

EMPLOYEE CONFIDENTIALITY AGREEMENT

Confidentiality/Privacy Agreement

In return for the opportunity to work for or do business with Dr. William Reid, I, _____, agree to the following regarding confidentiality and privacy:

1. All information which comes to my knowledge or attention, now or in the future, related to Dr. Reid, his patients or clients, his practice, or his affairs, including forensic cases, will be kept strictly confidential. It will not be divulged except to persons authorized by Dr. Reid to receive such information.

2. All stored information or records, whether in physical files, audio- or video disks, computer, or other media, will be protected against unauthorized access. Should a breach of protection or confidentiality occur, Dr. Reid will be notified within one calendar day of its discovery.

3. All stored information or records, whether in physical files, audio or video disks, computer, or other media, are Dr. Reid's property and will not be removed from the office without authorization. They will not be copied, nor will copies be removed, without authorization. Copies will be treated with the same care as originals.

4. Access to certain materials (such as patient records, forensic records, or "discoverable" and "work product" files) is governed by special legal provisions. I will be sensitive to those requirements, insofar as I am aware, or should be aware, of them, and will follow the law as best I can.

5. I understand that attorneys and other persons are often authorized to receive case-related information. I will take reasonable steps to verify their authorization before providing information or documents, and will refer questionable requests to Dr. Reid.

6. I understand that breaches of the letter or the spirit of this Agreement pose a danger to patient or client well-being, individual reputations and

interests, and the fair outcome of legal cases and, further, may be against the law.

7. This Agreement continues whether or not I continue to work for/with Dr. Reid, and extends indefinitely into the future.

8. I have had an opportunity to ask questions about any portions of the Agreement which I do not fully understand, and I have received a copy. I accept the fact that if I do not sign, and abide by, this Agreement, my employment and/or business relationship with Dr. Reid may be terminated immediately.

_____ Signature
_____ Printed name   _____ Date
_____ Witness for Dr. Reid   _____ Date

R 1

REPORT: TRIAL COMPETENCY (FITNESS TO PROCEED) (SIMPLE)

Hon. _____, Judge

_____ Judicial District Court

RE: **Report concerning A. B. defendant, <u>competency to stand trial</u>**
Cause No. _____ ([*state*] v. *A. B.*)

Dear Judge _____:

You have asked that I evaluate A. B. and report to you regarding (1) her competence to stand trial and (2), if not currently competent, whether or not there is a substantial probability that, with or without treatment, she will attain competence within the foreseeable future.

I am able to supply the comments and opinions below, based upon records and information received, personal examination, and my training, background, and experience. The methods used and materials reviewed are those routinely relied upon by forensic psychiatrists in matters such as this.

<u>OPINIONS</u>
The following opinions are offered to a reasonable degree of medical and psychiatric certainty, as I understand the meaning of that phrase. Please note that my opinions are not intended to usurp the authority of the trier of fact in actually determining competency.

> At the time that I saw the defendant, (*date*), Ms. B. knew, and appreciated, the nature of the charges against her, the legal processes in which she was and will be involved (including probable trial for [*charges*]), the participants in those processes, and their possible consequences. She was able to work with her attorney in her own defense with a reasonable degree of rational understanding

125

of the process and proceedings against her, and had apparently been doing so for several weeks without significant problems.

Ms. B.'s psychiatric condition and level of competency appear stable as of the date of my evaluation. It should be noted that she is being treated by Dr. _____ (a psychiatrist) and is taking psychiatric medication which improves her thinking and her contact with reality. If (a) she continues such treatment and medication, I have no reason to believe that her level of competence will deteriorate substantially between the time of my evaluation and the time of trial, assuming no extraordinary delay. If (b) she stops taking those medications, her level of competence could deteriorate within days or weeks, and she may or may not become incompetent to stand trial.

SOURCES REVIEWED/RELIED UPON

- Materials supplied by your office:
  (*list*)
- (*date*) Psychological testing done at my request by Dr. _____
- Interviews and examinations
  (*list*)
- My background, training, and experience in medicine, psychiatry, and forensic psychiatry

QUALIFICATIONS

I am a clinical and forensic psychiatrist with training and experience in medicine, psychiatry, and forensic psychiatry. My qualifications are further outlined in the *curriculum vitae* which has been supplied to your office.

R 2

REPORT: TRIAL COMPETENCY
(FITNESS TO PROCEED)
(COMPLEX)

NOTE: Most trial competence (fitness to proceed) reports are quite short. Some, however, are more complex and/or written to address expected criticisms by one of the parties. This one involved allegations of a capital offense, and prior competency hearings had been vigorously contested by the prosecution.

RE: **Report: Competency to Stand Trial**
    People of (state) v. *A.B.* (Cause No. _____)

You have asked that I once again evaluate A.B.'s competence to stand trial in the above matter, then report to you regarding my findings. I am able to provide the following opinions, which are offered to a reasonable degree of medical and psychiatric certainty. Please note that my opinions are not intended to usurp the authority of the trier of fact in actually adjudicating competency.

This report is predicated on my understanding of your recitation of the current (*state*) Penal Code, which states in part: ..., and on my understanding of relevant parts of the (*state*) Criminal Code which you supplied, which state, in part: ....

OPINIONS

1. <u>Competence to stand trial at the time of the most recent examination and testing (**date**)</u>. At the time that I most recently observed and interviewed the defendant in the _____ Jail (hereinafter "the jail"), and when relevant and important psychological testing was completed (*date*), **Mr. B. was not competent to stand trial.** That is, **as a result of his severe and chronic mental disorder, as expressed in current symptoms and significantly impaired thinking, the defendant was unable adequately to understand the nature of the criminal proceedings against him, in the sense**

127

that he did not adequately appreciate the criminal proceedings as they apply to him and would not be able adequately to understand, attend to, or assess the testimony of persons who may testify against him. In addition, the defendant was clearly unable to assist counsel in a rational manner in the conduct of his defense (see below).

This finding is consistent with information provided in his _____ Hospital records, with recent jail medical records, and with Dr. D.'s (*date*) report. It <u>disagrees</u> with the (*date*) competency report jointly prepared by social worker F. and psychiatrist H. of _____ State Hospital (see discussion below).

- During almost two hours of face-to-face, unchaperoned interview/examination on (*date*), in an interview room of the _____ jail, Mr. B. appeared improved since the last time we met (*date*), but still had very significant symptoms and signs of an acute psychotic disorder, which in turn interfered substantially with his ability accurately to perceive his charges and environment, to control his thinking process, or rationally to comprehend others' comments and testimony, particularly if required to do so in a trial setting over several hours or days.

  His "mental status examination" (clinical findings and reliable inferences based on his condition in the interview itself) indicated, among other things, clear evidence of several delusions (fixed, false beliefs), for example about "rays" from the walls, "cancer," the "agency," and people wanting him to take illicit drugs. He described (and the record corroborates) auditory (and perhaps visual) hallucinations (perceived sensory events that are not actually present, such as "voices" telling him to "sit very still"). His behavior implied psychotic preoccupation with internal stimuli (e.g., turning his head and staring inappropriately, apparently attending to voices or other stimuli that I could not hear or see). His responses also indicated other primitive, sometimes psychotic, defenses against unacceptable or very anxiety-producing thoughts or situations (e.g., frequent "thought-blocking," obsessive rocking at times, and odd staring at times). These are strong evidence of substantially impaired "reality testing," insight, concentration, and judgment, and are highly inconsistent with competence to stand trial.

  In spite of the above (but not implying competence), Mr. B.'s psychotic symptoms are not as severe as they were when I and others saw him in (*year*). He has responded to some extent to treatment with carefully chosen medication, but his response, as is the case for most schizophrenic individuals, is incomplete. He can, and does, get along reasonably adequately in superficial situations of following orders, asking for or obtaining simple items, etc. Like most other persons with schizophrenia, his illness does not affect his memory or general intellect; one would expect him to be able to read, use good vocabulary, carry out computations, etc., to the extent that he is not psychotically distracted by hallucinations, delusions, or severe withdrawal. However, <u>these do not imply competence to stand trial</u>.

His mental impairments are present all of the time, but some difficulties do not appear obvious unless brought out by such things as specific kinds of questions, emotion-laden topics (which may be specific to Mr. B. and poorly understood by others), mental stress (some idiosyncratic to Mr. B.) or fatigue. Nevertheless, those impairments are present and should be considered seriously when assessing his trial competency.

For example (without intending to be exhaustive):

(a) When asked about his trial and its potential consequences, he spoke of (*detailed description with quotes*).... He does not appear to consider, or mentally tolerate, alternative possibilities, or to consider that a reasonable jury could see things differently.

(b) Mr. B. referred several times during the interview to "rays" that were being used both at _____ State Hospital and currently in the jail to "help" him, "doing a lot of work on me ... I feel great," curing his (non-existent) "cancer."

(c) Upon more intimate questioning about why he behaved as he did, he eventually listed three somewhat bizarre reasons: (*details with quotes*).

(d) At various times, particularly when talking about topics that have special importance to him and to the alleged offense or trial, Mr. B. exhibited obvious signs of internal distress and mental defenses related to his schizophrenia, such as sometimes speaking in a particular halting manner that indicates "thought blocking" related to troubling thought content (e.g., when asked about _____), occasional compulsive rocking, a particular way of avoiding eye contact (seen several times during the interview), an odd closing of his eyes, and a belief that he has cancer (for which the "rays" are helpful). Although less impaired people also may show distress in situations such as this, his behavior was typical for and, in my opinion associated with, his psychotic illness (paranoid schizophrenia).

Mr. B. said that it is "tougher to keep it together" in jail than at (*hospital*). "I get interrogated here, through the walls."

That also "happened" at (*hospital*). When asked How?, he answered "...If you say something, the system hears it...Yesterday after I saw Dr. J., they [his auditory hallucinations] interrogated me for 30 minutes...(How?)... asking me to snitch...snitch on my [*deceased*] father...."

When asked how the voices sounded, he answered, "angry." When asked where the voices come from, he said (and indicated) a corner of his cell. I asked if there was a speaker in the cell, to which he replied, "There's nothing to see...." He didn't know whose voices they were; they change. He did not think they were associated with the custody staff or the police. Later in the interview, while talking about passing the time by reading a newspaper, he added that, "When the system comes on and wants to interrogate me, I open the paper." (Does that help?) "Yes." (How?) "...[it] gets my mind off the interrogation.... My head gets heavy and I read."

During much of this interchange, Mr. B. had his eyes closed, but was sometimes staring intently. When asked about his closed eyes, and whether or not he was "seeing" something as we talked, he said no, but "sometimes I close them and they stay shut." (This behavior began as he was becoming mentally fatigued and my questions were becoming more specific.)

Mr. B.'s mental condition and ability to attend to conversation deteriorated further as the interview continued beyond an hour and as the topics of discussion became more complex or anxiety-producing. This may have been associated with an unusual susceptibility to mild mental fatigue, but is probably related more to the topic or quantity of conversation, which appears to overwhelm his limited ability to manage his psychotic symptoms (which he often keeps to himself when he is less fatigued).

(e) Mr. B. was able to provide rote information about his charges and the general trial process and described "fake trials" during competency classes at _____ State Hospital. However, he appeared obviously and substantially impaired with regard to (i) his real appreciation of those things, (ii) his ability to address important issues with his lawyer before and during trial, (iii) his ability to tolerate the actual trial environment (that is, to remain attentive and accurate for hours, over days, when the trial is not "fake"), (iv) his ability to listen carefully to and rationally understand witnesses and other trial matters which are likely to trigger mental defenses that curtail his ability to participate rationally, (v) his ability to respond to witnesses' testimony and other trial matters, and (vi) his ability to respond <u>promptly</u> so that his response can be useful to counsel, particularly when mentally distressing topics are involved). He says it is "hard to pay attention, but (*his attorney*) won't let anything slip."

When I asked about or discussed court-related topics, Mr. B.'s thinking (as inferred through his speech and appearance) became more disorganized, often with longer pauses. He was able to recite his charges. When asked, he says that one possible outcome of a trial would be a sentence of "execute me 40 years from now," adding that "that's the way (*state*) does it . . . 40 years of appeals, then lethal injection." At some times, he said he does not need to return to _____ State Hospital, but at another point in the interview he said that it would be "fair" for the jury to return him to the hospital for "a couple of years . . . to stabilize me more."

He believes that (*his attorney*) is a good lawyer, and says he trusts him, but that a "guilty plea recommendation" (apparently meaning an insanity plea) would be bad advice. When asked more specifically about an insanity plea and what he thinks about it, Mr. B. paused, then answered in a vague and halting way, "might be . . . jury decides, right?" He was obviously confused, then said "I think (*his attorney*)'s gonna help with that." When asked who makes the decisions about his plea, he was silent for a long time, then asked quizzically "he (*his attorney*) can accept for me?"

- The few brief correctional staff observations reported over several months appear consistent with the above, and suggest that Mr. B. has been quite isolated during his current incarceration. Of all the correctional staff members interviewed by Detective K. and assistant prosecutor M. and listed in their (*date*) investigation report, two officers had no information or had not interacted with Mr. B. at all, two had interacted with him only once or twice, and two appeared to have observed or interacted with him from time to time (extent unclear). Most of the officers' statements appear to reflect superficial observations or interactions; none should be considered an "interview" or "examination." The observations generally note "almost always wrapped up in his blanket, lying on his bunk . . ." (Officer N.) and a little verbal interaction (most being simple requests, such as for a razor [Officer N.] and short verbalizations during his classification interview and routine jail evaluation [apparently responding to direct questions]).

Senior Officer O. stated that Mr. B. "spoke to the nurse and answered her questions" during his routine jail evaluation (which the officer apparently chaperoned), but it should be noted that <u>the official documentation of this event</u> (Jail Health Service Notes, (*date*), at Bates 000122) <u>contains the nurse's statement that he was "(u)nable to answer questions or provide any meaningful history</u>" (underlining mine; see below).

- Standard psychological testing was performed at my request by experienced psychologist and testing expert P., Ph.D., on (*date*). The primary test was a reliable, very well-validated and comprehensive "multiaxial" instrument (the Minnesota Multiphasic Personality Inventory, 2nd edition [MMPI-2]). That test provided additional, and additionally convincing, indication that Mr. B. is currently psychotic and cannot meet the criteria for trial competency. The test findings, carefully reviewed for validity given his criminal charges and diagnosis, indicate markedly aberrant thinking, a "psychotic process," high elevations of "paranoia" and "schizophrenia" indicators, and an extremely high paranoia subscale, all commonly seen in persons with paranoid schizophrenia (such as Mr. B.). The findings were consistent with "schizophrenic patients who experience confusion and internal distraction." Notably, the results indicate <u>low</u> antisocial tendencies and measures of anger, cynicism, and hostility. The test results were scored and interpreted by both a standard computerized scoring program and Dr. P. himself, using a standard interpretation manual.

  Dr. P's testing summary also notes that Mr. B. took much more than the usual time needed to complete the MMPI-2, and said that he could not administer a second test which had been scheduled, apparently because of Mr. B.'s inability to attend well to the task and/or mental fatigue. (Most people are able to complete both tests without incident.) This further suggests that Mr. B. would not be able to attend to, or respond adequately to, witnesses and other matters during trial.

- The clinical progress notes available from his current jail admission indicate that, during much of the time since returning to jail from _____ State Hospital, Mr. B. has been "unable to answer questions or provide any meaningful history" (quote from [*date*]). An antipsychotic medication (*name*) had been prescribed and has apparently been given to Mr. B. throughout his pre-trial incarceration.

2. <u>Diagnosis and extent of mental disorder</u>. Mr. B. has a severe and chronic mental disorder called Schizophrenia, Paranoid Type (DSM-IV-TR 295.30), which is currently symptomatic and in

only very limited and tenuous remission. This mental disorder (a) continues to markedly affect his thinking, behavior, and communication; (b) continues to be associated in Mr. B. with hallucinations and delusions (largely "hearing voices" and beliefs that others are threatening or doing things to him), even noting that he is improved over his condition some 15 months ago; (c) is still incurable; (d) has responded, to a limited extent, to appropriate medication and therapeutic milieu (the _____ State Hospital setting); and (e) has not responded sufficiently to treatment to render him competent to stand trial.

Mr. B.'s diagnosis, his limited improvement with certain treatments and supportive environments in the past, and his pattern of relapsing in the absence of antipsychotic medication have all been established over many years, by many clinicians, and were further established at _____ State Hospital. Most diagnostic entries in the record refer to Schizophrenia, Paranoid Type. The available medical record contains essentially continuous documentation of the above diagnosis, and his severe and chronic mental disorder, since (*date*).

3. **Regarding the possibility of malingering**: I found no indication that Mr. B.'s psychiatric symptoms and condition are malingered. His history and presentation are highly consistent with genuine illness and genuine impairment. That having been said, it may be noted that I have not performed any formal tests for malingering, nor has any other examiner so far as I know.

SOURCES REVIEWED OR RELIED UPON FOR THIS REPORT

- Materials supplied by your office:
  (*list*)
- Interviews, psychological testing, and professional conferences
  (*list*)
- Citations from the relevant professional literature
  (*list*)
- My background, training, and experience in medicine, psychiatry, and forensic psychiatry

QUALIFICATIONS
. . .

R 3

REPORT: CRIMINAL
RESPONSIBILITY (SANITY)

NOTE: The original consultation was for the presiding judge. This report was available to both attorneys and was eventually used by the defense.

RE: **Report concerning A.B., defendant, <u>sanity or insanity at time of incident</u>**
   Causes Nos. _____ and _____ (*[state]* v. *A.B.*)

You have asked that I evaluate A.B. and report to you regarding whether or not she met (*state*) criminal statute criteria for insanity at the time of the alleged acts described.

<u>OPINIONS</u>
I can offer the following opinion to a reasonable degree of medical and psychiatric certainty. Please note that my opinions are not intended to usurp the authority of the trier of fact in actually determining responsibility. The comments below assume that A.B. killed three of her children (S., T., and U.) and injured a fourth (R.) on (*date*) ("the acts").

> **It is my opinion that, at the time of killing three of her children and injuring the fourth, A.B. was suffering acute and profound symptoms of _____ (DSM-IV-TR ____), a severe mental disease. As a result or her immediate and severe symptoms, she did not know that her conduct was wrong.**
>
> With regard to the word "know" in the relevant insanity statute: Although Ms. B. was aware that she was killing or attempting to kill her children, that awareness should not be construed as any rational understanding of the wrongfulness, meaning, or consequences of her acts. The acts were committed within what was, for her, a completely separate, psychotic, and irrational version of "reality." That is, she had an irrational but deeply compelling belief, caused by her severe mental disease, that God was

instructing her to kill her children, and that doing God's will in this way was both right and necessary. At the time of the acts, that belief was so compelling and free of doubt that she was unable even to consider any conflict between God's instructions and the laws or rules of man.

The above opinion is based on a large number of highly consistent clinical, forensic, and scientific factors, virtually all mitigating in the direction of a finding of insanity at the time of the acts. Those factors may be summarized as

1. Substantial evidence that a severe mental illness (_____) existed at the time of the acts, as well as before and after them, whose acute symptoms in her case rendered her unable to know that her injuring and killing her children was wrong. That evidence includes, but may not be limited to, contemporaneous or near-contemporaneous videotapes, audiotapes, written transcripts of conversations, interviews, and observations; psychiatric and psychological examinations, physical evidence, and the defendant's unrebutted statements. All of these indicated and/or strongly supported the presence, during times relevant to the acts, of a compelling religious delusion which the defendant deeply believed represented reality and which was associated with visual illusions, brief auditory hallucinations, olfactory hallucinations, markedly inappropriate affect, and markedly inappropriate behavior.

2. Substantial evidence of undiagnosed _____, a severe mental illness, for several years before the acts.

3. Substantial evidence that after, committing the acts, Ms. B. was indifferent to what might happen to her at the hands of the police and the judicial system, caring only about God's wishes and her relationship with Him.

4. Credible evidence that Ms. B. believed that the consequences of refusing to do what she believed was God's will would be severe (for example, that the children would be killed in a more horrible way, and that their souls would be condemned to Hell).

5. Credible evidence that she felt no need for remorse for several weeks because of her delusional belief that she had done God's will, and because she expected her children to be "raised up" (to Heaven) on a particular date. After several weeks of psychiatric treatment, she began to feel doubts about her acts and the loss of the children, and became very depressed. Soon thereafter, psychiatric medication dispelled her religious delusion and she experienced great regret, loss, and remorse (which continue to the present) as she realized the true nature and consequences of her acts.

6. A noteworthy lack of evidence of any rational motive, any attempt to hide the acts from police, any attempt to evade capture or arrest, any

attempt to mislead officers or investigators, or other usual indicators of criminal intent. One may note that Ms. B.'s explanation of her behavior when her husband came into R.'s room as she was injuring her is credible, based on the presence of her delusional experience and motivation (which is not a "rational" motive).

7. A noteworthy lack of evidence of prior criminal or antisocial behavior, violent behavior or tendencies, or abuse of her children or others.

8. A noteworthy lack of evidence of voluntary intoxication.

9. A noteworthy lack of evidence of malingering. The possibility of malingering was carefully considered. The factors mitigating against malingering are substantial, including the evidence already mentioned above, the defendant's response to psychiatric treatment (including medication), and the many observations recorded and findings reached during jail monitoring, investigative questioning, psychiatric interviews, document review, and psychological testing.

SOURCES RELIED UPON

- Materials supplied by your office:
  (*list*)
- Report: _____, Ph.D., (*date*), concerning his psychological testing data and findings
- Interview of defendant A.B. (private, contact visit) (*date*), _____ Co. Jail interview room (3 hours, 25 min.)
- Interview/Conversations with Detective _____ (*date*) (about one hour total)
- Interview of C. B., (*date*) (about 45 minutes)
- Interview of Pastor _____, (*date*) (about one hour)
- Brief interview (telephone) of _____, Ph.D., (*date*)
- Visit to the incident scene, exterior and interior, with Det. _____ and C. B., (*date*)
- My background, training, and experience in medicine, psychiatry, and forensic psychiatry

QUALIFICATIONS

. . .

R4

REPORT: CRIMINAL DEFENSE, MITIGATION OF CHARGE OR SENTENCE

RE: *State of _____ v. B . . .*

Your client, Mr. B has admitted taking part in a shooting incident which took place on or about (*date*), in _____. He is charged with aggravated assault on a police officer and aggravated assault with a deadly weapon in that matter. You have asked for a report of my opinions regarding whether or not there were psychiatric factors involved in Mr. B.'s actions which might mitigate either his charges or his eventual sentence, should he be found guilty of a crime.

I am able to supply the opinions and comments below, based upon my review of the written and video materials provided (see list below); extended examination of Mr. B.; telephone interviews with his wife, mother, and sisters; review of the relevant psychiatric/psychological literature, and my training, background, and experience. The methods used are those routinely relied upon by forensic psychiatrists in matters such as this.

SUMMARY OF RELEVANT EVENTS

On (*date*), Mr. B., known to several officers as a supporter of local law enforcement, drove to the rear parking lot of _____ Police Department and parked some distance from the entrance. With several officers in the immediate vicinity, he stepped out of his car and fired a number of shots from a civilian-modified AR-15 rifle into the engine compartment and side of an empty patrol car. He then got back into his car and continued firing the rifle and a handgun in the general direction of the same empty patrol car. He did not hit any person, nor was any person ever in his line of fire.

Various police officers then shot at Mr. B. He did not return their fire. They approached his car to find him wounded in several places and unable to exit on his own. He surrendered without further incident. A search of his car revealed additional weapons and a large container of gasoline in the back seat.

137

EMS was called and Mr. B. was taken to _____ hospital. His blood alcohol concentration when he arrived at the emergency room was 0.17%. He underwent surgery and was hospitalized for 6 days, then was transferred to the infirmary unit of _____ jail.

FINDINGS AND OPINIONS
The following opinions are offered to a reasonable degree of medical and psychiatric certainty, given the information available to me at this time.

1. The clinical record, available behavioral history, and recent and current examinations of Mr. B. all indicate longstanding, substantial mental illness, including symptoms of significant depression and paranoia.

    Mr. B. had been noticeably depressed for some time before the shooting, had received antidepressant treatment, and at the time of the shooting was either not adequately responding to that treatment or was not participating in it as prescribed. He described sporadically taking psychiatric medications from his family physician, prescribed for regular use but taken only when he thought he needed them: antidepressants _____ and _____, _____ for sleep, and _____ for anxiety. He stated that he saw _____, M.D., some 10 or 12 years ago for antidepressant treatment. During the two years prior to the shooting, he had periods of very questionable judgment and what a relative described as markedly grandiose behavior. His judgment and insight have been sufficiently impaired at various times and his ability to seek and comply with treatment has been impaired. His wife stated that he has been "very paranoid" about seeing any mental health professional for years, and that he "doesn't believe in therapy."

    Mr. B.'s wife stated that prior to the shooting he was often pleasant at home, but when he was either depressed or intoxicated he would scream crazily at her, for example accusing her of poisoning his dogs, being a "whore," and deleting things from his computer. During those periods, she "worried about what he would do" (that is, that he might commit suicide).

    Mr. B.'s brother described an event about a month prior to the shooting in which Mr. B.'s wife came home to find Mr. B. in a battle helmet and bullet-resistant vest. According to his wife, he thought she might be bringing someone home to harm him. (See comments below about the results of the police search of his residence.)

    In addition to his well-documented depression and grandiose and paranoid characteristics (which meet clinical criteria for a diagnosis of severe mood disorder), Mr. B. has had abnormal personality traits since late adolescence which both impaired his social and interpersonal functioning and rendered him more than usually vulnerable to loss and humiliation. Those traits and other conditions associated with poor insight and judgment predispose him to social and vocational problems (such as marital discord, poor judgment, and business failure). When problems occur, those traits and conditions make him prone to react poorly to them (cf. his humiliation at needing money, vague fears of others harming him or his wife, building bulletproof barriers in his home, obsessively digging an underground structure for "emergencies," being markedly fragile in the face of his wife's threats to leave him, and marked fear of abandonment and divorce). His wife was worried that he would become further depressed and harm himself if she left him.

There is ample evidence to suggest previous suicidal thoughts, and perhaps attempts. The record indicates at least two recent single-vehicle accidents which may have been either suicide attempts or "parasuicidal" behavior (behavior associated with suicidal thoughts). Some time before the shooting, he asked his parents to remove him from their wills, implying that he believed he was not going to be around for very long.

Several of Mr. B.'s close relatives have, or had, significant psychiatric disorders, some commonly associated with increased suicide risk. (Persons whose close relatives have serious depression or other significant mood disorders are at substantially higher risk than other people for a similar illness.) All family members described his father as having had significant mood instability, grandiosity, and irritability. One sibling has been hospitalized for depression and possibly "manic" symptoms. Two others have been treated for depression.

Uncontroverted reports from Mr. B., his mother, and his sisters describe his father as very abusive, both mentally and physically. Mr. B.'s childhood development was immersed in his father's virtually continuous, very harsh criticisms and predictions that he would never be successful at anything. His father punished him severely for small infractions in ways that are consistent with brain damage (e.g., shaking him very hard and throwing him against a wall).

When I examined Mr. B., he was superficially cooperative and oriented, not acutely psychotic or severely depressed, telling his story in an often rambling, somewhat grandiose and pathologically self-centered manner. He insisted that the shooting incident happened in a certain way in spite of knowing about video evidence that contradicted some of his statements. For example, he said he walked up to an officer's car, with the officer in it, and fired bullets into the door and engine, then walked back to his own car to wait for the officer to come and kill him. (Police video indicates that he remained in or near his car, and that the officer was not in the patrol car at which he fired.) *He expressed disappointment that the officers had not killed him* (see below).

2. **It is more likely than not that Mr. B. was impaired by significant mental illness at the time of the (*date*) shooting, and during the several days and weeks prior to it.**

    Mr. B.'s description of the events is highly consistent with acute depression and suicidal thoughts, made worse by alcohol intoxication. The officers' reports and incident video, although not specific with regard to mental symptoms, do not rebut that likelihood. The medical record and descriptions by others (notably his wife and a sister) indicate a chronic depressive, perhaps bipolar ("manic-depressive") condition. Although I was not present, there is ample reason to assume that those symptoms, consistently observed by others hours before the shooting, were present on the night of the shooting. Indeed, they had apparently been present to some extent for weeks before the incident.

3. **Mr. B. was also impaired by alcohol intoxication at the time of the shooting (see _____ trauma center record).** That intoxication appears to have been voluntary but, more likely than not, it added to a previously existing state of impaired judgment and insight which was a result of his mental illness.

    Mr. B. often drank heavily during the prior few weeks, becoming noticeably intoxicated about three times a week and on weekends, according to his wife, and drinking "lots of beer" when working on his underground shelter.

4. **The shooting is consistent with a wish to harm himself which, in turn, is consistent with his recent losses and a severe depressive condition.**

    Mr. B.'s behavior at the scene is highly consistent with a plan to have himself killed by police (so-called suicide by cop). His statements about the incident and the events just prior to it further support that premise. He was carrying four firearms in the car (two handguns and two rifles, plus extra clips); he was apparently holding a handgun when an officer walked very close to his driver-side window just prior to opening fire. He appears to have had ample opportunity to shoot (and likely kill) several officers in the parking lot, *but did not do so*. Although he owned bullet-resistant vests and a helmet, he was not wearing either during the shooting, nor was any body armor or other protective material found in his car. The car itself was not particularly heavy and was not outfitted in any protective way (e.g., with armor). Most notably, the gasoline in the back seat suggests much more danger to Mr. B. than to anyone else.

    Mr. B.'s statements to EMS personnel after being shot several times, apparently in a state of significant trauma with no indication of guile, indicate that he expected to be killed (see EMS record).

Mr. B.'s explanation of the shooting is that it was a "suicide by cop gone wrong." The way in which he describes his behavior and motivation suggest a paranoia and grandiosity which is uncommon in ordinary defendant statements (for example, saying he expected to make a hero of an officer in return for being cleanly killed and denying that there was ever any danger to the officers or others because, he stated, he is an excellent marksman).

5. **I am unable to discern any likely rational motive for Mr. B.'s actions other than self-destruction (see above).**

Two other considerations of motive were particularly considered:

(a) One interviewee told me that Mr. B. was sometimes frustrated with the local police coverage of his business several years before the shooting. However, most statements to me by him, his wife, and his siblings indicated that this was an anomaly, and that he had great respect and appreciation for law enforcement. Four days before the shooting, he noticed two empty police cars beside a roadway and called 911 out of concern that the officers might be injured or in trouble (see 911 record of *date*).

(b) Some prosecution observers apparently believe that the underground structure he dug obsessively for months has characteristics of a so-called bunker (from which one might indirectly infer an assaultive motive). Mr. B. consistently, over many months before the shooting, described the digging project as a "shelter" (see statements by family, wife, and neighbors). Whatever its purpose(s) to him, the process of his digging the "shelter" (and his obsession with it) appears outlandish and to some extent irrational (and tend to support mitigation rather than exacerbation of his charges).

Mr. B.'s mother and siblings describe similar structures that he built when he was a child, and note that he immersed himself in such projects to control stress and anxiety. His wife describes his work on the present structure in a way that is highly consistent with obsessive behavior to reduce anxiety. The best psychiatric interpretation is probably that his incessant thoughts and work on the project, for hours at a time at all hours of the day and night, were an obsessive way to keep psychological symptoms (such as depression or anxiety) at bay, and at worst represented a kind of break with reality clinically described as "manic" or "delusional."

The kinds of weapons and materials found in the home are unusual, but do not necessarily indicate an assaultive motive. They are consistent, in my experience, with inordinate concern about one's safety (cf. the amount of ammunition, high-capacity magazines and taped magazines, bullet-resistant vests, air filtration masks). Note that a month or so before the shooting, he appeared frightened that his wife might bring someone home to harm him, and he was found wearing a helmet and bullet-resistant vest.

Although many of the weapons and materials in the home are consistent with aggressive as well as protective purposes, I saw no indication in the records or other information available to me that Mr. B. had planned or carried out any assaults on other persons prior to the (*date*) shooting. His wife described his going to a shooting range from time to time; there is no indication of other practicing or firing of the weapons. Proof of the legitimacy of his firearm purchases (receipts, etc.) was kept in a binder, and most of the weapons were kept in a gun safe (where they were found during the search of his home). He had a concealed carry permit. I have seen no indication that any of his firearms was automatic or otherwise required "class-3" federal licensure. He, his mother, and his sisters reported that gun ownership has been common in the family for generations.

6. The records and other information available to me suggest that unless he was intoxicated or experiencing significant mood symptoms (such as depression or possibly hypomanic symptoms), Mr. B. generally avoided confrontation, was thoughtful of others and of his animals, and cared for and supported disadvantaged family members (e.g., an uncle). Although he had periods of screaming and accusations when symptomatic, his wife states that he never physically harmed her. Even after the considerable abuse he suffered at the hands of his father, and his father's abandonment both in childhood and after Mr. B.'s arrest, he expressed sympathy for both his father and mother when his father died a few weeks later.

7. Another psychiatrist, _____, M.D., examined Mr. B. at the _____ County Detention Center for purposes of diagnosis and treatment. I concur generally with Dr. _____'s clinical findings and treatment recommendations (see Dr. _____'s [*date*] report).

SOURCES RELIED UPON

(*list*)

R 5

REPORT: NGRI RELEASE, DEFENSE

RE: Matter of A.B.

You have asked for a report which summarizes my findings regarding Ms. B.'s readiness for discharge to outpatient treatment. After (a) review of materials provided by your office and gathered from C. State Hospital (CSH); (b) review of my several past interviews and evaluations of Ms. B.; (c) a further interview of Ms. B. on (*date*); (d) discussions with Dr. D. (her attending psychiatrist), E.F., M.D. (on-site CSH forensic psychiatrist-evaluator), Dr. G.H. (Ms. B.'s inpatient and proposed outpatient psychotherapist), and I.J., M.D. (a forensic psychiatrist who has evaluated her several times since her arrest); and (e) review of the relevant professional literature, I am able to provide the opinions and comments below.

The methods used and materials reviewed are those routinely relied upon by forensic psychiatrists in matters such as this. All opinions are expressed to a reasonable degree of medical certainty, and in this case also to a higher, "clear and convincing" level, given the information available to me at this time.

FINDINGS AND OPINIONS

1. **Ms. B. does not present a measurable danger to the public.** I found no indication of either current or future danger to others in my review of CSH records, extended interview of Ms. B. herself (*date*), discussions with facility clinical staff and administration, and review of independent evaluations (including my own past examinations). (See, e.g., Dr. D.'s extensive inpatient evaluation of (*date*), and the list of materials reviewed and persons interviewed at the end of this report.)

   Ms. B.'s killing of her children was the product of a then severe mental disorder which has been successfully treated, has been in complete remission for several years, and can convincingly be expected to remain in remission (see clinical opinions and comments below). Further, Ms. B. has changed a great deal, in the direction of lack of dangerousness, during the past 10 years, both with respect to her mental illness and with respect to her general characteristics and life.

2. **Ms. B.'s clinical condition is stable, and is safely and effectively treatable on an outpatient basis.** She has been essentially symptom-free for many years, and has demonstrated emotional health and resilience that indicate she will continue to be so. She has not shown signs or symptoms of the psychosis she experienced in (*year*) for over eight years.

   Ms. B.'s diagnosis, which has been significantly refined since her trial, is now established as "major depressive disorder" (DSM-IV-TR 296.36). That condition was very severe on (*date*), with then psychotic features and probably post-partum onset. Her illness is now, and for years has been, in complete remission. (Major depressive disorder usually responds well to adequate treatment.) Her "Global Assessment of Functioning" rating (DSM-IV-TR "Axis V") has been 85–90 ("absent or minimal symptoms . . . good functioning in all areas") for many years as well. Her clinical course has been what one would expect for such a patient (with better improvement than most). *Ms. B. has remained in the hospital far longer than would have been the case had she not been under a criminal court commitment* (average hospital stays for persons with her diagnosis are usually measured in days, or a few weeks, not years).

   While at CSH, Ms. B. has experienced many of the large and small losses and frustrations that we all encounter in life, including a divorce and the deaths of close relatives. She reacted to those events in ordinary ways; her overall condition did not deteriorate significantly at any time, and she did not "relapse" or exhibit any signs of danger to others.

   In addition, of course, Ms. B. has dealt with extraordinary experiences, such as having killed her own children, having been prosecuted and tried for murder, having been "psychotic" (significantly out of touch with reality) at that time because of severe and undiagnosed post-partum depression, leaving her previous church, and being in a psychiatric hospital for many years. She long ago volunteered for tubal ligation in order to reassure herself and others that she would not have more children. Over time, she has responded well to treatment and has developed ways of dealing with those painful losses and memories. Once again, she has not exhibited any signs of danger to others during this long personal and therapeutic process.

3. **Ms. B. has reached maximum benefit of inpatient treatment.** She improved clinically, psychologically and behaviorally in large increments during her first several months of treatment (starting before her trial), continued to make steady progress after her psychosis cleared, and has been on a "plateau" of maximum hospital benefit and essentially normal functioning for well over two years.

Ms. B. was initially sent to the _____ unit of _____ State Hospital on (*date*) after being found Not Guilty by Reason of Insanity (NGRI). After a short time and extensive evaluation, a _____ Dangerousness Review Board determined that she did not represent a danger to others and she was transferred to C. State Hospital (CSH, a medium- and low-security forensic hospital). At CSH, she progressed to the "high-functioning" unit and then to a new unit designed for the very highest-functioning, least dangerous patients. That unit is not locked and provides a living experience which is as close as feasible to ordinary community living. She continues her medication, continues to participate in group and individual psychosocial treatment and therapeutic activities, began (and continues) insight-oriented psychotherapy, and has for several years assumed a reliable leadership role in her unit's "community." She has made excellent use of her time in both therapeutic and other ways, for example earning a bachelor's degree online from _____ College. Relatives and at least one friend visit her regularly; she spends time with them at the CSH on-grounds visitor center, sometimes spending the night there.

While at CSH, Ms. B. has gotten as much "real life" social and community experience as has been allowed by the Court. She has a regular, paying job on the grounds, participates actively in her unit "community," has formed appropriate relationships among other high-functioning patients, and is often a model for lower-functioning ones. She experiences the ordinary joys, sadnesses, enthusiasm, and frustration of ordinary life; neither her clinical condition nor her behavior has ever suggested danger to others.

4. **Ms. B.'s proposed discharge and aftercare plan is excellent, and exceeds both necessary safety considerations and clinical treatment expectations.**
    The CSH staff, Ms. B., her clinicians, and her family have been planning her transition to community living and aftercare for well over a year. Arrangements have been made with _____ County mental health services for extensive follow-up in their program, which has considerable experience with persons found not guilty by reason of insanity (NGRI), including patients who have killed others. Ms. B. will continue to take a monitored, injected "depot" form of medication (_____) every two weeks (which eliminates the need to remember daily pills for that primary medication and assures treatment compliance), as well as a second, oral medication (_____). She will not only be required to make the routine clinic visits expected of all such patients, but will visit the clinic more often in order to receive her injections.
    In addition, Ms. B. will continue her insight-oriented psychotherapy with Dr. H. (who practices in _____ and comes to CSH a few days

a week). She has made excellent use of this extraordinary opportunity, and she and Dr. H. have developed a plan to continue the therapy indefinitely after her discharge.

Ms. B. has specific plans for housing, work and community transition. If the Court approves, she will live in a small home beside responsible relatives, in a moderately rural area on the outskirts of _____. She is aware of the possibility that other people might seek her out or even harass her, and plans to live inobtrusively. She has applied for employment, apparently with a good chance of acceptance. Her family is providing her with a reliable car and funding for many of her needs until she can begin work.

5. **Separate from the above, the cost of continuing to house and treat Ms. B. in an inpatient setting (such as CSH) is far higher than the cost of outpatient treatment.** The cost of CSH inpatient care (essentially for "housing" at this point, since all of her clinical treatment can be given as an outpatient) is hundreds of dollars per day. If she is allowed discharge to community living and care, those costs will decrease dramatically, and most will be borne by Ms. B. herself.

I expect to testify to the above in more detail at Ms. B.'s (*date*) hearing, and expect that the various clinicians and CSH staff who are called will provide testimony which is highly consistent with these opinions.

SOURCES RELIED UPON

- Materials supplied by your office, including current and recent facility records, the original criminal proceeding prior to my report dated (*date*), and pre-trial examinations/interviews
  (*list*)
- Materials supplied by C. State Hospital
  (*list*)
- Interviews and examinations
  (*list*)
- Additional (*year*) interviews
  (*list*)
- Professional literature reviewed
  (*list*)
- My background, training, and experience in medicine, psychology, psychiatry, and forensic psychiatry, and health-care administration

QUALIFICATIONS
 . . .

R 6

REPORT: PERSONAL INJURY DEFENSE (PTSD) (WITH TREATER–EXPERT CONFLICT)

Preliminary Report (amended): Matter of A.B. Cause no. _____ : _____
et al. v. _____ Company
_____ Judicial District Court, _____ County, _____

You have asked that I supply a preliminary report that summarizes my findings, within the nature and scope of my expertise, after review of the records you have supplied and a brief Internet search. The methods used and materials reviewed are those routinely relied upon by forensic psychiatrists in matters such as this. Information developed and/or received in the future may suggest additions or changes to the opinions below and could mitigate either for or against the defendants' case; thus I reserve the right to change or add to this report should further relevant information become available.

It should be noted that I have not been permitted to examine Mr. B., nor to talk with people whom he might have brought to an in-person evaluation. In addition, the records supplied lacked several items which would be important to making professional inferences about Mr. B.'s psychiatric/ emotional complaints (see Findings and Opinions, below). You have told me that no other records are available to you at this time.

Brief Summary of Events. Mr. B. was a passenger in a vehicle carrying workers to a job site on the afternoon of (*date*), when the vehicle was struck by a slow moving (apparently about 10 MPH) train. Although there were apparently no severe injuries, several workers sustained injuries of some kind and were taken to _____ Medical Center for further assessment and possible treatment. Mr. B., who was ambulatory after the collision, was among them. He was examined and released with prescriptions for _____ and instructions to see a general physician, Dr. C., within a day or two. He apparently did not see Dr. C. but instead saw D.E., M.D., to whom he was referred by his lawyer three days later. He has continued seeing Dr. E. for evaluation and treatment, as well as various other physicians (often at Dr. E.'s referral), to the present.

Around (*date*), Dr. E. recommended that Mr. B. see a psychiatrist and referred him to Dr. F.G., whom he first visited on (*date*) and saw twice more over the next two months. Dr. G. diagnosed post-traumatic stress disorder (PTSD) and prescribed low doses of an antidepressant (_____, sometimes effective for anxiety as well), which he apparently took for about one month before discontinuing it on his own.

There are several indications in the record that weekly counseling was recommended and may have taken place (see e.g., Dr. E.'s note of [*date*], p. 4); however, I found no record of the counseling itself or of the name of the person to whom he was apparently referred.

There are several indications in the record that psychological testing was recommended and/or "pending" (see e.g., _____ 0036); however, there is no record of any psychological testing, or of the person to whom he may have been referred for testing and test interpretation, or of what psychological tests were contemplated.

Dr. G. apparently re-evaluated Mr. B. in (*date*) (see _____ Medical Center billing sheet); however, no notes or report of that evaluation are in the records supplied to me.

Mr. B. was referred to psychiatrist L.M., M.D., in mid-(*year*). Dr. M. diagnosed "_____" and continued the prior PTSD diagnosis (perhaps by history rather than based upon the new examination). Dr. M. prescribed medications consistent with his new diagnosis (_____, _____); his last two notes indicate that Mr. B. responded well and improved considerably.

A few months after the accident, Mr. B. experienced a very substantial emotional trauma and loss (*dates*). His daughter, B.B., was severely injured in an automobile accident that also injured Mr. B. himself (who sustained minor injury). The daughter died a few days later. That fact is very briefly recorded in Dr. M.'s (*date*) initial psychiatric interview of Mr. B., but I do not find it anywhere else in the records supplied which are dated after the daughter's death. In particular, I found no documentation that any mental health professional or other person assessed Mr. B.'s reaction to the loss of his daughter, treated him for it, considered it in the context of his post-accident symptoms and complaints, etc.

FINDINGS AND OPINIONS

The following opinions are offered to a reasonable degree of medical or psychiatric certainty, given the information available to me at this time.

1. So much relevant information is lacking in the available record that, based on that record, no reasonable and ethical forensic psychiatrist or other mental health professional can form opinions to a reasonable degree of medical or psychiatric certainty regarding Mr. B.'s emotional condition now or in the past, or any element of causation, with respect to the train-vehicle accident. In some

matters in which information is incomplete, one can express some opinions in a context of professionally and ethically required *caveats* and disclaimers. In this case, however, it would be improper, and outside professional practice standards, to form professional opinions with regard to such things as (without intending to be exhaustive)

- the presence or absence of accident-related post-traumatic stress disorder or any other psychiatric diagnosis at any time, either immediately after the accident or in some "delayed" form, or the presence or extent of psychiatric/emotional symptoms which may not have reached the level of "diagnosis";
- the adequacy and completeness of evaluation(s) purporting to make such diagnoses;
- the effectiveness of treatments applied to such symptoms or diagnoses, to the extent they exist(ed);
- the course, remission, exacerbation, or prognosis of such symptoms or diagnoses, to the extent they exist(ed);
- the extent to which any such symptoms or diagnoses, to the extent they exist(ed), may or may not be related to the accident on (*date*);
- the extent to which the (*date*) death of Mr. B.'s daughter, assumed to have been a very substantial emotional event, is responsible for emotional or psychiatric symptoms which might be confused with symptoms caused by the earlier event.

2. **The following items or information lacking in the records supplied are important to the lack of ability to render opinions about the above.** Some are referenced in the available records but were apparently not supplied to you. Others may or may not exist, but are nevertheless important to arriving at reasonable opinions regarding psychiatric/psychological effects, if any, on Mr. B. related to the (*date*) incident. Those missing and/or omitted items include, but may not be limited to,

- reliable information about Mr. B.'s pre-accident history, including psychological, social, vocational, family, and medical information (cf. suggestive notations in Dr. M.'s (*date*) evaluation);
- records of competently administered and interpreted psychological testing;
- detailed records of mental health counseling;
- a detailed description/report of Dr. G.'s (*date*) evaluation;
- corroborated information regarding where Mr. B. was sitting in the vehicle;

- reliable information regarding the effect of, and Mr. B.'s reactions to, the accident which killed his daughter on (*date*) (cf. symptoms described in Dr. M.'s [*date*] notes);
- reliable information regarding other psychologically significant events that have occurred since (*date*);
- detailed and corroborated information regarding Mr. B.'s day-to-day life, general activities, and abilities outside medical settings (e.g., at home);
- results of the two drug screens performed at the _____ emergency room visit on the day of the accident at issue (see _____ Medical Center billing sheets), and any other tests for substance abuse.

3. The inability to perform an in-person examination of Mr. B., with relevant psychological testing, is another factor that limits the offering of psychiatric opinions.

4. Some parts of the available psychiatric record have been misconstrued and/or contain inaccurate information (some apparently from Mr. B. himself).

First, Dr. N.O.'s two comprehensive treatment and evaluation notes from (*date*) ("_____ Pain Management"), refer to evaluation and treatment by psychiatrist Dr. M. (see Dr. M.'s notes of [*dates*]) and state (apparently erroneously) that Dr. M. only "prescribed medications for PTSD." However, **Dr. M.'s notes indicate diagnosis of, and treatment (prescriptions) for,** _____ (_____ and _____), which he diagnosed in (*month, year*) and ratified as a separate diagnosis in subsequent notes. _____ may be prescribed for some anxiety syndromes, but is used primarily by psychiatrists for _____. On the second of the three visits to Dr. M. (*date*), PTSD is not mentioned and _____ is the sole diagnosis entered. It should be noted that, although Dr. M.'s notes should not be considered exhaustive with regard to the entire question of emotional damage, _____ **is not caused by external trauma, but by neurochemical dysfunction unrelated to events such as the collision which has been described.**

Second, Mr. B. apparently told Dr. M. (or Dr. M. inferred) that he had sustained some sort of head injury in the accident (see p. 3 of his [*date*] evaluation); however, there is no indication elsewhere in the record, including the emergency room reports, of any allegation of head injury. This apparently led Dr. M. to infer a "cognitive disorder due to closed head injury" which is not supported by the record.

Third, Mr. B. apparently told Dr. M. (or Dr. M. inferred) in early (*year*) that he had been losing weight (weight changes are sometimes associated with psychiatric symptoms). However, I can find no indication that this was the case. The record indicates a stable weight of about 240 pounds through (*year*) (see, e.g., Dr. E.'s records; two weighings elsewhere indicated 245 and 250 pounds) and 240 pounds on (*date*).

Fourth, two of Dr. G.'s evaluations include the comment that Mr. B. gained weight after his accident; however, the available record indicates otherwise (see above).

5. The most recent psychiatric evaluation and treatment notes suggest that Mr. B.'s mental condition improved substantially with treatment for (*mental illness unrelated to the accident*) (see Dr. M.'s records of ____, ____, and ____). Those notes should not be considered exhaustive with regard to the entire question of emotional damage, however.

6. Contrary to Dr. G.'s and others' comments and inferences that Mr. B. has/had no psychiatrically relevant history other than the accident, Dr. M.'s psychiatric evaluation of (*date*) cites the very significant death of his daughter in (*month, year*), as well as a pre-existing propensity to "cut up animals" when angry. These notes underscore the importance of obtaining and reviewing additional, and reliable, social, vocational, family, and psychological information about Mr. B. before offering opinions about the extent of his emotional response to the accident.

7. The life care plans developed for plaintiff (e.g., the "revised" plan dated [*date*] by ____, life care consultant) do not anticipate any expenses for psychiatric or psychological care, counseling, etc.

8. To the extent that Mr. B.'s treating clinicians may offer opinions or opinion testimony, I am concerned about the substantial potential for conflict of interest between the role of treating clinician and that of opining expert.

    The relevant professional literature in psychiatry and psychology is very clear that having a treatment relationship with a person (who is then called one's "patient" or "client") interferes substantially with one's ability to provide credible opinions to a court, and *vice versa*. This potential for interference occurs whether or not the treatment relationship was in the past or is continuing, and applies particularly when one anticipates future care of the person. It includes both conscious and unconscious factors in the clinician. In some cases, such interactions can reach a level at which professional ethics become an issue (such as, but not limited to, when payment depends on the outcome of a case). For further discussion of this topic, one may refer to the following, among other references: . . .

151

SOURCES REVIEWED/RELIED UPON

Written materials supplied by your office as follows, represented as all available and relevant:

(list)

Review of relevant professional literature

See above.

My background, training, and experience in medicine, psychology and psychotherapy, psychiatry, and forensic psychiatry

R 7

REPORT: CLINICIAN–PATIENT SEX, PLAINTIFF

NOTES: Some of the wording in this report ("reckless," "indifferent") reflects an intent to support opinions of "gross negligence" in addition to "ordinary negligence."

The use of conditional phrases such as "to the extent that" in this and some other reports (particularly preliminary or pre-suit reports) is a way of commenting on topics for which there is incomplete information in the record, allowing for criticism if it is found to be warranted but not opining on something for which there is insufficient evidence. If and when additional information becomes available, the conditional phrasing should be corrected in whatever way is consistent with the new data.

RE: **PRELIMINARY REPORT:** *A.B.* v. *C.D. et al.*

You have asked for a report which summarizes my findings after review of the materials you provided. I am able to supply the opinions and comments below, based upon those materials and my training, background, and experience. The methods used and materials reviewed are those routinely relied upon by forensic psychiatrists in matters such as this. It should be noted that I have not personally examined the plaintiff, Ms. B., and that this report relies heavily on the accuracy of Ms. B.'s own statements. Although I do not believe that a personal examination is necessary for the rendering of the opinions below, such an examination could yield relevant information not obtainable elsewhere in the record. Competent persons who have examined her and followed her care are likely to be in a better position than I to enumerate her damages and discuss her progress toward alleviating them.

Should additional information cause me to change or add to my opinions, I will communicate with you promptly. I reserve the right to supplement this report as necessary should additional, relevant information become available in the future.

FINDINGS AND OPINIONS

The following opinions are offered to a reasonable degree of medical and psychiatric certainty given the information available to me at this time and assuming that information accurately represents the facts in this matter. Please note that, although the following wording is often in the present tense, all of the statements and opinions below apply the relevant U.S. standard of care as it existed in the 1980s through (*date*), unless otherwise stated.

With regard to C.D., M.D.
Standard of Care and Breaches Thereof

1. **The relevant standard of care requires that psychiatrists refrain from sexual activity with patients or former patients.**

   The presence of a "doctor–patient relationship" includes any period in which a physician sees a patient clinically, examining, interviewing, advising, prescribing, making clinical or therapeutic recommendations, following care, representing to her that he is doing any of those, and the period after prescribing during which the patient is expected to take the prescribed medication, unless care has been appropriately terminated or transferred to another clinician.

   The record indicates that A.B. was a patient of Dr. D. during her inpatient treatment at E. (*dates*), apparently for some period after that, and perhaps continuously until at least (*date*). Ms. B. has stated on many occasions that she was seeing him for what she was told was "treatment" until (*date*); I have seen no independent corroboration of that statement. It is clear that she was his patient on and for some time after (*date*), since he prescribed medication for her on that date.

   Assuming reasonable accuracy of Ms. B.'s statements, Dr. D. engaged in extensive and repeated sexual activity with his patient, Ms. B., while she was experiencing substantial psychiatric symptoms, during her inpatient and outpatient treatment, in more than one location, and represented his actions as therapeutic and part of her treatment. Such behavior by a psychiatrist falls below the standard of care and, further, is intentional, reckless, beyond the bounds of decency, indifferent to his patient's well-being, and abusive.

2. **The relevant standard of care requires that psychiatrists refrain from activities that they know, or should know, exceed reasonable boundaries of care to the detriment of patients and/or the processes of diagnosing, treating, managing, or protecting patients.**

   In addition to the alleged sexual activity, Ms. B. states that Dr. D. gave her many gifts (some quite personal), telephoned her a great many times (perhaps hundreds), sometimes followed or observed her from afar, and drove by her home, all for reasons unrelated to reasonable patient care, over many years ending in (*date*).

To the extent that the events occurred as Ms. B. describes, Dr. D. knew or should have known that (a) his sexual activity with his patient Ms. B., (b) his misleading her about her treatment, (c) his significant breaches of other reasonable boundaries of clinical care during treatment (above), and (d) his continuing engagement in those activities over years of purported treatment while she was his patient were all detrimental to Ms. B.'s well-being, including, but not necessarily limited to, her diagnosis, treatment, symptom alleviation, and care management.

Such behavior by a psychiatrist falls below the standard of care and, further, is intentional, reckless, beyond the bounds of decency, indifferent to his patient's well-being, and abusive.

3. **The relevant standard of care requires that, insofar as is feasible, psychiatrists place their patients' interests above their own.**

To the extent that they occurred as described by Ms. B., Dr. D.'s sexual behavior, his misleading her about her treatment, his lack of useful treatment, the extraordinary length of time in which he engaged in the above activities, his warning or threatening her with regard to her revealing his actions, and his exhortations to keep his behavior a secret from persons likely to be able to help her were all intended to further his own interests at the expense of her interests and well-being. Dr. D. clearly knew or should have known that fact. Such behavior by a psychiatrist falls below the standard of care and, further, is intentional, reckless, beyond the bounds of decency, indifferent to his patient's well-being, and abusive.

4. **The relevant standard of care requires that psychiatrists not mislead patients regarding their care by claiming or representing that sexual or other significant "boundary crossing" behavior is a part of legitimate treatment.**

Ms. B. states that Dr. D. represented to her that his various sexual acts and other inappropriate acts in which he engaged Ms. B. were clinically sound and necessary for her mental health and therapeutic progress.

To the extent that Ms. B.'s statements are reasonably accurate, Dr. D. knew or should have known that this was not true, that the behaviors he ordered or requested of her would harm his patient and interfere with her clinical progress, that Ms. B.'s judgment and mental condition were such that he could strongly influence her to comply with his harmful requests, and that such representations were likely to strongly influence Ms. B. to comply with harmful requests.

Such behavior by a psychiatrist falls below the standard of care and, further, is intentional, reckless, beyond the bounds of decency, indifferent to his patient's well-being, and abusive.

5. **The relevant standard of care requires that a psychiatrist not engage in treatment, or lack of treatment, which he knows or should know is likely to harm a patient, to interfere significantly with legitimate treatment, or unreasonably to delay or impair opportunity for improvement.**

   To the extent that Ms. B.'s statements are reasonably accurate, the behaviors in which Dr. D. engaged under the guise of treatment (including, but not limited to, his warnings, threats, and exhortations about not revealing his behavior) (a) could not have helped Ms. B., (b) were virtually certain to harm her, and (c) delayed or prevented her seeking or receiving important help and treatment from others. Dr. D. clearly knew or should have known those facts. Such behavior by a psychiatrist falls below the standard of care and, further, is intentional, reckless, beyond the bounds of decency, indifferent to his patient's well-being, and abusive.

   To the extent that Dr. D.'s decision not to prescribe psychotropic medication for Ms. B. was intended to increase or maintain her vulnerability to his advances, that action (or inaction) was intentional, reckless, indifferent to her well-being, and abusive.

6. **The relevant standard of care requires that a psychiatrist take immediate mitigating action, such as seeking consultation or referral, when he or she knows, or should know, that his or her treatment is harming a patient. Further, once a psychiatrist recognizes, or should recognize, that his or her treatment or other behavior is harming or probably harming the patient, the standard requires stopping that treatment and behavior. In matters of sexual behavior with patients, the care of the patient should be transferred to a more appropriate clinician at once, in a way designed to minimize further harm to the patient and to allow prompt and proper care.**

   Assuming reasonable accuracy of Ms. B.'s statements, Dr. D. knew or should have known of the harm he was causing to her (including, but not limited to, the harm of keeping her from receiving potentially effective treatment). Nevertheless, he did not refer her to another clinician, nor did he recommend that she seek additional psychiatric treatment. Dr. D. not only failed to stop his treatment of Ms. B. but also failed to do anything which might have minimized further harm and delay of her care. Such behavior falls below the relevant standard of care. If his purpose in not referring her for effective treatment was to hide his own behavior, to further that behavior, or to increase or maintain her vulnerability to his advances, then his behavior was intentional, reckless, beyond the bounds of decency, indifferent to his patient's well-being, and abusive.

7. The relevant standard of care requires that a psychiatrist not delay the proper care of a patient by pursuing harmful, ineffective, or otherwise negligent care, and that a psychiatrist recognize that such delay is in itself likely to harm his or her patient.

Assuming reasonable accuracy of Ms. B.'s statements, (a) Dr. D.'s failure to instigate and continue effective treatment after his sexual behavior with Ms. B. began, (b) the permanent interruption of useful treatment from him after that behavior began, and (c) his failure to refer or recommend her to a competent clinician all created and unreasonable delay in her receiving the care she needed.

8. The relevant standard of care does not recognize patient participation in doctor-patient sexual activity as a defense to the doctor's negligence, recklessness, or indifference.

The American Psychiatric Association's annotations of the American Medical Association *Principles of Medical Ethics*, the great bulk of the relevant professional literature, state statutes of which I am aware, and other accepted iterations of the standard of care on this topic all agree that patient participation, even patient willingness, does not excuse a psychiatrist or psychotherapist from his or her duty under the standard, from responsibility for breach of it, or from damage reasonably caused by such breach.

9. The relevant standard of care recognizes that the sexual exploitation of patients who are particularly vulnerable is even more serious than exploitation of those who are less vulnerable.

The standard recognizes that many factors affect a patient's vulnerability and potential for damage, including the seriousness of the patient's impairment, the patient's ability to understand the harmfulness or inappropriateness of the activity, the extent to which the patient is led to believe the activity is "therapeutic," the patient's ability to resist inappropriate advances, the forcefulness and physical intrusiveness of the activity, the amount of emotional influence or force used by the perpetrator, the duration of the activity, the frequency of the activity, the chronicity of the activity, the extent to which therapeutic intimacy and trust are betrayed by the activity, the patient's ability to recover from damage related to the activity, the patient's opportunity to recover, the extent to which the clinician limits the patient's ability and opportunity to escape or recover from the activity, attitudes of the patient's family and friends who become aware of the events, and the manner in which post-activity matters are handled (including level of remorse, repentance, or accepting responsibility by the clinician; quality of post-activity counseling and other treatment; and the rigors and embarrassments of discovery, complaint, investigation, or lawsuit processes).

Assuming Ms. B.'s statements are reasonably accurate, Dr. D. deliberately chose a patient–victim who was severely mentally ill, required inpatient care and frequent therapy visits, had obvious personality characteristics which made her substantially more vulnerable to his influence than most other patients, and had "transference" characteristics within the doctor–patient relationship which made her unusually prone to accept his behavior, influence, rationalizations, exhortations, and/or intimidations. His taking advantage of those vulnerabilities, especially in light of her high potential for substantial damage, fell below the relevant standard of care and, further, was intentional, reckless, beyond the bounds of decency, indifferent to his patient's well-being, and abusive.

Damage and Causation Related to Dr. D.

Sexual activity by a psychiatrist with a patient is almost always damaging to that patient in some way. The likely level of damage depends upon a number of factors, including those enumerated in item 9, above.

I am unable to provide a complete and detailed recitation of damages in this report. I am able to outline areas in which it is reasonable to infer damage from the available record, and refer the reader to qualified clinicians and/or experts who have directly examined Ms. B. (or will do so) and have carefully assessed her life during and since the events which transpired prior to (*date*).

Relying on the records provided and assuming the accuracy of Ms. B.'s statements, it is more likely than not that Dr. D.'s intentionally negligent, reckless and abusive care damaged her by:

10. **Delaying and preventing adequate treatment of her pre-existing mental condition**, thus fostering and perpetuating painful symptoms of severe depression, emotional instability, suicidal behaviors and impulses, anxiety, social and relationship dysfunction, limited enjoyment of life, and other symptoms and conditions which are likely to have responded, at least in part, to adequate treatment.

11. **Delaying and preventing any treatment of the mental conditions and other damage caused by Dr. D.'s behavior and her relationship with Dr. D.**, thus fostering and perpetuating additional post-traumatic symptoms of depression, emotional instability,

suicidal behaviors and impulses, intrusive memories, social dysfunction, limited enjoyment of life, guilt, shame, anxiety, and other
symptoms and conditions for which the delay in treatment is likely
to have decreased opportunity for and extent of improvement.

12. Exposing her to conditions and behaviors that harmed her
emotionally and had a high risk of harming her physically,
including (but not limited to) exacerbating her earlier symptoms,
increasing her suicide risk, and exposing her to risk of sexually trans-
mitted diseases.

13. Delaying and impairing her ability to form successful, stable,
and rewarding relationships with men; to marry successfully;
and to create and maintain a healthy family environment.
Assuming the facts of Dr. D.'s behavior as described by Ms. B., there
is substantial likelihood that the conditions of this case (that is, the
combination of Ms. B.'s pre-existing condition, Dr. D.'s behavior,
and Ms. B.'s foreseeable reactions to that behavior) have damaged
Ms. B.'s mental condition, treatment, treatment response, relationships, continuing emotional development, and general well-being.
That damage should be weighed against reasonable expectations of
clinical and social problems attributable to her pre-existing condition, had it been treated in a way consistent with the standard of care
between (*dates*).

With regard to E. Medical Center and its related facilities and entities
("E.")
Standard of Care and Breaches Thereof

14. The relevant standard of care requires that a facility such as E.
reasonably prevent its staff, including voluntary physician staff,
from engaging in sexual activity with patients.
    To the extent that Dr. D.'s behavior with Ms. B., or other indices
of inadequate or inappropriate care, were reasonably knowable or pre-
ventable by E. while patients such as Ms. B. were being treated by E.
employees or medical staff and/or in its facility, and it did nothing
substantial to stop or prevent that condition, E. fell below the
standard.

15. The relevant standard of care requires that a facility such as
E. reasonably attempt to ascertain that clinical activities by
members of its medical staff and/or in its facility meet the standard of care and are free from behavior such as that alleged of
Dr. D. in this lawsuit.

To the extent that E. failed to create and maintain reasonable and effective credentialing and privileging procedures, quality assurance/improvement activities, peer review, abuse and neglect policies and procedures, procedures for recognizing and investigating clinician impairment and incompetence, and similar policies and/or procedures designed reasonably to discover and correct problems in patient care and safety while patients such as Ms. B. were being treated by its employees or medical staff and/or in its facility, it fell below the standard.

To the extent that E. failed to create and maintain professionally expected policies and procedures designed to discover, investigate, report, and/or monitor problems related to the clinical competence, patient safety, clinically relevant character or morals, and similar problems of its clinicians, including Dr. D., while patients such as Ms. B. were being treated by its employees or medical staff and/or in its facility, it fell below the standard.

To the extent that E. became reasonably aware, or should have become aware, of any significant suggestion that Dr. D. was engaging in inappropriate behavior with patients, or was significantly clinically impaired, and did not act properly on such suggestion(s), it fell below the standard.

16. **The relevant standard of care requires that, if a facility such as E. becomes aware of real or suspected problems with patient treatment, patient safety, or clinician behavior, it must instigate protective, reporting, investigatory, and/or corrective actions as soon as feasible, in a reasonable effort to protect patients and staff and address the causes of those problems. Further, the facility must require that its medical staff act in ways consistent with the foregoing.**

There is ample indication that E. and/or its senior administrators were aware, at various times, of substantial problems with Dr. D.'s behavior. For example, (a) F.G., M.D., testified that he was present at an E. meeting at which "H.I." began to speak about Dr. D., apparently regarding concerns about sexual behavior with patients. Dr. D. pre-empted I.'s comments by reading a letter purportedly from his lawyer which threatened and intimidated I. and the group into saying and doing nothing (G. deposition pp. 20–21, [*date*]). (b) A Ms. J. sent a letter to the then administrator of E. (a few years before) complaining about Dr. D., who she alleged sexually assaulted her, among other allegations. Ms. J. was told that E. was investigating Dr. D., but was never contacted further or notified of any outcome. (I found no record of any such investigation.) Ms. J. also reported her allegations to the (state medical licensing agency), who investigated and eventually censured Dr. D. (J. affidavit). (c) <u>Dr. K.</u>, a former E. Executive Committee member and former president of E.'s medical staff, said that Dr. D., acting during a meeting in his then role as president of E. medical staff, publicly discarded a complaint related to sex between a physician and a patient, saying "Here's the best way to handle this crap" (or similar words).

To the extent that E. knew, should have known, or reasonably suspected that any of Dr. D.'s patients was being subjected to sexual activity, being assaulted or neglected, or was otherwise at unacceptable risk of harm or inadequate care by his hand, and then failed to instigate adequate protective, reporting, investigatory, and/or corrective actions as soon as feasible, E.'s inaction fell below the relevant standard of care and, further, was intentional, reckless, beyond the bounds of decency, and indifferent to its patients' well-being.

17. The relevant standard of care requires that a facility such as E. have <u>policies and/or procedures</u> in place which are sufficient to recognize and deal properly with reasonable signs that the activities alluded to in this lawsuit above may be occurring. Those policies and/or procedures must mandate employee and medical staff reporting of suspected significant infractions and provide an acceptable method of investigation and/or reporting to relevant entities such as facility supervisors, administrators, peer review and credentialing bodies, and (for matters of patient abuse or neglect at least) government agencies.

To the extent that E. did not have and follow such policies and procedures while patients such as Ms. B. were being treated by its employees or medical staff and/or in its facility, it fell below the standard.

18. The relevant standard of care requires that a facility such as E. adequately <u>orient, educate, and/or train</u> its employees and medical staff in order reasonably to protect patients from prohibited sexual activity, sexual and other assault or abuse, neglect, inadequate care, care likely to do harm, and other prohibited or harmful events. Such events include, but are not limited to, improper, inadequate, and/or harmful behaviors by staff (including medical staff, contracting clinicians, and other persons working in the facility or under its aegis).

To the extent that E. failed to provide such orientation, education, and/or training as indicated given the role and level of various employees and practitioners, it fell below the standard. For example, and without intending to be exhaustive, (a) to the extent that nursing and other unit staff were not trained and encouraged to recognize and report reasonable signs of poor patient care and patient

161

abuse and neglect, including sexual abuse, it fell below the standard; and (b) to the extent that there were not reasonable and sufficient opportunities and encouragements in place at E. through which anyone who observed or suspected poor patient care, neglect, or abuse (including sexual abuse), could report and/or seek help without fear of retribution, it fell below the standard.

19. The standard of care requires that a facility such as E. require its employees and medical staff to <u>report</u> observations or reasonable suspicions of staff or clinician sexual activity with patients, sexual and other forms of assault or abuse, patient neglect, inadequate care, and/or care likely to harm patients to appropriate internal and/or external parties such as supervisors, administrators, and public agencies.

   To the extent that E. or any member of its staff knew or reasonably suspected that Dr. D. or any other person on its medical staff or under its aegis was engaging in sexual activity or other assaultive, abusive, or neglectful behavior with any of its patients and that knowledge or suspicion was not reported to the appropriate party(ies), it fell below the standard.

Damage and Causation Related to E.
Assuming reasonable accuracy of Ms. B.'s statements, adherence to the standards enumerated above increase the likelihood that E. could have prevented Dr. D.'s negligent and harmful behavior or, in the alternative, discovered, corrected, or mitigated it, thus preventing or decreasing the damage to Ms. B. To the extent that E. fell below those standards, the opportunity for such prevention, discovery, correction, or mitigation decreased.

SOURCES RELIED UPON

- Written materials as follows, represented to me as all relevant and available from your office at this time:
  (*list*)
- American Medical Association *Principles of Medical Ethics*, original and as annotated for use by psychiatrists by the American Psychiatric Association, 1980s, 1990s, and post-2000 editions
- My background, training, and experience in medicine, psychology, psychiatry, and forensic psychiatry

QUALIFICATIONS
. . .

R8

REPORT: MALPRACTICE, PLAINTIFF (COMPLEX, DOCTOR AND HOSPITAL)

NOTE: Many jurisdictions require that plaintiffs' reports in malpractice cases, particularly pre-suit reports or affidavits, address all elements of the tort of malpractice (duty, breach of duty, damage, and causation). Some states, such as Texas, are very picky. Be certain that each of these is addressed as required; failure to do so in detail can cause a suit to be dismissed or never filed, regardless of its factual merits. That's what makes this report seem long and redundant.

RE: **Preliminary Report: *A. et al.* v. *Dr. B. and C. Medical Center* (re: D., deceased)**

You have asked for a report of my preliminary opinions regarding Ms. A.'s care by Dr. B. and C. Medical Center prior to her death. I am able to supply the opinions and comments below, based upon the materials you have provided, review of relevant professional literature, and my training, background, and experience. The methods used are those routinely relied upon by forensic psychiatrists in matters such as this. Note that additional information could change or add to these opinions; should that become the case, I will communicate with you promptly.

FINDINGS AND OPINIONS
The following opinions are offered to a reasonable degree of medical and psychiatric probability given the information available to me at this time.

STANDARD OF CARE AND BREACHES THEREOF

1. **Many duties related to the standard of care (hereinafter "the standard") are predicated on the existence of a physician-patient and/or facility-patient relationship.** The record clearly indicates the presence of such relationships between C. Medical Center and Ms. D., and between B., M.D. ("Dr. B." in much of the record) and Ms. D. Such a relationship existed with various other clinicians as well.

2. The standard required, among other things, that C. Medical Center accept certain responsibilities for Ms. D.'s care, custody, and safety while she was a patient there, including providing adequately trained, licensed, and competent staff; management or elimination of reasonably recognizable safety risks; adequate monitoring of the patient and her inpatient environment; discharge planning; and appropriate privileging, credentialing and monitoring of clinicians (including Dr. B.) who practice in the hospital.

3. The standard required that, prior to discharging Ms. D., Dr. B. adequately assess her condition and the knowable risks of sending her to a setting (her home) which, Dr. B. knew or should have known at the time of her (*date*) discharge, lacked professional monitoring, observation, protection, evaluation, care or treatment (and in which obvious implements of suicide would foreseeably be available) before coming to a conclusion that the patient was ready for discharge and ordering discharge.

Dr. B. and C. Medical Center fell below the relevant standard when they discharged Ms. D. (or, in the case of C. Medical Center, allowed her to be discharged without apparent question or protest, or adequate discharge investigation and planning) under the conditions described above. Both Dr. B. and C. Medical Center were aware, or should have been aware, of those conditions on the morning of (*date*), of the unacceptable risk of suicide associated with her discharge, and of the inability of her home environment to provide the clinical and protective measures that Ms. D. required.

Dr. B.'s actions and statements, as reflected in both the available record and her own depositions (*dates*), indicate a remarkable lack of proper assessment, care, clinical judgment, and knowledge of several well-established principles of clinical psychiatry as of (*date*), when she was treating Ms. D. All of those were important to Ms. D.'s safe and adequate treatment.

Risk Assessment. Dr. B. failed to perform an adequate predischarge risk assessment (or virtually any risk assessment) or to give adequate attention to the ominous symptoms, behaviors, and statements that were observed just hours and days earlier, and for which no reliable evidence of positive and consistent change existed (see, e.g., chart progress notes of late [*date*] and early [*date*]: "You overdosed me!," severe swings of emotion ["lability"], threats to kill staff, wishing she had died from her inpatient overdose, wishing to die after she returned from intensive care, and orders to keep the patient within "line of sight" of staff and in a hospital gown up until the moment of discharge).

The standard required, among other things, that before assuming that Ms. D. was ready for discharge on (*date*), Dr. B. not rely simply on a patient statement and a brief interview in order to assess the patient and her risk. **The standard and accepted psychiatric procedures are very clear that relying on statements such as those Dr. B. described in order to decide that Ms. D. was improved, reliably improved, and sufficiently free of suicide risk, is both inadequate and dangerous.**

Examples of common, easily available, and clinically routine actions which could have contributed to a useful pre-discharge risk assessment procedure (and which, more likely than not, would have indicated far greater risk in Ms. D.) include (but are not necessarily limited to) careful chart and prior record review, more competent and extensive interview/examination, reasonable discussion with the treatment team, interviews with family members, consultation with a second psychiatrist or a psychologist, relevant psychological testing, exploration of whether or not firearms and other common instruments of suicide were easily available to the patient and, particularly, extended observation of the patient's behavior and treatment response (that is, keeping her in the hospital longer, either voluntarily or involuntarily), all followed by adequate consideration of the results when discharge was eventually contemplated.

Unfortunately, Dr. B. fell below the standard in that she failed to order, and/or adequately consider, any of the above before assuming that her patient was significantly improved, clinically and behaviorally stable, and safe for discharge. Dr. B. failed to evaluate or observe Ms. D.'s condition and progress for an adequate length of time and under conditions other than "line of sight" restrictions in a hospital gown, and failed adequately to assess her response to treatment, including her response to the medication which had very recently been prescribed. Neither consultation with another clinician nor psychological testing was apparently considered.

Reliance on medication. Contrary to Dr. B.'s assumption (voiced during her deposition), Dr. B. should have known that the primary medication she prescribed to stabilize Ms. D.'s mood and alleviate her psychosis (*medication*) (a) is very often ineffective or only partially effective for patients such as Ms. D. and (b), even when it is effective, usually takes weeks to show the desired response (see, e.g., [*reference*], below, as well as standard psychiatric and psychopharmacology texts). The same principles apply to the other medications Dr. B. prescribed for her primary symptoms (_____, _____). This information is common and required knowledge among practicing psychiatrists.

The ways in which a psychiatrist can meet the standard of care vary with individual patients, reasonable clinician preference, treatment availability, clinical and other findings, and reasonably knowable future conditions. Dr. B. did not avail herself of any of the above routine ways of assessing patients such as Ms. D., or consider them (so far as the record shows), or even know (as the standard requires) how to interpret and prioritize adequately the very limited information she says she used in order to assume that Ms. D. was safe and reliably stable for discharge.

Length of stay. The standard of care required far more inpatient psychiatric observation and treatment than Ms. D. received after her intensive care (ICU) treatment. Regardless of how many days of additional observation and care may eventually have been indicated, and the specific elements of that observation and care, discharging Ms. D. less than 30 hours after she was released from the ICU, and just a few hours after the ominous statements, behaviors, and conditions documented in her chart (see above), was virtually *per se* below the standard.

Reliance on patient statements. Dr. B. further fell below the standard in that she relied primarily (virtually exclusively, according to her deposition) on the patient's own statements (e.g., that she would not kill herself) to assume that Ms. D. was "more stable in mood ... Not suicidal or homicidal" at the time of her discharge order. Dr. B. knew, or should have known, that (a) it was highly unreasonable and unsafe to assume dramatic, stable improvement so quickly given Ms. D.'s history, condition on admission, behaviors, and stormy hospital stay; (b) it was similarly unreasonable and unsafe to assume dramatic, stable improvement the day after the patient returned from intensive care treatment for a very recent, very severe overdose; (c) suicidal patients very often try to mislead clinicians as a result of their mental illness, their wish to die, and other factors, in order to gain discharge from the hospital; (d) Ms. D., as a result of her mental illness and/or other factors, was already known to have grossly misled hospital staff and clinicians while at C. Medical Center and purposely placed herself in danger of dying; and (e) patients such as Ms. D. cannot be expected reliably to assess their own conditions or "predict" their suicidality and future behavior even when they are trying to communicate honestly (which honesty must not be assumed in Ms. D.'s case). On the day of her discharge, Dr. B. knew, or should have known, that Ms. D.'s diagnoses, current and very recent symptoms, and very recent behaviors clearly indicated that she was not a reliable judge, reporter, or arbiter of her own condition or safety.

4. The standard required that relevant C. Medical Center behavioral health unit staff, and perhaps other staff, question or protest clinical care and discharge decisions that they knew

or reasonably should have known were substantially outside adequate and safe psychiatric procedures.

C. **Medical Center** fell below the standard in that members of the C. Medical Center unit behavioral health staff, and perhaps other staff, knowing or being required to know that discharging Ms. D. on (*date*) was premature and highly dangerous, and further knowing that they had a duty to question or protest questionable clinical care (either directly or by reporting their concerns to superiors), **failed to raise any question or protest either to Dr. B. or to other C. Medical Center staff who could have intervened.** Dr. B. stated in her deposition that, had staff questioned the discharge, she would have reconsidered.

5. **The standard required that Ms. D. not be discharged home if her risk to herself still required "line of sight" observation and a hospital gown for her protection.**

Ms. D.'s very close inpatient monitoring on (*dates*), with Dr. B.'s order and knowledge, included remaining in a staff person's "line of sight" until the moment of her discharge. Dr. B.'s deposition comment that she inadvertently left those precautions in place notwithstanding, the record is clear that those precautions were indicated the evening before her discharge and on the morning of (*discharge date*) as well. No staff person documented any suggestion or belief that those extraordinary precautions should be lifted. If one assumes, reasonably in my opinion, that the precautions were a result of both Dr. B. and the hospital staff recognizing marked risk in Ms. D., and notes the absence of any documented contemplation by hospital staff or Dr. B. of lifting those precautions, one must conclude either that Ms. D. was discharged while Dr. B. and the C. Medical Center staff considered her a very substantial risk, or that neither Dr. B. nor the C. Medical Center staff adequately considered the fact that the patient was on such precautions when discharged.

Dr. B. thus fell below the standard in discharging Ms. D. prematurely and without adequate assessment.

C. **Medical Center** fell below the standard by allowing the discharge to occur without question or protest, knowing that Ms. D. was still considered at high risk and required substantial monitoring for that risk, and further knowing that they had a responsibility to question or protest apparently substandard clinical care.

6. **The standard required that, before agreeing to discharge Ms. D., Dr. B. reasonably establish that sufficient and reliable positive change and decrease in risk had occurred since her admission, in order reasonably to establish stable clinical**

improvement and reduce her risk of post-discharge severe or catastrophic deterioration to an acceptable level.

Upon admission and during her hospital stay, Ms. D. was described in the record as being acutely and markedly mentally ill, as chronically mentally ill, as at very high risk of killing herself (particularly) or harming others, as functioning at extremely low levels (cf. her exceedingly low admission "Global Assessment of Functioning" [GAF], defined in the current edition of the American Psychiatric Association *Diagnostic and Statistical Manual* [DSM-IV-TR] [p. 34] as having "Persistent danger of severely hurting self or others . . ." [underlining mine]), and as being very impulsive and unstable.

During her brief hospitalization, and within 1–2 days prior to discharge (sometimes only hours), Ms. D. exhibited severe symptoms (e.g., severe depression, marked lability of mood, suicidal thoughts and threats, treats to others), engaged in very dangerous behavior (her in-hospital overdose), and expressed obvious intent to commit suicide.

Dr. B. fell below the standard when she nevertheless discharged Ms. D. without reasonable evidence of substantial and stable improvement, and without reasonably reliable evidence of acceptable and stable decrease in her symptoms and her very high risk of self-harm.

Dr. B. documented an estimate of the patient's Global Assessment of Functioning (GAF) of "55–60" at discharge. That estimate is completely without support in the record. ("55–60" is defined in DSM-IV-TR as having "moderate" symptoms or difficulty, and is just short of a level of "some mild symptoms . . . but generally functioning pretty well.") It should be said that the GAF is a summary estimate which, although fairly reliable between qualified raters, varies somewhat among them; nevertheless, such a finding, and such a marked change from the earlier level (especially noting her potentially lethal overdose in the hospital and the GAF recorded on [*date*]), is simply not credible. The record is clear that Ms. D. did not show nearly enough evidence of the stable symptom remission and reliable risk reduction that is required for discharge, and indicates that Dr. B. fell below the standard in discharging her.

C. Medical Center staff fell below the standard by allowing the discharge to occur without question or protest, knowing (or being required to know) that they had a duty to question or protest obviously substandard clinical care.

7. **The standard required that C. Medical Center perform a thorough search for items which might threaten her health or safety, or that of others, when admitting Ms. D., particularly after she was found to have surreptitiously brought a**

weapon onto the inpatient unit (discovered the day before her in-hospital overdose).

The standard requires a search of patients such as Ms. D. when they are admitted to units such as the C. Medical Center psychiatric unit. Such a search must be adequate to discover such obvious and dangerous contraband as a knife or a large number of pills hidden among cosmetics. In addition, Ms. D. was known, or should reasonably have been assumed, to be paranoid, to be severely depressed, to have thoughts of suicide and harming others, to have a history of suicidality, and to be clinically and behaviorally unstable. Discovering that she had secretly brought a weapon onto the unit further established the likelihood of her having other dangerous items (such as the pills with which she overdosed the next day) and the importance of searching her and her surroundings.

C. Medical Center fell below the standard when it failed to search Ms. D. and her belongings adequately.

8. To the extent that Ms. D. requested discharge on the morning of (*date*), the standard required that Dr. B. make substantial effort to prevent that discharge. Such effort should have included strongly advising her to stay or be transferred to another clinically suitable inpatient facility. Had Ms. D. refused, Dr. B. should have attempted involuntary detention using standard emergency detention procedures.

First, there is no documentation in the available record, except for Dr. B.'s comments after the patient's suicide, that Ms. D. actually requested discharge on (*date*). One would expect to find clear documentation in the chart if such a request had taken place, particularly for a patient such as Ms. D.

Second, assuming for the sake of argument that she requested discharge on (*date*), there is no indication that Ms. D. would not have remained in the hospital had she been encouraged to stay.

Third, the standard of care requires psychiatrists and hospital staff to question requests for discharge by patients such as the one Ms. D. allegedly voiced on (*date*), and strongly to encourage them to remain in the hospital. Many patients such as Ms. D. respond well to such encouragement, take it as a sign of concern by doctor and staff, accept the importance and implied authority of such encouragement when it comes from a clinician or nurse, and/or realize that, if they do not remain voluntarily, emergency detention procedures may be employed. There is no indication that either Dr. B. or any C. Medical Center staff member even advised Ms. D. to stay, much less strongly encouraged her to stay.

Fourth, the record indicates that Ms. D. almost certainly met criteria for emergency detention on (*date*), and that an emergency detention certificate would have been easily supportable. Nevertheless, Dr. B. either failed reasonably to recognize that fact or ignored that routine avenue for protecting patients such as Ms. D.

9. The standard requires that patients such as Ms. D. not be precipitously discharged without, among other things, appropriate discharge planning, including reasonable attempts to communicate with relevant members of the patient's family. Both Dr. B. and C. Medical Center were aware, or should have been aware, of several family members with whom communication would be helpful: Her sister (who had brought her to the hospital), her twin brother, her parents (with whom she was living), and another sister (who came to the hospital when she was to be discharged). Nevertheless, there was apparently no significant communication, or effort at communication, with any of those persons by either Dr. B. or C. Medical Center.
Both C. Medical Center and Dr. B. fell below the standard in this regard.

There is indication in statements by _____ (see her written statement and her deposition), with corroboration in _____'s and _____'s depositions, that her sister (and perhaps her parents) immediately expressed their disagreement with the discharge decision to the psychiatric unit staff, strongly recommended that it be reconsidered, and asked that those concerns be conveyed to a person who could reconsider the discharge. The record indicates that the staff person with whom (*patient's sister*) spoke failed to convey, or to try to convey, that important information and request either to Dr. B. or to nursing superiors.

Dr. B. has referred to the concept of patient privilege as a reason for not contacting other persons in order to get potentially important clinical information about the patient's history and condition (see her deposition). Those comments fail to suggest any reason that the standard of care could not be met, since (a) Ms. D. had provided written authorization for communication with her siblings and parents; (b) psychiatrists and hospital staff persons can easily obtain important collateral information merely by engaging in a "one-way" conversation with a cooperating relative, in which the relative is asked for information but none is divulged by the clinician or staff person; (c) even patients who have refused authorization (not the case for Ms. D.) often change their minds if the importance of family contact is explained to them; and (d) when the situation is as serious and dangerous as it was for Ms. D. on the dates in question, reasonable caregivers carefully weigh issues of confidentiality against those of danger to the patient and routinely document those efforts. There is no documentation in Ms. D.'s record of any attempt to communicate with her family or prior caregivers. Finally, (e) when (*sister*) arrived at the C. Medical Center unit on (*date*), the staff person willingly discussed a few things about Ms. D. (e.g., giving the sister the weapon that had been confiscated).

Had family members (such as _____, _____, _____, _____, and/or _____) been contacted and appropriately interviewed, it is more likely than not that one or more would have provided information which would (or should) have added to Dr. B.'s and C. Medical Center's concerns about Ms. D.'s condition and risk (such as, but not necessarily limited to, information about past suicide attempts, recent talk of suicide, recent purchase of a gun, and pending legal problems).

10. The standard requires that reasonable effort be made to obtain information about the past psychiatric history, including hospitalization and treatment history, of patients such as Ms. D.

    Ms. D. had been psychiatrically hospitalized many times prior to her final admission. At least four of those hospitalizations were at C. Medical Center, two within the past two years. Three were under Dr. B.'s own care and one under the care of a Dr. _____. Dr. B.'s admission notes documented that Ms. D. had a "very complicated history."

    So far as I can ascertain, past C. Medical Center and _____ records, which should have been quickly and easily obtainable and contained relevant information (such as prior suicide attempts, diagnoses and treatments), were never requested. _____ hospital records, which included at least one involuntary hospitalization, were not requested either.

11. The standard requires that clinical and nursing staff of hospitals such as C. Medical Center, when they suspect or become aware of unreasonable or dangerous patient care, promptly report, question, and/or protest that care to an appropriate person without delay.

    Relevant members of the nursing staff at C. Medical Center knew, should have known, or should reasonably have suspected, that Ms. D. was far from being well enough for discharge on (*date*). Those who were in a position to observe Ms. D.'s condition and behavior should have questioned Dr. B.'s discharge decision, either to Dr. B. herself or to a facility superior. There is no indication in the available record that any such reporting or questioning took place.

12. To the extent that a C. Medical Center clinical staff person, or a clinical staff person acting on behalf of C. Medical Center, was made aware of the very significant clinical or safety concerns voiced by (_____) at the time of discharge. Regardless of

whether or not the discharge had been administratively completed, but assuming the patient was still within the hospital, the staff person who received the information from (*sister*) should have reported, or vigorously attempted to report, those concerns to an appropriate person without delay.

The failure to report, or vigorously attempt to report (_____)'s concerns by such a staff person was a breach of the applicable standard of care.

13. With additional regard to the standard of care for C. Medical Center, I have reviewed the (*date*) report by nursing expert _____. She opines, and I concur, that the standard of care required the following of the C. Medical Center nursing staff on (*dates*), and that their absence fell below the standard. (Items in parentheses are my additions.)

(a) Thorough search of Ms. D. and her belongings upon admission to the psychiatric unit, removing all (reasonably knowable) potentially dangerous items, including medications. The hospital nursing staff breached this standard by failing to perform an adequate search of Ms. D.'s belongings and failing to take the medication which would have been found from her.

(b) Contact Dr. B. and inform her of the family's concerns (as iterated in _____'s [*date*] interview with [*decedent's relative*] and in [*relative's*] deposition) about taking Ms. D. home. C. Medical Center fell below the standard by not accomplishing such contact or reasonably attempting to do so under time-critical discharge circumstances.

(c) Be aware that, until clearly shown otherwise, it was unsafe to discharge Ms. D.

(d) Communicate to Dr. B. the recommendation that Ms. D. not be discharged as Dr. B. contemplated, and that any pending discharge order be rescinded.

(e) If efforts to reach Dr. B. were unsuccessful, or if Dr. B. failed to reconsider discharge, report the nursing staff concerns to an appropriate nursing supervisor and request his or her assistance.

_____ further opines that, if such action did not stop Ms. D.'s release, the standard required that the C. Medical Center nursing staff or an appropriate supervisor alert the relevant chief of service or chief of staff to their strong concerns about Ms. D.'s discharge.

To the extent that the C. Medical Center nursing staff proceeded with Ms. D.'s discharge in spite of reasonable opportunities to question or protest it, C. Medical Center fell below the standard of care in that its nursing staff failed (as applicable) to contact Dr. B. and convey the information received and their concerns, and/or to contact an appropriate nursing supervisor or the chief of service or staff to convey the information received and their concerns.

14. The standard of care, strong iterations of medical and psychiatric ethics, routine hospital procedures, and perhaps statute all require that physicians such as Dr. B. refrain from altering medical records in the ways that have been described, and admitted, by Dr. B. at least in part (see her deposition).

    I have rarely seen more serious examples of inappropriate, unethical, and apparently self-serving medical records alterations than those which appear in this matter. My faith in Dr. B.'s credibility and ethics is eroded further by the fact that she denied changing the record until she was presented with proof during her deposition (at which time she realized, apparently, that the discrepancies in the record were incontrovertible).

15. To the extent that any administrative or financial factor significantly affected Dr. B.'s decision to discharge Ms. D., and/or affected C. Medical Center staff behavior in failing to protest the discharge, succumbing to that influence by either Dr B. or C. Medical Center staff was below the standard of care.

    That is (and notably without evidence in the record to date), if Ms. D., a severely ill and at-risk patient, was discharged prematurely because of a lack of insurance, insufficient prospects of payment, potential adverse effect on hospital utilization statistics, or something similar, then any person who ordered or significantly effected her premature discharge fell below the standard.

DAMAGE AND CAUSATION

Dr. B.'s failures to meet the applicable standards of care, individually and collectively, described in the items above, foreseeably led to (i.e., were a significant cause of) Ms. D.'s suicide some 24 hours after she was discharged from the hospital, and to resulting damage to Ms. D.'s family members. (Note that I have not personally examined any party in this matter, but it is reasonable to assume substantial damage to at least some family members.) If Dr. B. had not fallen below the standard of care, then the following, to a reasonable degree of medical and psychiatric certainty (more likely than not), would have been the case:

1. Ms. D. would not have committed suicide on or about (_____). She would have remained in the hospital, receiving treatment, protection, and observation to monitor her condition and treatment response,

until her risks had decreased sufficiently to allow reasonably safe discharge and outpatient follow-up. Had she remained in the hospital with adequate monitoring, her probability of killing herself would have been substantially lower than that outside the hospital, since she would have had the benefits of a protective and observing environment, a professional staff, and a therapeutic milieu.

2. Based upon both my own experience and studies in the professional literature of reasonably similar patients after inpatient treatment, it is statistically more likely than not that Ms. D. would have remained alive for many years.

3. Ms. D.'s psychiatric condition would have improved and—separate from the issue of suicidality already addressed—her psychiatric condition would have become less painful and damaging, assuming the benefits of a professional inpatient staff, a protected environment as she was improving, a therapeutic milieu, adequate medication, and adequate attention from a psychiatrist and other clinicians. Ms. D.'s diagnosis (irrespective of which particular one in the record was most nearly accurate) and mental condition were serious, but treatable, and in her case had responded to treatment in the past. Most patients similar to Ms. D. eventually leave the hospital and function reasonably well in the community; her own past history contained long periods of adequate functioning outside the hospital.

C. Medical Center's failures to meet the applicable standards of care described in the items above with regard to Ms. D.'s care, her discharge from the hospital, C. Medical Center's interactions (or lack of interactions) with Dr. B., and C. Medical Center's failure to respond adequately to (*relatives'*) warnings and concerns, individually and collectively, foreseeably led to (i.e., were a significant cause of) Ms. D.'s suicide within 24 hours after her discharge.

For example, had C. Medical Center nursing staff appropriately protested what they knew or should have known was Ms. D.'s premature discharge, Ms. D. would more likely than not have remained in the hospital and not committed suicide on or about (_____) (see rationale herein). Similarly, had C. Medical Center nursing staff adequately communicated (_____)'s warning and concerns to Dr. B., an appropriate supervisor, and/or the chief of service or chief of staff (and assuming there would have been time to interrupt Ms. D.'s leaving), Ms. D. would more probably than not have remained in the hospital and would not have committed suicide on or about (_____).

Note that Dr. B. said in her deposition (p. 91) that she expected C. Medical Center staff to notify her if they had any concerns about the discharging ("we're a team"). Dr. B. further stated that, if a family member picking up a patient told a C. Medical Center staff member that he or she was concerned about the discharge being unsafe, she (Dr. B.) would " would expect someone to tell me" (underlining mine). Dr. B. also stated that, if staff had questioned her discharge of the patient, she (Dr. B.) " would have considered it very carefully, . . . postponed discharge if there were the smallest concern" (underlining mine) (B. deposition, pp. 91–93).

With regard to the in-hospital overdose and its sequelae, C. Medical Center's failures to meet the applicable standards of care, individually and collectively, described above, with regard to searching Ms. D. and her belongings, led to substantial suffering in Ms. D., a significant threat to her life, treatment in the hospital intensive care unit, interruption of her psychiatric care, and contribution to her mental stress and deterioration. That is, if C. Medical Center had not fallen below the standard of care, it is more likely than not that the pills would have been found and taken from Ms. D., preventing her overdose and its associated damage.

SOURCES RELIED UPON

- Written materials, represented as everything relevant and available from your office:
  (*list*)
- Relevant references in the professional literature
  (*list*)
- My background, training, and experience in medicine, psychiatry, forensic psychiatry, residential care, and mental health administration.

QUALIFICATIONS
. . .

R9

AFFIDAVIT: MALPRACTICE, PLAINTIFF PRE-SUIT

NOTE: The format for affidavits and other legal forms should ordinarily be provided by the attorney. Some wording may be completed by the attorney in consultation with the expert, but the expert must understand and approve all content attributed to him or her before signing ("executing") the affidavit. Pre-suit expert opinion formats and requirements vary among states. When in doubt, ask.

IN THE PRE-SUIT SCREENING OF CLAIMS
PURSUANT TO _____ X., as Personal Representative of the ESTATE OF Y., Plaintiff, v. Z. Hospital and A., M.D, Defendants.

<u>AFFIDAVIT OF WILLIAM H. REID, M.D., M.P.H.</u>

STATE OF TEXAS   )
) SS:
COUNTY OF LLANO   )

BEFORE ME, the undersigned authority, personally appeared this date WILLIAM H. REID, M.D., M.P.H., who, being duly sworn by me under oath, states as follows:

1. I, WILLIAM H. REID, M.D., M.P.H., am over the age of 18 years and am otherwise *sui juris*.

2. I am a medical doctor licensed to practice medicine in the States of Texas, Illinois, Nebraska, New Mexico, Louisiana, California, and Minnesota. I am Board Certified in general psychiatry and forensic psychiatry and certified by the American Psychiatric Association in psychiatric administration and management. I am currently clinical professor of psychiatry at the University of Texas Health Science Center in San Antonio, Texas. I am also adjunct professor of psychiatry

at Texas A & M College of Medicine and Texas Tech University School of Medicine.

3. A copy of my current *curriculum vitae* is attached to this Affidavit as Exhibit "1".

4. I have reviewed the following medical records and documents relative to the care and treatment of Y.:

   (a) Medical records of Y., including Z. Hospital admission of (*date*);
   (b) Investigation report and related materials of _____ Police Department, Case No. _____; and
   (c) Autopsy report prepared by Associate Medical Examiner _____, M.D.

5. I am familiar with the standard of care for hospitals and health-care professionals in the clinical diagnosis, evaluation, treatment, and monitoring of hospitalized psychiatric patients.

6. It is my opinion, within a reasonable degree of medical probability, based solely on the materials reviewed and listed in Item 4 and subject to amendment if additional or contradictory information becomes available, that Z. Hospital, by and through its officers, directors, agents, and/or employees, real or apparent, deviated from the prevailing professional standard of care for hospital inpatient psychiatric care in that:

   (a) It failed to attend properly to the risks associated with new inpatients (i.e., Mr. Y.) who are acutely mentally ill, have a significant history of substance abuse, and are unfamiliar to the hospital, its staff, and the admitting physician;
   (b) It failed to attend properly to the risks associated with patients (i.e., Mr. Y.) who are known, or should be known, to have acute symptoms, behaviors, and/or conditions reasonably associated with, among other things, significantly impaired judgment, impulsive behavior, severe alteration in thought process, and substantial risk of suicide. "Attending to" such risks includes, but may not be limited to, appropriate monitoring and other protective measures in the absence of (but pending) physician notification and orders.

7. It is my further opinion, within a reasonable degree of medical probability, based solely on the materials reviewed and listed in Item 4 and subject to amendment if additional or contradictory information becomes available, that A., M.D., deviated from the prevailing professional standard of care for psychiatric physicians in that:

177

(a) He failed to order, or otherwise reasonably to assure, appropriate monitoring and/or suicide precautions for a new, acutely mentally ill inpatient with a significant history of substance abuse, who was unfamiliar to him, the hospital, and its staff;

(b) He failed to attend properly to the risks associated with patients (i.e., Mr. Y.) who he knew, or should have known, had acute symptoms, behaviors, and/or conditions reasonably associated with, among other things, significantly impaired judgment and impulsive behavior, severe alteration in thought process, and substantial risk of suicide. "Attending to" such risks includes, but may not be limited to, providing orders for appropriate monitoring and other protective measures.

8. It is my further opinion, within a reasonable degree of medical probability, based solely on the materials reviewed and listed in Item 4 and subject to amendment if additional or contradictory information becomes available, that Y. sustained significant and permanent injuries, ultimately resulting in his death, which very probably would not have occurred if medical diagnosis, evaluation, treatment, and/or monitoring by the above health-care facility and/or physician had met the relevant standard(s) of care.

9. I have never been disqualified as an expert witness nor, to my knowledge, has any of my opinions ever been disqualified in a court of law.

FURTHER AFFIANT SAYETH NAUGHT.

WILLIAM H. REID, M.D., M.P.H.

The foregoing Affidavit was acknowledged before me on this _____day of _____, 20xx by WILLIAM H. REID, M.D., who is personally known to me or who has produced as identification and who did/did not take an oath.

NOTARY PUBLIC, State of Texas

Typed, Printed or Stamped Name of
Officer Taking Acknowledgment

My commission expires:

R10

LETTER/REPORT: MALPRACTICE, PLAINTIFF PRE-SUIT, LACK OF CAUSATION

NOTE: In a few states, pre-suit letters and reviews are sometimes viewed by lawyers as almost pro forma. Experts should take them seriously, however, and never opine criticism where none should exist. This is an example of a matter that, in my opinion, did not meet criteria for filing a malpractice action.

RE: **A.B. (deceased)**

Thank you for sending the records concerning **Mr. B.**, the gentleman who committed suicide on (*date*). I have reviewed them in some detail in an effort to determine whether or not the information in the records appears sufficient to sustain a malpractice action against C., D. hospital/program, E. Hospital, and/or F. Mental Health Center.

I must report that although there were some episodes of likely negligence, in my opinion, there was not sufficient negligence or sufficient indication of *causation* to allow me to swear in the necessary affidavit that I have reasonable medical certainty that negligent acts by any of the potential defendants were a direct cause of Mr. B.'s death on (*date*).

As you know, a malpractice action requires that the plaintiff prove four things, each to a "preponderance" or "more likely than not" burden: That the defendant(s) had a duty to adhere to the relevant standard of care, that the duty was breached by the defendant(s) (e.g., through negligent acts), that the plaintiff (patient, Mr. B.) was damaged, and that the damage was a direct result of the breach of the standard (causation).

There is no doubt that each of the potential defendants had a level of duty to Mr. B. There are indications of breach of duty (negligence) within some parts of the record. Mr. B. and his family clearly sustained great damage (that is, he died by his own hand and the family suffered substantial loss). I am not able, however, to link his death to the probable negligent acts of the potential defendants with "reasonable medical certainty" (more likely than not; the level of certainty required by the affidavit). That is, any items of negligence do not, to a preponderance of the available evidence, appeared materially to have caused Mr. B.'s death. In addition, there appear to be so many interim and intercurrent events between the acts of the potential defendants and Mr. B.'s eventual death that I cannot say that one or more of the defendants "caused" his death.

I understand the pain and loss that has been sustained by Mr. B.'s family, and I have dealt many times with the sadness and frustration family members experience when a loved one commits suicide. Trying to make some sense of the events; wrestling with facts, feelings and theories about what happened or might have happened; and eventually finding closure are enormous tasks. I can only offer a bit of uninvited, general advice to those who must bear this burden: Suicide is the cruelest of deaths. The feelings do not pass quickly. Nevertheless, family members should try hard to understand that the suicide was not their fault, and it does not reflect any prediction or prophecy for their own futures.

Your retainer more than covered the time expended in my review and preparation of this letter. The remainder will be returned, along with an itemized, paid statement and the records you forwarded, within the next week or so.

Sincerely,

R11

REPORT: MALPRACTICE, PLAINTIFF (COMPLEX)

NOTE: This report contradicts my usual preference for brevity, and may appear quite redundant. Many jurisdictions require that plaintiffs' reports in malpractice cases (particularly pre-suit and federal case reports) exhaustively address all elements of the tort of malpractice (duty, breach of duty, damage, and causation). Some state requirements are extremely specific. Failure to meet those requirements can cause a suit to be dismissed or never to be filed, regardless of its merits.

RE: Matter of B., deceased

Dear _____:

You have asked for a report which summarizes my preliminary findings after review of the materials you provided. I am able to supply the opinions and comments below, based upon those materials and my training, background, and experience. The methods used are those routinely relied upon by forensic psychiatrists in matters such as this. It should be noted that I have never examined Ms. B. and have not spoken with any of the parties to this matter. Should additional information become available which changes or adds to the opinions below, I will communicate with you promptly.

FINDINGS AND OPINIONS
The following opinions are offered to a reasonable degree of medical and psychiatric certainty (that is, more likely than not), given the information available to me at this time.

Standard of Care

* The applicable standard of care ("the standard") requires, among other things, that a hospital and/or independent health-care professional who accepts the care of a patient such as Ms. B. on (*date*) offer such assessment, diagnosis, care, monitoring, supervision, protection, and

181

follow-up planning as meets the patient's reasonable needs for care and safety, insofar as feasible and those needs are known or reasonably able to be known under the circumstances. The standard requires that, if the hospital cannot meet those needs, reasonable effort be made to transfer the patient or otherwise to meet the standard. _____ Medical Center, _____ Hospital, and Dr. D., at various times relevant to this matter, accepted the care of Ms. B. and thus assumed the duties associated with that acceptance.

- Much, but not all, of the hospital's and clinician's duty under the standard is predicated on the formation of a clinician–patient or hospital–patient relationship. The records reviewed clearly establish such a relationship with the facilities discussed below, and with Dr. D.
- Other duties owed patients such as Ms. B. include, but are not limited to,

  (a) Adequate assessment, including, but not limited to, review of reasonably available historical information, obtaining information from reasonably available prior clinicians and treatment facilities, and specific, competent assessment of suicide risk. "Adequate assessment" is not limited to initial admission examinations; the standard requires continuing assessment as clinically indicated throughout hospitalization and, especially, when contemplating discharge. In general, more serious (or potentially serious) presenting conditions require more comprehensive assessment and more caution in discharge planning and discharge itself.

  (b) Adequate care, including type of care, competence in rendering care, physical setting for care and patient safety, resources devoted to care, and time allowed for care and reasonable alleviation of symptoms and of risk.

  If the hospital and/or clinician knows, or reasonably should know, that the patient requires care that it cannot provide, that fact should at least be communicated to the patient and/or family along with recommendations for better care. In general, and especially in critical cases such as those involving a suicide attempt, the hospital and clinician are required reasonably to attempt to transfer the patient to an appropriate setting, or otherwise to provide an avenue for the patient to obtain that care.

  (c) Reasonable awareness by an admitting physician of the limitations of the facility to which he/she admits patients. The standard also requires that an attending clinician reasonably recognize when his patient is not able to get necessary care in the current facility. In either case, the standard requires the clinician to (1) provide information to the patient and/or family about getting the needed care, (2) recommend other care or care settings, and/or (3) assist with transfer or some other mechanism in order to get the necessary care.

(d) Adequate monitoring of condition and care after admission, such as monitoring and assessing treatment response and performing appropriate assessment (including assessment of change, stability, and suicide risk) prior to discharge.

(e) Adequate documentation of assessment and care, including relevant positive and negative findings, potentially relevant items not able to be assessed, participation in treatment activities, and the relevant content and results of interviews and treatment activities. This includes, but is not limited to, discussions about important clinical or disposition issues and justification for important treatment, management, or discharge decisions.

(f) Adequate opportunity for, assessment of, and documentation of treatment response, including allowing appropriate time and monitoring for medication effects to occur.

(g) Adequate consideration of clinical condition, patient stability, and risk prior to discharge.

(h) An adequate balance of patient autonomy and clinical assertiveness. The standard does not allow patients such as Ms. B. to substitute their own preferences for a hospital's or clinician's knowledge or duty of care without substantial evidence that the patient's preference meets the standard expected of the doctor and hospital. Although patient consent is required for most care, the standard requires that the clinician and hospital not allow the patient or spouse to dictate care when the patient's/spouse's wish is counter to what the clinician or hospital reasonably believes is necessary. For example, if a patient demands discharge, the hospital and attending clinician must (1) take reasonable steps to assess whether or not discharge is safe and clinically appropriate; (2) if not, make reasonable effort to encourage the patient to stay; (3) if the patient insists on leaving, carefully consider whether or not involuntary detention is indicated; and (4) if not, make it clear to the patient (and family, as appropriate) that the discharge is against medical advice.

(i) Adequate planning for follow-up care, including reasonable consideration of safety, clinical need, and the relative benefits and risks of different discharge plans.

Breaches of the Standard of Care

- Based on the information available to me, it was virtually *per se* negligent for Dr. D. to discharge Ms. B. voluntarily to a setting with little or no professional supervision or attention after less than 48 hours in the hospital. Many of the comments below about breach of the standard address whether or not there was, or reasonably might have been, some acceptable reason for his ordering Ms. B.'s discharge under the then existing circumstances. In my opinion, there was none.

(a) Dr. D.'s, and perhaps other staff's, negligent failure reasonably to attempt to get potentially important clinical information from prior treaters, particularly considering the fact that Dr. D. had never seen the patient prior to her admission, yet knew that other, local clinicians had been treating her (see Dr. D.'s deposition, pp. 51–55, 77).

Initial assessment by Dr. D. and others clearly established that Ms. B. had substantial need for competent inpatient assessment, treatment, and protection from the suicidal impulses associated with her severe (but treatable) mental illness. Her diagnosis was known, and known to be associated with substantial risk of deterioration and harm to herself. Her very recent suicide attempt was established as a serious effort to take her own life; a continuing wish to die was recognized; and her overall functioning was gauged on admission as extremely poor (e.g., a global assessment of functioning [GAF] of 10, among the lowest seen in psychiatric practice), including a serious suicidal act in which she both expected to die and was disappointed that she did not die. Nevertheless, and knowing that the patient had been treated during the recent past by other clinicians, Dr. D. failed to contact, or to try to contact, any of them for information about his patient's history, recent condition, treatment efforts and responses, concerns about her safety, and the like.

(b) Dr. D.'s and other Hospital staff's negligent failure to perform an adequate suicide risk assessment when contemplating discharge, and discharging the patient without a current, adequate suicide risk assessment, particularly considering the fact that Dr. D. had never seen the patient prior to her admission, had no information from her other clinicians about her past history, and chose not to obtain any consultation from a colleague before deciding to discharge her. There is no evidence in the record of a comprehensive suicide risk assessment on the day of discharge, or on the afternoon before, or of any consultation with the treatment team or professional colleagues (see Dr. D.'s deposition, p. 77). Although there were some comments from the patient that she felt better, there is no indication that most of the significant suicide risk factors had changed since her admission, that her statements were reasonably weighed for reliability, or that she could reasonably be protected from those that had not changed after she was discharged.

(c) <u>Dr. D.'s negligently failing to recognize the seriousness of Ms. B.'s condition, the substantial risks (including suicide risk) associated with it, and the need for more than very short-term, superficial care.</u> To the extent that Dr. D. actually believed that his patient was <u>not</u> ill enough to require inpatient care after less that 48 hours, or that her suicide risk was <u>not</u> still substantial less than 48 hours after her potentially lethal suicide attempt and her statement that she was sorry she hadn't died, his belief connotes a negligent error in clinical judgment. There is nothing in Dr. D.'s notes to suggest that the patient's underlying condition had changed prior to discharge, and nothing to suggest that she was protected against a rapid recurrence of her serious suicide attempt.

The only narrative nursing notes in the inpatient record which describe the patient's appearance and behavior, written the afternoon before Ms. B.'s discharge, state that, although she is planning for discharge the next morning, she "verbalizes little insight," "displays very poor self-esteem," "maintains [a] superficial demeanor," and is "reclusive," staying in her room much of the time. She was offered a few supportive group activities during the one full day she spent in the Hospital; she declined all but one, apparently a bingo game.

Dr. D.'s discharge summary states that Ms. B.'s mental status upon discharge had improved over that found on admission; however, his statement that her thought content was "free of lethality" cannot be verified, and rests solely on the patient's own statements (see Dr. D.'s deposition, pp. 89–91, and see below for comments about the unreliability of patient statements). Similarly, to the extent that she told him that she "contracts for safety and identifies a safety plan," such utterances or promises are not considered reliable by reasonably trained and experienced psychiatrists,[1] nor does the inference that she seemed "future oriented" or was "taking detailed notes" suggest, in itself, substantial decrease in risk. Dr. D. states in the discharge summary that her insight and judgment are intact, but does not indicate any foundation for that comment (especially given the ominous events of two days before and the nurse's note just a few hours before discharge). There is (1) no suggestion of change in Ms. B.'s risk factors (or reliable change in the <u>effect</u> of those which cannot change, such as her history of suicide attempt) and (2) no statement that reliably indicates that any

---

1 There is a substantial professional literature which strongly recommends against relying on patient promises or "contracts." References can be provided upon request.

improvement in mental status was reasonably expected to be stable over the coming days or weeks.

Dr. D.'s impression that the patient's husband's receiving a large salary bonus substantially (and *per se*) lowered her suicide risk (deposition p. 61) is very likely wrong, negligent, and would not be made by other reasonably trained and experienced psychiatrists.

The assertion that Ms. B. improved from functioning in the very lowest range of the professionally accepted "Global Assessment of Functioning" (GAF) scale (estimated by Dr. D. on admission as "10" of a possible 100) to a moderately impaired level of "55" in less than 48 hours, and the further implied assumption that the improved level was stable and reliable, requires documentation which is lacking in the record, since such rapid improvement occurs rarely in patients such as Ms. B. Her illnesses, and most of their symptoms, would not reasonably be expected to dissipate and remain quiescent after only 48 hours of limited treatment.

(Note that, contrary to Dr. D.'s comments that GAF is irrelevant to assessment or care [deposition, p. 80], GAF is described in the professionally accepted diagnostic nomenclature as "the clinician's judgment of the individual's overall level of functioning. This information is useful in planning treatment and measuring its impact, and in predicting outcome."[2] It is considered "an integral part of the standard multiaxial psychiatric diagnostic system.")[3]

(d) To the extent that they did so, Dr. D.'s and the Hospital's apparent negligent emphasis on the patient's perceived privacy concerns, business status, and work schedule when planning or carrying out clinical treatment and patient management. Although Dr. D. stated that Ms. B.'s concerns about privacy did not affect his discharge decision (deposition, p. 99), there is indication in both the hospital record and elsewhere in his deposition that her job status interfered with her being treated as a routine patient. If so, and assuming that interference was one of the reasons she received overly brief and superficial care, voluntarily allowing such interference was below the applicable standard of care.

2 American Psychiatric Association (2000) *The Diagnostic and Statistical Manual of Mental Disorders*, 4th Edition, Text Revision. Washington, DC: American Psychiatric Association, pp. 32-35.

3 Moos, R. H., et al. (2002) Global assessment of functioning ratings and the allocation and outcomes of mental health services, *Psychiatric Services* 53(6): 730-737.

Dr. D. states that the patient was given a pseudonym ("Ms. _____"). He used her statements that her career might suffer as reason not to pursue further hospitalization or intensive outpatient monitoring and treatment. Some of Dr. D.'s office records are apparently redacted to disguise her identity (cf. p. _____, apparently completed at Dr. D.'s office by the patient herself).

Dr. D. states in his deposition (e.g., pp. 98, 104) that he was influenced by the patient's statement that certain kinds of care would interfere with her work. Although it is reasonable to consider patients' wishes and preferences when planning or recommending care, Dr. D.'s contemporaneous documentation in the medical record indicates that he either did not know the appropriate care for his patient or inappropriately allowed extraneous factors to influence his choice of care. Note that I am not implying here that he should have "forced" certain specific modes of treatment, but rather that there is no indication in the Hospital record that he ever recommended them, or even considered them. He states at deposition that he had offered therapy appointments, other counselors, and partial hospitalization, but that she declined (deposition, p. 104). He states that he suggested, and told her she "ought" to attend, partial hospitalization, etc. (pp. 105–106), but there is no documentation of either discussion in the medical record. The question of whether or not Dr. D. should have considered involuntary treatment is discussed separately below.

(e) <u>Dr. D.'s negligently failing to consider and reasonably seek important avenues of treatment for the patient's severe condition.</u> To the extent that Dr. D. recognized the seriousness of Ms. B.'s illness and the substantial risk associated with her condition, and to the extent that his deposition statements about the lack of available treatment at _____ are accurate, the record indicates that he did nothing to pursue getting necessary outside care for Ms. B. If, for example, he knew or believed that _____ Hospital was merely a very short-term facility that provides only superficial care (see his deposition, pp. 65, 83, 115), then he was obligated to try to find and recommend a more appropriate facility (just as cardiologists or oncologists routinely guide severely ill heart or cancer patients to treatment centers that offer specialty care). There is no indication in the record that Dr. D. did so, or that he even considered such action.

Similarly, when Ms. B. requested discharge the day after her suicide attempt, the standard of care required that he strongly encourage her to stay or to be transferred to a safe and therapeutic setting. The record indicates that he did not. When the patient further requested discharge, he should have strongly considered pursuing involuntary hospitalization. There is no indication of such consideration in the record. (Such discussions and considerations are routinely carefully documented by psychiatrists, since they are important clinical events and have obvious implications for safety, future care, and risk management.)[4]

Hospitals have a routine procedure for discharge "against medical advice," but Dr. D. does not allege that he discharged Ms. B. against medical advice. His deposition statement that some of his actions were designed to foster a therapeutic alliance with her is worth considering, and the <u>principle</u> is valid, but in this instance acute care and safety for Ms. B. were more important. Reasonable physicians must not allow the "doctor–patient relationship" to be used to extort bad care from the doctor.

(f) <u>Dr. D.'s negligently allowing his severely ill patient to be hospitalized in a setting which he knew to be unlikely to be able to provide the necessary treatment opportunities</u>. To the extent that _____ Hospital was an inappropriate hospital for Ms. B., and that Dr. D. knew that it was merely a very short-term facility that provides only superficial care (as he indicates in his deposition, pp. 76, 86, 124, 125), he should have carefully considered hospitalizing her elsewhere. Dr. D. stated in his deposition that he did not have admitting privileges at other hospitals in the area. Assuming that was the case, he could, for example, easily have attempted to find a colleague in a different facility who could take over the patient's care. <u>The standard does not allow limitations of Dr. D.'s hospital privileges to force his patient to receive care at an inappropriate facility</u>.

(g) <u>The Hospital's negligently accepting a patient for whom it knew, or should have known, adequate care was likely to be beyond its usual treatment procedures</u>. To the extent that _____ Hospital does not offer adequate care for patients such as Ms. B. (as Dr. D. indicates in his deposition), it appears that the Hospital represented itself to the patient (and perhaps to Dr. D.) as able to provide adequate and competent care when it knew it would not. For example, if the Hospital's policy, expectation, or routine was to keep patients for only 48 hours, then the Standard requires that it either not knowingly accept patients such as Ms. B. or be able to provide some reasonable avenue to further necessary care. Similarly, if it is Hospital policy not to offer meaningful

4 Motto, J. A. (1999) Critical points in the assessment and management of suicide risk, in D. G. Jacobs (ed.), *The Harvard Medical School Guide to Suicide Assessment and Intervention*. San Francisco: Jossey-Bass, p. 232.

psychotherapy or counseling, then it should not knowingly accept patients such as Ms. B. unless arrangements can be made to provide commonly recommended care.

(h) Dr. D.'s negligently assuming that less than 48 hours of weekend hospitalization at _____ Hospital produced so much improvement in Ms. B. that she had moved from a very high risk category to a low one, and that any such improvement was stable. Neither the record nor Dr. D.'s deposition provides any indication that Ms. B.'s serious mental illnesses had improved, or that her symptoms had substantially abated, or that any such improvements could reasonably be expected to be stable. Dr. D. is correct when he says (in deposition) that suicide is generally unpredictable, but, as reasonably trained and experienced psychiatrists know, that is exactly why it is important to be very cautious with risk assessment and clinical risk management. He agrees that Ms. B. had a great many significant risk factors for suicide, some of which act synergistically to increase risk even further, but he appears not to have considered the additional, substantial risk factor of unstable or unpredictable psychiatric symptoms.

Given a patient who is being treated for depression and anxiety by other clinicians who then becomes extremely symptomatic and almost dies by her own hand, a mere two days of weekend hospitalization is far too little to establish whether or not her acute symptoms have improved and stabilized and so to be able reasonably to assume that she will be safe if discharged. In discharging Ms. B., Dr. D., relying in part on the Hospital's assessment and treatment team, failed to note substantial and foreseeable risk and "predicted" that she would be safe outside a hospital and make acceptable clinical progress. Dr. D. acted on that "prediction" and ordered the patient's discharge in the face of a great deal of known, or indicated, substantial risk. He had almost no information about her likely response to the new medications, about whether or not her condition (if truly improved) was likely to be stable outside a hospital, or about whether or not she was still harboring thoughts of suicide.

(i) Dr. D.'s negligently relying on the patient as the primary source of information about suicide risk. Reasonably trained and experienced psychiatrists know, or should know, that patients are very often unreliable when describing their suicide risk. For example, (1) many patients who have recently attempted suicide still want to kill themselves and thus refrain from telling their doctors because they would be stopped. (2) Many suicidal patients refrain from telling their doctors about continuing suicidal thoughts or plans because they want the option of considering suicide outside a supervised setting. (3) Suicidal thoughts and impulses are often unstable; although a patient may not want to kill himself at the moment (e.g., while in the hospital), he or she may foreseeably become suicidal again after returning to the environment in which the prior plan or attempt occurred. (4) Patients often do not understand their own illnesses, the waxing and waning of their symptoms, and whether or when the symptoms will return. It is the clinician, not the patient, who must try to assess the risk, based on knowable factors. Patients who attempt suicide may be intelligent and articulate, but their insight about suicide risk is very often limited, and they may not cooperate with clinicians' efforts to help them.[5] (5) Even when patients can (or are willing to) provide good information, clinicians may do incomplete interviews or ask about suicidality in ways the patient doesn't understand.

When potentially important collateral information is available from family, past clinicians, or other sources, the Standard requires reasonable effort to obtain it. The Standard further requires that, when there is reason to be concerned but collateral information is not readily available, the clinician should exercise caution in an effort to protect the patient while the risk is further assessed by other means and/or treatment is carried out which is reasonably expected to reduce the risk.

When asked in his deposition about patients' lying about, or misunderstanding, queries about their suicidal thoughts (pp. 126–129), Dr. D. says he has never seen any professional literature about suicidal patients' not telling the truth. In fact, reasonably trained and experienced psychiatrists know that the topics of not relying on the patient alone and seeking collateral information to assess risk are stressed in psychiatry training programs and very common in the general psychiatry literature.[6, 7]

(j) The Hospital's negligently failing to provide therapeutic activities during Ms. B.'s inpatient stay. There is no indication in the record that the Hospital provided significant counseling or

---

5 See case examples in Motto, J. A. (1999) Critical points in the assessment and management of suicide risk, in D. G. Jacobs (ed.), *The Harvard Medical School Guide to Suicide Assessment and Intervention.* San Francisco: Jossey-Bass, pp. 232-233.

6 American Psychiatric Association (2003) *APA Practice Guideline for the Assessment and Treatment of Patients with Suicidal Behaviors*, pp. 4, 5, 28 (also published as a special supplement to the *American Journal of Psychiatry*, 2003).

7 Jacobs, D. G., *et al.* (1999) Suicide assessment: an overview and recommended protocol, in D. G. Jacobs (ed.), *The Harvard Medical School Guide to Suicide Assessment and Intervention.* San Francisco: Jossey-Bass, p. 22 (see also p. 27, which defines "severe risk" of suicide as "behavior with suicidal intent and moderate to high lethality").

psychotherapy. It is reasonable to assume that much of the first day or two of hospitalization may be consumed with assessment; however, Dr. D. states in his deposition that _____ Hospital had little to offer a patient such as Ms. B.; it appeared in some ways to be merely a domicile for her.

(k) There is no indication that Dr. D. or other Hospital staff or consultants attempted to assess Ms. B.'s response to the treatment offered (essentially medication alone) prior to her discharge to a virtually unmonitored, unsupervised setting. The extraordinarily short length of her hospital stay made it impossible to assess accurately whether or not the antidepressant medication prescribed was likely to be effective. Dr. D. knew, or should have known, that medications such as _____ are often ineffective for patients such as Ms. B., and, when they are effective, require up to several weeks to assess treatment response. Further, it is difficult to assure that they will be taken as directed after discharge (see his deposition, p. 107). It is unreasonable for him to state that he had time to evaluate whether or not her medications were working by the time she was discharged (p. 148), except to the extent that the _____ (an anti-anxiety drug) has a rapid effect and that some potential side effects of the antidepressant _____ might have been observed at the early date and low dose before she was discharged. The _____ was given only in small doses while she was in the Hospital; the increase to a hoped-for therapeutic dose was to occur after discharge.

Dr. D. correctly notes that _____ has a rapid anti-anxiety effect; however, there was no time, and apparently no effort, to determine whether or not the patient's significant anxiety symptoms were reliably controlled or that any improvement was likely to continue after discharge. Medications such as _____ are symptomatically and temporarily effective; they do not address underlying causes of anxiety.

(l) Dr. D. and the Hospital treatment team negligently failed to establish that any improvement the patient may have shown would be stable after discharge to her previous environment, a setting in which she would be virtually unmonitored and unsupervised and not see any clinician for over two weeks (Dr. D.'s deposition, p. 123). Dr. D. and the Hospital staff failed to consider that much of the patient's appearance was likely to be related to temporary, superficial factors such as brief respite and getting a good night's sleep. They negligently and erroneously assumed that, just because she may have looked better in some ways, the underlying factors in her illness, particularly her suicide risk, were also better; that any improvement was stable and reliable improvement; and that her risk of deterioration and/or harming herself was low. To act as they did based on those assumptions was negligent and below the standard of care.

(m) <u>Dr. D.'s negligently failing to monitor Ms. B. appropriately while waiting for treatment to take effect and/or ascertaining that the treatment was *not* effective.</u> There was no reliable indication that Ms. B.'s illnesses, or her risk of suicide, had changed significantly at the time of her discharge, or that any reliable mechanism for monitoring treatment effectiveness, patient condition, or suicide risk factors was in place upon discharge. No professional monitoring or supervision was arranged or anticipated. Even the patient's husband, who cannot appropriately be given the responsibilities of a trained, experienced mental health professional, could not be with her continuously. Given her very serious symptoms and life-threatening behavior, most or all of that monitoring should have been in a controlled setting.

(n) <u>There is no indication in the available record that Dr. D. took reasonable steps to assess whether or not discharge was clinically appropriate on (date), that he made sufficient and reasonable effort to encourage Ms. B. to stay or to secure other appropriately safe and competent care, that he carefully considered whether or not involuntary hospitalization was indicated, or that he made it clear to the patient and her husband that the discharge was against medical advice.</u> Dr. D. stated at deposition that he did not press the patient to stay because he wanted to preserve the doctor–patient relationship (p. 182), even though he did not plan to see her until over two weeks later. There is no documentation of appropriate clinical deliberation in the record; the record thus indicates a failure either to recognize, or firmly to encourage, necessary care and monitoring.

Damages

- Ms. B. committed suicide by hanging herself on (*date*), just after discharge from inpatient care.
- There was very likely pain and suffering associated with the immediate cause of her death.
- She suffered very substantial depression and anxiety between her hospitalization and her death. Some of those symptoms would, more likely than not, have been alleviated had she received adequate assessment and treatment during her hospitalization and had she received additional, competent care (such as extended hospitalization).
- Although I have not examined her child, _____, or reviewed any records regarding her, it is reasonable to assume that she experienced great trauma upon discovering Ms. B.'s body, and that the ongoing sequelae of that trauma, and of her mother's suicide, are substantial.

- Although I have not examined her husband, or reviewed any records regarding him, it is reasonable to assume that he has been substantially damaged by the loss of his wife, and by the fact that her death was a suicide, and that those damages will continue for an extended period.

Causation

The instances of negligence described above were substantial causes of the damages described above. Without listing each and every point to be made:

- The brevity of Ms. B.'s hospital stay prevented more complete assessment of her condition and risk, limited necessary treatment, and curtailed necessary assessment of treatment response. Had those things occurred and been within the standard of care, it is more likely than not that Ms. B.'s risk of suicide would have been substantially decreased and she would not have killed herself on (*date*).
- Dr. D.'s inadequate assessment of and/or appreciation of Ms. B.'s suicide risk and risk of clinical deterioration (associated with, among other things, suicide risk) negatively affected his care, treatment, protection, and guidance of his patient and (at times) her husband. Had his assessment been adequate and his appreciation of her situation been reasonably accurate, it is likely that he would have made a much greater effort to decrease that risk (e.g., by pressing for a longer hospital stay and other treatments and protections to reduce her risk). Given the foregoing, it is more likely than not that her risk of suicide would have been substantially decreased and she would not have killed herself on (*date*).
- In the alternative, and assuming Dr. D. did appreciate the great seriousness of the situation and the risks associated with the various breaches of the Standard already described, his negligent failure to address the factors already mentioned caused a lack of otherwise reasonably attainable care and protection. Had she received some reasonable combination of that care and protection (that is, had her care risen to the applicable standard), it is more likely than not that she would not have committed suicide on (*date*).
- To the extent that Dr. D. is correct in his description of the Hospital as a place in which patients such as Ms. B. cannot expect necessary care, treatment, and protection even though the Hospital accepted her for care, and to the extent that such a factor was important in his discharge decision and recommendations to the patient, the lack of availability of adequate care in the Hospital contributed substantially to Ms. B.'s risk. It is more likely than not that the Hospital's not meeting the standard of care in this way (described by Dr. D.), and Dr. D.'s decision not to make reasonable attempts to move his patient to a

place of adequate care, <u>and</u> the lack of communication to the patient and her husband about those limitations contributed substantially to the inadequacy of Ms. B.'s care and to increasing substantially her risk of suicide.

- The precipitousness of discharge and lack of close monitoring and follow-up contributed substantially to Ms. B.'s suicide risk, and thus to her suicide on (*date*). Less than 48 hours after her near lethal suicide attempt on (*date*), she was sent from 24-hour monitoring by mental health professionals in a clinical environment directly to a dangerous environment with <u>no</u> professional monitoring (cf. Dr. D.'s deposition statement, p. 104; <u>it simply cannot be stated that her home was, in his words, a "safe place to go"</u>). It is more likely than not that the lack of adequate monitoring and reasonable protections for a longer time, while assessing possible treatment response and assisting with important psychological issues, contributed substantially to her risk of suicide and to her death on (*date*).

SOURCES RELIED UPON

- Written materials, represented as everything relevant and available from your office:
  (*list*)
- Limited review of professional literature regarding suicide assessment, risk, "global assessment of functioning" (GAF), and other topics.
- My background, training, and experience in medicine, psychiatry, mental health care administration, and forensic psychiatry.

QUALIFICATIONS

. . .

R 1 2

REPORT: MALPRACTICE,
DEFENSE (COMPLEX, FACILITY)

NOTE: This report is on behalf of the government and a government facility, not the physician defendant per se. In this case, the facility wanted to distance itself from the behavior of its staff clinician.

RE: **PRELIMINARY REPORT:** *B.B.* v. *A.A., M.D., and the United States of America* (Case no. _____)

You have asked for a report which summarizes my findings after review of the materials you provided. I am able to supply the opinions and comments below, based upon those materials and my training, background, and experience. The methods used and materials reviewed are those routinely relied upon by forensic psychiatrists in matters such as this. Any additional information received in the future may or may not suggest additions or changes to the opinions below.

FINDINGS AND OPINIONS
The following opinions are offered to a reasonable degree of medical or psychiatric certainty, as I understand the meaning of that phrase, given the information available to me at this time.

1. It is not *per se* below the standard of care for a psychiatrist to examine his or her patient physically. Psychiatrists are fully trained medical doctors. Physical examination by a psychiatrist is within the standard of care when clinically indicated and appropriately performed. Partial examination, for example of parts of the body related to suspected medication side effects, is common in psychiatric practice. Complete physical examination is unusual in most U.S. psychiatric settings, but acceptable (and may be routine) in some others.
2. There is no indication in the available record that the Veterans Administration in any way authorized Dr. A. to perform physical examinations for other than legitimate purposes and using legitimate clinical procedures, or that it encouraged or condoned the

inappropriate behaviors attributed to Dr. A. Similarly, there is no indication whatever that the sexual behaviors alleged of Dr. A. should be considered in any way a part of his employment or of his specific or discretionary duties.

3. The standard of care regarding organization supervision of employee physicians generally does not require close supervision of licensed physicians once they have been properly credentialed and privileged. Most psychiatric and general medical care is necessarily provided in private. It is unreasonable to compromise the need for patient privacy in the conduct of medical and mental health care without adequate cause.

4. Item (_____) of _____'s memorandum should not be construed as creating, or necessarily reflecting, either VA policy and procedure or some "standard of care."

   That portion of _____'s memorandum refers to one of many items discussed at a general meeting. It notes that the "allegation regarding MHC staff" was not discussed. The memo (a) does not create VA policy regarding chaperones during physical examinations, (b) does not necessarily refer to any existing VA policy, (c) refers to "complete" physical examinations, (d) is apparently not intended to imply final or definitive action (cf. "will work with ... to clarify"), and (e) does not create, or necessarily reflect, a "standard of care" for psychiatrists.

   I have not been supplied with, nor am I aware of, any official VA policy or procedure regarding chaperone requirements for physical examinations of male patients by male physicians which existed prior to the events alleged by Mr. B.

5. Although I do not necessarily believe that all facts described by Mr. B. are accurate, the following comments about damage assume for the sake of argument that the alleged events occurred substantially as he described them in his various statements (including his _____ written statement to the VA OIG and his criminal trial testimony).

   (a) The record indicates that any mental damage caused to Mr. B. is likely to be slight and time limited. There is no indication of any disability or significant symptoms that can reliably be attributed to actions by Dr. A. or the Veterans Administration. There is no reliable indication that his pre-existing and previously compensated service-connected disability has been significantly worsened by the alleged experience with Dr. A. All available records suggest that Mr. B. functioned at least reasonably well during and after the period in which the alleged events were occurring. See, e.g., Dr. _____'s (*date*) note which describes him as "doing well," with a "Global

Assessment of Functioning" of 70 (defined by the American Psychiatric Association DSM-IV-TR as "some mild symptoms . . . but generally functioning pretty well").

It should be noted that I have not had an opportunity to interview Mr. B. These opinions and comments are based on the available record, including Mr. B.'s testimony and other statements.

(b) **Neither the contemporaneous medical record nor the post-complaint record available to me contains any suggestion of significant damage from any alleged behavior of Dr. A. or the VA.** There are brief allusions to anger, but even these appear related largely to how "he only learned about (Dr. A.'s charges) from the newspaper." Mr. B.'s psychological condition appears to have remained essentially constant at the level described before the alleged events.

(c) Mr. B. filed for an increase in his service-connected disability on _____. At that time, he had a longstanding disability rating related to general medical problems. A 10% depression disability rating was awarded, effective _____, based on his military service and predicated on "mild or transient symptoms" and the fact that he was receiving medication (AAA 5723). Mr. B.'s stated reason for requesting the rating was post-traumatic stress disorder associated with military service (see, e.g., _____, AAA 5884). There is no indication that this 10% disability award was related to damages from any action of Dr. A. or the VA.

(d) There is no indication that Mr. B. has sought evaluation or treatment outside the VA for psychiatric symptoms, or that he has received any form of counseling or therapy for any condition that might reasonably be related to the events alleged.

(e) There is no indication in the record, either prior to the _____ Report of Contact or anytime thereafter, that Mr. B. was, or is, reluctant to use the _____ VA clinic services (either psychiatric or general medical). Indeed, he has made frequent visits for general medical services and kept most or all psychiatric appointments throughout this period.

(f) Again assuming for the sake of these comments that the events occurred essentially as alleged, it should be pointed out that **certain characteristics of such events are associated with fairly good emotional outcome in victims generally.**

   (i) Mr. B. was a competent adult at all times relevant to these events, with considerable life experience, access to help and support, the ability to respond and defend himself against this kind of behavior and, in all likelihood (based in part on his own statements), knowledge that Dr. A.'s behavior was inappropriate (in contrast to naive, psychotic, or incompetent persons or children who lack such experience and opportunity, which would be associated with greater damage).

(ii)   Mr. B.'s experiences with Dr. A. were very occasional and sporadic, a few events of allegedly inappropriate conduct of physical examinations and one reference to possible anal penetration over about three years. This should be contrasted with situations of frequent and chronic abuse, which are associated with greater damage.

(iii) Mr. B. described Dr. A.'s behavior as nonviolent and relatively non-aggressive (in contrast to violent, aggressive, or physically intimidating behaviors, which are associated with greater damage).

(iv)   Mr. B.'s complaints were taken seriously by the VA (see, e.g., the Report of Contact by Mr. _____ and the _____ note by Dr. _____) and by law enforcement (in contrast to victims who experience disbelief or lack of support from others, which is associated with greater damage).

(v)   Mr. B. came to know that other patients had described similar experiences and were involved in the investigations and criminal charges (in contrast to victims who feel alone in their experience, which is associated with greater damage).

(vi)   Major parts of the case were resolved with Dr. A.'s conviction (in contrast to victims who perceive that their perpetrators receive no consequences for their transgressions, which is associated with greater damage).

(vii) Once he voiced his complaint, Mr. B. had rapid access to administrative and psychological support. In addition, he had—and used—ready access to mental health clinicians other than Dr. A. at the VA clinic both before and after he voiced his complaint (e.g., Dr. _____, Mr. _____). This is in contrast to patients/victims whose support and treatment is delayed, which is associated with greater damage.

(g) With regard to **prior or intervening conditions which may affect his current condition**, Mr. B. has experienced many large and small traumas and crises over the period before, during, and after Dr. A.'s alleged actions. It is reasonable to assume that many factors other than Dr. A.'s behavior contribute to any mental symptoms he may currently describe. For example, his father died (*date*) (AAA 7286). At his (*date*) session with Dr. _____, he expressed loss about that as well as concern that he might be treated unfairly regarding his inheritance. By (*date*), he continued to be depressed about his father's death. On (*date*), he was described as "in remission," with no new psychological issues since his last visit. (See related comments below.)

One must also consider the likelihood that the lawsuit itself increases Mr. B.'s attention to lawsuit-related thoughts and symptoms.

(h) **With regard to Mr. B.'s ability to recognize and respond to Dr. A.'s alleged behaviors, and his emotional condition during and soon after the events,** the record contains no reliable suggestion that he was substantially damaged or impaired. I found no indication in the record that he would have been constrained by either the VA or some psychological condition from complaining about or questioning Dr. A.'s care when he first experienced discomfort with it. The record suggests that Mr. B. has been assertive with other doctors (including psychiatrists) in appealing his VA compensation, asking for changes in care or medications, etc. In addition, Mr. B. has been examined by many physicians, including psychiatrists, over several decades. It is reasonable to assume that he is familiar with the general process and expectations.

Dr. _____'s comments that Mr. B. had "certain specific vulnerabilities" in seeing a physician appear to be greatly overstated (see his [*date*] plaintiff's expert report). The pre-existing "long-standing post-traumatic stress disorder" Dr. _____ mentions has never been sufficient to impair Mr. B.'s function by more than 10% (and generally has been seen as non-disabling); it is unrelated to the topic of the current alleged trauma. There is no indication in the record that it is relevant to any damages stemming from Dr. A.'s alleged behavior. His "stressful parental divorce at age 10" is an unfortunate but very common experience which is not implicated in the record, or shown to any reasonable degree of medical certainty to be related, specifically or otherwise, to any notable vulnerability in Mr. B., much less to any damage from the alleged behavior of Dr. A. Similarly, citing his relatively mild general medical problems as associated with increased vulnerability in the matter at hand is irrelevant, in my opinion. Indeed, **the record suggests that the various "vulnerabilities" mentioned by Dr. _____ are more appropriately seen as intervening sources of symptoms, rebutting or diluting allegations that any current symptoms are a result of Dr. A.'s alleged behavior.**

(i)   Finally, the record does not support Dr. _____'s contention that Mr. B. was constrained from reporting earlier by Dr. A.'s alleged position of authority, or by some implied ability of the VA clinic to affect his disability status or have him hospitalized (see Dr. _____'s [*date*] report). There is no indication in the record that Mr. B. did not fully understand that both he and Dr. A. were civilians and that Dr. A. was merely a staff physician like all the others he had seen over the years. Although it is true that physicians generally have an authoritative position in doctor–patient relationships, it is a mistake to construe that role as overwhelming or greatly controlling the behavior of adult, competent males in situations such as this. Further, it is likely (and at least uncontradicted in the record) that Mr. B. was quite familiar with VA disability procedures, understood that his disability determination was permanent, and had every opportunity to be aware of posted notices and rules encouraging patients to report suspected abuses by VA staff.

SOURCES RELIED UPON

- Written materials as follows, represented to me as all available from your office:
  (*list*)
- My background, training, and experience in medicine, psychology, psychiatry, and forensic psychiatry, and health-care administration

QUALIFICATIONS
. . .

CASES IN WHICH I HAVE TESTIFIED DURING THE PAST FOUR YEARS
. . .

R13

REPORT: MALPRACTICE, DEFENSE (FACILITY), FORENSIC PRACTICE STANDARDS

RE: Preliminary Report: *A.B.* v. *C. Medical Center (dba D. Hospital)*
No. CV ____; ____ Judicial District, County of ____, ____

You have asked for a report which summarizes my preliminary findings with regard to the above matter, with particular reference to (1) C. Medical Center's (C.'s) hiring, credentialing, and supervision practices and responsibilities; (2) Dr. E.'s expert report on behalf of the plaintiff; (3) the presence or absence of voluntariness or responsibility associated with Ms. B. with respect to her relationship with Dr. F.; and (4) the issue of possible damages to Ms. B. as a result of Dr. F's and/or C's actions. I am able to supply the opinions and comments below, based upon the materials you have provided and my training, background, and experience. The methods used to arrive at the opinions are those routinely relied upon by forensic psychiatrists in matters such as this. It should be noted that I have not examined the plaintiff, A.B. Should additional information become available which changes or adds to the opinions below, I will communicate with you promptly.

FINDINGS AND OPINIONS
The following opinions are offered to a reasonable degree of medical certainty, as I understand the meaning of that phrase, given the information available to me at this time.

1. C.'s hiring and credentialing practices regarding Dr. F. easily met the applicable standard of care. Further, there was absolutely no requirement that C. individually monitor Dr. F.'s patient interactions, either as part of a routine for all new physicians or as a special procedure for him in particular.

   The C. application, investigation, and hiring procedures described in the records available to me reflect common procedures that are widely accepted in other, similar health-care facilities and are quite consistent with the accreditation requirements of the Joint Commission on Accreditation of Healthcare Organizations (JCAHO), by which C. was accredited at all times relevant to the events in question. Further, the record indicates that those procedures were carried out to an extent well within the applicable standard of care (e.g., verification of credentials, checking pertinent references, background searches, and other measures).

The results of those procedures and searches indicated, to any reasonable observer, that Dr. F. had successfully completed a respected and fully accredited U.S. university residency program in psychiatry, was well qualified for independent patient care, and was highly recommended by senior clinicians and supervisors who had personally observed his work and training over the past two years.

Contrary to the plaintiff's allegations, Dr. F. was reasonably known to C. as a very well-trained, fairly experienced psychiatrist. In addition to his early medical training in _____, he had several years of psychiatric experience in (*country*), some of which was apparently in a supervised training setting and some with independent responsibility for patients and hospital units. After finishing his accredited registrar experience there (equivalent to residency training in the U.S.) and qualifying for membership in the Royal College of Psychiatrists, he completed an <u>additional</u> period of U.S. residency training at _____ University, apparently as part of U.S. license and certification requirements. In short, Dr. F. had far more psychiatric training than most U.S. medical school graduates when he started work at C., including a great deal of both supervised and independent clinical experience.

Nothing in the records I have reviewed suggests that C. had any reason to doubt Dr. F.'s abilities, clinical performance, or ethics in patient care during the times before and during his apparent exploitation of Ms. B. Separate from his eventual reprehensible behavior with this patient, Dr. F.'s written clinical workup of Ms. B. suggests a good evaluation, with clinical acumen and uncommonly complete documentation.

The one report in the record of inappropriate contact with a staff member (not with a patient), described as "harassment" by plaintiff's expert Dr. E., appears to be an example of C.'s prompt and firm response to discovering such behavior—a strong warning with the expectation that, if the behavior occurred, again he would be terminated—consistent with the hospital's policies and procedures, and in turn well within administrative standards. This incident with another staff member <u>did not</u> dictate any special monitoring requirement for Dr. F.'s patient care. I know of no facility within my experience which has restricted or more closely supervised the patient care of a physician based solely on such an event/complaint, nor have I heard of any instance of such an action.

Finally, the plaintiff's various comments (Second Amended Complaint) that C. should have specially monitored and/or supervised Dr. F. because he was a "young psychiatrist ... away from his wife and his home country," or that C. "did not do a complete background investigation ... of ... a foreign national who had recently immigrated to the United States," are so fraught with error and basic misunderstanding as to be virtually incredulous and sometimes completely frivolous. The adequacy of C.'s investigation and credentialing is described above. With regard to some of the other comments in the Complaint, no hospital credentialing standard, accreditation requirement, accepted professional or administrative practice, or scientific or social study, to my knowledge, suggests that any physician applicant with Dr. F.'s then known credentials requires *per se* special "supervision," "professional direction," or "guidance" (quotes from the Complaint) simply because he immigrated from _____ two or three years before, is away from his spouse, or is purportedly "young" (being in his late 30s when he applied for privileges at C., with many years of medical and psychiatric training and experience).

2. **Dr. E.'s (*date*) opinion letter contains a number of errors and misunderstandings of the applicable standards, and of C.'s duties and potential breaches under those standards. Dr. E. also misunderstands and/or misrepresents any applicability of my writings to this lawsuit.**

Without attempting to be exhaustive in my criticism of Dr. E.'s opinions, or to attack him in *ad hominem* fashion, it is important to point out, for example, that Dr. E.'s opinions regarding a duty owed of "carefully monitor[ing] and supervis[ing] Dr. F.," etc., are not based in the reasonable and accepted practices of other, similar facilities, or in any accepted mental health administration references or other literature with which I am familiar. His allegation that C. "failed to act on reasonable signs of abuse or clinician impairment" is without adequate foundation, based on the records I have reviewed (see above regarding the staff contact episode).

The presence or absence of specific C. policies for physicians regarding avoiding exploitation and sexual behavior with patients is irrelevant to Dr. F.'s actions, and irrelevant to any damage suffered by Ms. B. as a result of them. That is, the responsibility in this matter lies with Dr. F., not with facility policy. Although I have not seen the C. or D. Policy and Procedure Manual (nor does Dr. E. list it among the items he has reviewed), it is fair to say that (a) the presence or absence of any specific policy about sex with patients is completely irrelevant to whether or not Dr. F. knew his behavior was unethical and reprehensible; physicians, including psychiatrists, are fully aware of that fact. (b) Dr. F. was provided with written statements about C.'s expectations when hired (although even that is superfluous given his clear knowledge that his eventual actions were wrong). (c) There is every reason to expect that the mere existence of a policy against doctor–patient intimacy and exploitation, to the extent that none did exist in writing at C., would have no bearing on the behavior of the kind of person Dr. F. eventually proved to be.

I have not been supplied with C. staff training logs or curricula (and do not know whether or not Dr. E. reviewed them); however, there is no indication in the records I reviewed that Dr. F. exhibited any behaviors during the relevant period that would, or should, have raised concerns that he was exploiting a patient. (The staff contact episode, and C.'s handling of it, is addressed above.)

The (*date*) memorandum referred to by Dr. E. is not evidence of any failure on the part of C., nor does it suggest any breach of C.'s duty under the applicable standard, nor does it represent a causative link with any damage that may have been suffered by Ms. B. The date of the memo clearly indicates that it was not available to anyone, much less C. management, during the times relevant to Dr. F.'s unethical behavior. Once the memo, its content, and its implications were discovered by C., C. took very rapid and definitive action to investigate, and then to stop, Dr. F.'s care of C. patients. The record indicates that he was terminated within two weeks. C. did exactly the right thing just as soon as its management knew, or reasonably should have known, that something was amiss.

Dr. E.'s statement that my publication "Organizational liability: Beyond *respondeat superior*" supports his opinions is erroneous. A part of that article refers to psychiatrist sex with patients (p. 260); however, the portions to which Dr. E. alludes refer to "potential areas of vulnerability" involving negligent credentialing, incomplete references, inadequate supervision or monitoring (when supervision or monitoring is reasonably known to be required—not the case for Dr. F. during the period in question), not acting on reasonable signs of abuse or relevant impairment (not applicable to this case), inadequate staff training when relevant (not applicable in this case), and inadequate policies and procedures when relevant (not applicable in this case). Of course, the article does not establish a standard of care, nor does anything in it imply a breach of duty on the part of C. (A copy of that article is appended to this report.)

With regard to Dr. E.'s allegations of damage to Ms. B., I do not have what he describes as a lengthy discussion of damages allegedly caused by "the acts and omissions of Dr. F. and the hospital," and so cannot comment on those statements at this time. I do not know what Dr. E. has reviewed, nor do I know whether or not he has examined Ms. B. (if he has not, then his letter lacks the ethically required disclaimer). My own discussion of damages follows below.

3. <u>Without meaning to diminish Dr. F.'s role and responsibility for his behavior</u>, it should be pointed out that the record indicates considerable voluntary participation on Ms. B.'s part—e.g., meeting him outside the office, paying for the motel room, inviting him into her home, deciding not to report him—regardless of any so-called power differential between doctor and patient.

Ms. B. had considerable experience with physicians and other clinicians, including psychiatrists, by (*date*). She had worked in clinical settings for years, had experienced unethical sexual behavior from a physician and contemplated reporting him (but did not), and had been seen in a number of mental health settings in which she was exposed to doctors, counselors, and other patients. Her statements to clinicians indicate that she was aware that she had been physically and sexually exploited in the past, and apparently was able to recognize the effects of that past exploitation.

According to her deposition, Ms. B. told at least five people about her intimate relationship with Dr. F. between the beginning of the sexual behavior in (*date*) and her sister's confrontation of him in (*date*) (her sister, her aunt, two friends, and another patient, to whom she did not give the doctor's real name). She concealed the unprofessional relationship from C. and its staff throughout that several-month period and complimented them on her care on the psychiatric unit. Although she often sought out others for support and attention, the record indicates that, during most of the eight months between (*dates*), she was quite capable of recognizing the inappropriateness of F.'s behavior, resisting his advances and her own sexual impulses, seeking another psychiatrist or psychotherapist, and/or reporting Dr. F., should she have chosen to do so.

4. Although I have not examined A.B., and an examination could possibly change or add to the following opinions, the record available to me strongly implies (a) that Ms. B.'s psychiatric condition in the months and years after the events in question has been no worse, or not substantially worse, than her condition before the events <u>and</u> (b) that any additional symptoms she may have suffered during the several years since the events in question are very likely to have been caused by, or at least greatly affected by, the many other stressful experiences she described both before and after her interactions with Dr. F.

The medical record indicates that Ms. B.'s clinical and social prognosis prior to seeing Dr. F. was guarded at best, and probably poor. The statements in some of the discharge summaries of her many psychiatric hospitalizations that her prognosis was "good" appear to misunderstand the patient's actual experience over those years. The rest of the pre-(date) record is quite consistent in its descriptions of her chronic "borderline" personality traits, frequent severe clinical deterioration which interfered with her day-to-day life and often required hospital care, frequent poor social and family functioning (often with inability to live alone), and symptoms so severe and/or unstable that she resorted to self-injury and suicide attempts on several occasions. Descriptions of her post-event functioning—including specific recordings of her "global assessment of functioning" (GAF)—do not suggest a worsening of her overall condition, or any worsening due to her relationship with Dr. F.

It is impossible reasonably to link the majority of Ms. B.'s post-event problems primarily to Dr. F.'s unethical behavior and their non-professional relationship. First, few (perhaps none) of her post-event symptoms appears clearly associated with either his behavior or the relationship. Although there has been mention of potential difficulty with her accepting other clinicians or forming a therapeutic relationship since the events, this appears to be overstated by the plaintiff. She has had good access to care, and has an ongoing relationship with a psychiatrist[1] whom she saw before the events. It is very likely that her _____ disorder and her personality traits are far greater impediments to care and treatment relationships than are the events with Dr. F.

Second, it is likely that Ms. B.'s opportunity for treatment when she was seeing Dr. F. was indeed compromised by his unprofessional behavior; however, she did not perceive this as a clinical problem during most of that time (according to her deposition), and it does not appear to have affected her long-term prognosis. She reports in deposition that her aunt and sister perceived her as doing better while seeing Dr. F. (pp. 72–73).

Third, since seeing Dr. F., Ms. B. has experienced a number of events which would be expected to have adverse effects on her function and psychiatric condition, including the discovery of her colon cancer with lymph node invasion, her cancer treatments (major surgery, radiation, and chemotherapy), her sister's illness, trouble with her son (which she vaguely described to clinicians as "very bad news," precipitating her [date] overdose), her divorce, and other apparent family problems and issues. Some of these events were/are quite serious; none was associated with Dr. F. Ms. B. stated in her deposition (p. 79) that her cancer has caused far worse difficulties than have her psychiatric symptoms.

Fourth, it is fair to implicate the lawsuit itself in the exacerbation, and perhaps the creation, of at least some of Ms. B.'s symptoms.

---

1 It might be noted that her current psychiatrist, and one with whom she worked before (date) as well, is an immigrant who graduated from a non-U.S. medical school, qualities which the plaintiff has criticized in Dr. F. and raised as "red flags" for C.

While it may be said that the lawsuit would not exist without Dr. F.'s reprehensible behavior, it is my general experience, supported by the professional literature, that the process of being a malpractice plaintiff often contributes to keeping symptoms prominent, delays the resolution or amelioration of those symptoms, and creates pressing expectations in the plaintiff that he or she must continue to suffer whatever has been alleged in the (generally lawyer-composed) complaint.This statement should not be construed as an opinion that the plaintiff is malingering, but rather that lawsuits themselves are stressful and interfere with care and prognosis.

SOURCES RELIED UPON

- Written materials, represented as everything relevant and available from your office
  (*list*)
- Reid, W. H. (2004) Organizational liability: beyond *respondeat superior*, *Journal of Psychiatric Practice*, 10(4): 258–262
- My background, training, and experience in psychiatry, mental health care administration, and forensic psychiatry

QUALIFICATIONS

. . .

R14

REPORT: MALPRACTICE, DEFENSE (CLINICIAN) (ALLEGED FETAL DAMAGE FROM MEDICATION)

RE: **PRELIMINARY REPORT:** *A.B.* v. *USA* (No. _____)

You have asked for a report which summarizes my findings after review of the materials you provided. I am able to supply the opinions and comments below, based upon those materials and my training, background, and experience. The methods used and materials reviewed are those routinely relied upon by forensic psychiatrists in matters such as this, and are based on the national standard for similar matters in forensic psychiatry. Additional information received in the future may suggest additions or changes to the preliminary opinions below; I thus reserve the right to supplement this report as necessary.

It may be noted that my opinions are limited to my areas of expertise and do not purport to comment definitively with respect to obstetrics, prenatal development, or the nuances of pharmacologic toxicity to a developing fetus.

NARRATIVE
In (*month, year*), unknown to her psychiatrist (Dr. D.) or her obstetrics/gynecology providers (Dr. F. and nurse practitioner H.), A.B. became pregnant while being prescribed _____ for her acute and chronic psychiatric symptoms. She had been pregnant in (*year*), suffering a miscarriage in (*month, year*), and had apparently told Ms. H. that she wanted to become pregnant quickly after the miscarriage (but had never been more specific).

On (*date*), Dr. D. saw Ms. B. in the course of her ongoing psychiatric care for "_____ with psychotic features," which had led to her being hospitalized with very serious symptoms some two years before. He documented that she had had the miscarriage and was "now much more depressed." He wrote that her response to (*medication*) had been inadequate and she needed a trial of _____, "esp(ecially) in view of weight gain" about which she expressed concern (see also Dr. D.'s earlier clinical notes.) At that time, he was also prescribing _____, apparently for anxiety or sleep. Ms. B. was scheduled to see Dr. D. again in four weeks but did not keep the appointment (see clinic records, B. 0024-25 and elsewhere).

Ms. B. next saw Dr. D. about two months later (*date*) and was described as "very depressed, angry all the time, . . . stressed out . . . , bad arguments with _____. Having thoughts of suicide and cutting but hasn't done so. Cries or lashes out at times, and feels like going to _____ (hospital)."

On that visit, Dr. D. recorded anxiety and . . . "Depression score 'extreme'." He added "_____" to her diagnosis of _____ with psychotic features. At that time, Dr. D. prescribed _____ and _____ for her unstable and worsening symptoms. He discontinued the _____ and _____. She was scheduled to return in two weeks (B. 0020).

On (*date*), apparently unrelated to pregnancy or any knowledge of pregnancy, and without any mention of wanting to become pregnant, Ms. B. spoke with Dr. D. by telephone about discontinuing the (*medication*) and substituting _____ because she feared gaining weight. She had apparently researched the drug and its side/adverse effects. After some discussion, Dr. D. recommended she stay on the _____, continue to take _____, and call him back in a week. Ms. B. agreed to take the _____ for another week and call back, but there is no record of a return call. Ms. B. states, and there is documentation in the record, that she discontinued the _____ on her own initiative around (*date*) (but see below).

On (*date*), Ms. B. saw nurse practitioner H. because she suspected she was pregnant. Her pregnancy test was positive that day, after having been negative on (*date*) (Bates 0134,136). Ms. H.'s notes and her and Dr. F.'s depositions suggest that conception occurred about (*date*), with the earliest outward indication (a missed menstrual period) no earlier than (*date*). Ms. H. states, and the record indicates, that she discussed medication effects with Ms. B. at the (*date*) visit, and told her that, if a developmental defect were to occur, whatever its cause, it could already have happened (i.e., much earlier, or even before she knew she was pregnant; see, e.g., H. deposition, p. 53). An appointment was made for Ms. B. to see obstetrician/gynecologist Dr. F. on (*date*).

There are somewhat unclear statements in Ms. B.'s (*date*) deposition asserting that she called Dr. D. "as soon as I thought I was pregnant," and that Dr. D. called her back, "told me to stop the _____," and told her that the other medication would "be okay." The comments are further confusing in that she also said she had been trying to reach him for about two weeks prior to that conversation and, when he called her back "around that time," she told him she was pregnant (see e.g., B. deposition, p. 54). (It appears that Ms. B. may be mixing memories of her [*year*] pregnancy in these statements; cf. Dr. D.'s [*date*] note indicating such a call and discontinuing _____ [Bates 0338].)

Ms. B. did not keep her next scheduled appointment with Dr. D. (*date*), and there is no documentation of subsequent contact with Dr. D. until (*date*), at which time she told him she was five months pregnant.

Obstetrician Dr. F. saw Ms. B. (*date*). Per his deposition, Dr. F. discussed her _____ prescription with her, including benefits and risks, and
recalls indicating to her that the benefits made the _____ worthwhile. He
"had faith in" Dr. D.'s psychiatric abilities and his judgment that she
needed the medication, and stated at deposition, "I didn't have a problem
with _____, based on my experience in the past with it." Dr. F. did not
contact Dr. D. (F. deposition pp. 20, 22, 40).

There is no indication in the written record that Ms. B. ever told Dr. D. that
she was trying to become pregnant, or that Dr. D. reasonably had access to such
information prior to (date). Understanding that she was beyond her first trimester
at that point (date), Dr. D. did not change her prescription.

Some or all of Ms. B.'s prescriptions were filled at (large discount store),
where she was working before and during part of her pregnancy. She states
that she did not discuss her medications with any pharmacist. The record
does not indicate whether or not she worked in the pharmacy area, nor does
it indicate whether or not the prescriptions were dispensed with the kinds
of patient information sheets that are commonly provided to patients.

At some later point in the pregnancy, Ms. B.'s unborn child (now "R.")
was found to have (anatomical abnormalities), for which she has received
post-natal surgery and other medical care. Ms. B. alleges, in part, that
Dr. D.'s prescribing of _____ was negligent, and that negligence caused
her daughter R.'s abnormalities.

FINDINGS AND OPINIONS

The following opinions are offered to a reasonable degree of medical or
psychiatric probability, based on the national standard of care in same or
reasonably similar circumstances, given the information available to me at
this time, and assuming that information is an accurate representation of
the facts in this matter.

1. **Prior to (*date*) Dr. D. did not know, and could not reasonably**
    have known, that Ms. B. was pregnant. (See above for foundation.)
    By the time Dr. D. became aware of Ms. B.'s pregnancy, it had
    progressed well beyond the first trimester (that is, beyond the period
    of primary genesis and early development of an infant's _____
    structures, so far as I understand and without asserting additional
    expertise in fetal development).

2. **Dr. D. properly considered the benefits and risks of the medi-**
    cations he prescribed for Ms. B., including _____, particularly in
    light of Ms. B.'s severe mental illness, current and potential symp-
    toms, and their attendant risks. Dr. D.'s prescribing was a matter of
    clinical judgment, which he exercised appropriately.

3. There is significant risk to an unborn child if one does *not* ameliorate severe psychiatric symptoms in a patient such as Ms. B., including increased risk of psychosis (lost contact with reality), suicide or suicide attempt, other self-injury, inadequate self-care, decreased insight, impaired judgment, and impulsive behavior.

4. Dr. D. adequately considered Ms. B.'s participation in her own care, and her expressed wishes regarding her medication, when prescribing for her. (See above for foundation.)

5. The applicable standard of care did not require Dr. D. to substitute, or attempt to substitute, nonbiological treatments (such as psychotherapy or some other form of "counseling" or psychosocial intervention) for Ms. B.'s medication, particularly given her diagnosis and his lack of awareness of her pregnancy.

   It is unreasonable to believe, much less assume, that psychotherapy or "counseling" treatments for Ms. B. (i.e., nonbiological or non-pharmacologic treatments) would have been significantly effective for Ms. B.'s severe mental illness during the period contemplated.

   Intensive psychotherapeutic and psychosocial intervention may assist some patients with stabilization and/or behavior control, but (1) it is unreasonable to assume or predict that they would have adequately controlled the symptoms of _____ disorder and _____ traits in Ms. B.; (2) intensive psychotherapeutic and/or psychosocial treatment is difficult to implement for, and generally not rapidly available to, patients such as Ms. B.; (3) even when nonbiological treatments are reasonably able to be substituted for previously effective medications, the standard of care requires careful transition and close monitoring of symptoms, a procedure which takes weeks to implement, as the medication is slowly decreased; and (4) based on her prior records—and separate from whether or not it may have helped—it appears unlikely that Ms. B. would have been willing and/or able to participate meaningfully and consistently in such counseling or psychotherapy if it had been offered (cf. her missing scheduled appointments with Dr. D. and appointments for lab tests [Bates 062, 72, 177, 230], and declining Dr. D.'s earlier referrals for counseling).

6. Dr. D. did not fall below the applicable standard of care by prescribing _____ for a woman of childbearing age such as Ms. B.

   The fact that a female patient is of childbearing age should be considered when prescribing many medications; however, just as for nonpregnant patients, consideration of adverse effects should be reasonably tempered by the known or reasonably knowable level of risk, the severity of the potential adverse effect, the likelihood of the potential adverse effect, diagnosis, the acuity and significance of the patient's symptoms, the reasonably foreseeable consequences of *not* prescribing, the patient's current and past treatment response, and the patient's competent decisions regarding the prescription when provided adequate knowledge about risks and benefits. Both the clinical record and the various depositions in this matter indicate that Ms. B.'s mental illness was severe, symptomatic, at times dangerous, and required vigorous attempts at clinical control.

7. **Dr. D. was entitled to rely upon Ms. B. to tell him if she was pregnant or trying to become pregnant.** The record indicates that Ms. B. knew that some medications increase risk of damage to an unborn child, and knew she should notify her doctor. For example, she called Dr. D. in (*month, year*) to tell him she was pregnant (Bates 0395; her earlier pregnancy, at which time he discontinued her _____ prescription).

8. **The risks of treatment with _____ during pregnancy appear to have been overstated by the plaintiff.** Without implying that I am an expert in the effects of medications on embryologic or fetal development, it is reasonable to point out that _____ monotherapy (i.e., not taken with other, similar medications) does not appear to be, or to have been reasonably known to be, as dangerous for unborn children as the plaintiff represents, either before or since (*dates*).

A U.S. Food and Drug Administration (FDA) "FDA Alert" issued in (*month, year*) drew attention to "preliminary data," from one pregnancy registry out of many, of a "possible" association between first trimester _____ monotherapy and _____ abnormalities. That alert stated quite specifically that "the (abnormalities) were few . . . . Other pregnancy registries of similar size have not replicated this observation . . . . The clinical significance of this preliminary report is thus uncertain." It also stated, in part, that the alert reflected a "preliminary analysis," and that the "FDA is considering, but has not reached a final conclusion about, this information." According to the FDA sheet, and assuming (solely for the sake of argument) that the reported frequency of (abnormalities) (5 in 564 pregnancies, or about 8.9/1000) were replicated and reliably associated with _____, the increase in (abnormalities) over "mothers not taking _____" would be between 4.1 and 17.8 times (the general population frequency being 0.5/1000 to 2.16/1000).

The FDA "preliminary report" appears not to have been borne out in other registries or subsequent surveys or research studies. Although that publication states that the FDA "intends to update this sheet when additional information or analyses become available," *no further updates or alerts have been issued by the FDA*. So far as I know, *the manufacturer's package insert information* for (all years since the event), as found in various iterations of the *Physicians' Desk Reference* (see, *e.g.,* pp. _____ in the 2010 edition or p. _____ of the 2011 edition) and routinely supplied or summarized with consumers' medications, *does not contain a warning about (this) or related abnormalities.*

My independent searches of the U.S. and international professional literature (National Library of Medicine/PubMed), performed on *(date)* and *(date)* and combined with articles and abstracts provided by your office, failed to reveal a pattern of special findings or warnings to suggest increased _____ risk *vis-à-vis* (this abnormality). Indeed, those reviews suggest that _____ is safer than many (perhaps most) medications in its class. For example, a 2010 article in *Contemporary OB/GYN: Translating Science into Sound Clinical Practice* states, in part (with original source citations not footnoted here),

> "Final data from the International _____ Pregnancy Registry covered 2,444 women and 2,492 pregnancy outcomes...."[7] The rate of major defects associated with first-trimester exposure to _____ was 2.2% for monotherapy...(By comparison, the incidence of birth defects in the general population is about 3%.)[8]...Data from the North American AED registry suggested a possible link between first-trimester _____ exposure and (this abnormality). However, no such association was found in a large case-control study"[9] (Abel D.E. [2010]. Medication safety during pregnancy, *Contemporary OBGYN* 65[10]:30–41)

See also, e.g., Cunnington M., Tennis P., International _____ Pregnancy Advisory Committee (2005), "_____ and the risk of malformations in pregnancy," *Neurology* 64(6):183 (NOTE that this author was affiliated with GlaxoSmithKline at the time of publication.); Ornoy A. (2006), "Neuroteratogens in man: an overview with special emphasis on the teratogenicity of antiepileptic drugs in pregnancy," *Reproductive Toxicology* 22(2):214–226; and Shor S. *et al.* (2007), "Teratogenicity of _____," *Canadian Family Physician* 53(6):1007–9 (all published prior to Ms. B.'s pregnancy with R.);[1] as well as a scholarly interchange concerning one of the articles cited

---

1 Only those studies and treatises published prior to *(date)* would seem relevant to allegations of negligence; those published after that time may be relevant to allegations of causation.

by plaintiffs and published as Hunt S.J. *et al.* (2009), *Neurology* 72:1108–1109.

9. **Ms. B. sought, and apparently found, information regarding some side effects and adverse effects of her various medications** (cf. her comments about weight gain and requests to change medications to avoid it). She was aware of at least some easily accessible resources for information about adverse medication effects.

10. **Dr. D. obtained adequate consent before prescribing for Ms. B.**
   Plaintiff's expert Dr. O., in his *(date)* preliminary report, errs in his discussion of consent in the context of Ms. B.'s prescriptions. Dr. O. opines that there is no documentation of "Informed Consent," and further implies that this alleged lack precluded Ms. B.'s receiving adequate information about ____, which might (or might not [parenthetical comment mine]) in turn have caused her to discontinue or avoid it.
   On the contrary, there <u>is</u> information in the record and in subsequent depositions indicating that Ms. B. did consent adequately to her various prescriptions from Dr. D., including ____, and did have or receive adequate information about them from several sources at various times. In that regard, one should note the difference between consenting to a *treatment* (i.e., a treatment to be administered by a clinician) and accepting a *prescription* which is part of overall treatment, with the information to decide whether or not to take it (i.e., the medication is not to be administered by a clinician, and the patient chooses to take each dose). Ms. B.'s situation is an example of the latter. That is, her medications were prescribed by Dr. D. and apparently taken later.
   There is no indication in the record that the level of discussion with Dr. D. was inadequate. In addition to whatever doctor–patient interchanges occurred, there is evidence that Ms. B. examined Internet resources about side- and adverse effects. Further, it seems likely (although I do not know) that she received written information about adverse effects from her pharmacist every time the prescriptions were filled.
   To the extent that Ms. B. received written medication information from her pharmacist, I do not know whether or not that information contained any warning about (fetal deformities) as of *(dates)*; however, current package insert information for that medication does not (consistent with current FDA requirements and prescribing recommendations).
   Without meaning to appear harsh, The record is clear that Ms. B. discussed weight gain with her psychiatrist, and in that regard chose, at times, not to take medications that he prescribed for her. It is fair

to say that Ms. B. knew that some medications can affect an unborn child, that she should notify her prescribing physicians if she was trying to become pregnant (or believed she was pregnant), that she could choose not to take the medication if she was trying to become pregnant (or believed she was pregnant), and that she could obtain further information about risks or concerns from Dr. D. and/or a number of other sources.

Finally, the applicable standard of care did not, and does not, require <u>written</u> consent prior to prescribing outpatient medications such as those prescribed by Dr. D..

SOURCES RELIED UPON AND FOUNDATIONS FOR THE ABOVE OPINIONS

- Written materials as follows, provided by your office (NOTE that some records which appeared limited to topics outside my expertise were not reviewed):
  (*list*)
- Review of relevant professional and prescribing literature
  (*list*)
- My background, training, and experience in medicine, psychiatry, and forensic psychiatry

QUALIFICATIONS AND PUBLICATIONS

. . .

CASES IN WHICH I HAVE TESTIFIED DURING THE PAST FOUR YEARS

. . .

R15

REPORT: ACCIDENTAL OVERDOSE VS. SUICIDE

NOTE: This case involved the death by overdose of a military veteran who had been treated for PTSD, extensive substance abuse, and antisocial behavior. There was a lot of conflicting information about his military experience and later symptoms and substantial indication that he had misrepresented his symptoms, largely to obtain narcotics, at least some of the time. Most of the extensive narrative summary has been redacted.

RE: **PRELIMINARY REPORT:** *A.B.* v. *USA* (Case No. _____)

You have asked for a report which summarizes my findings after review of the materials you provided. I am able to supply the opinions and comments below, based upon those materials and my training, background, and experience. The methods used and materials reviewed are those routinely relied upon by forensic psychiatrists in matters such as this, and are based on the national standard for similar matters in forensic psychiatry. Additional information received in the future may suggest additions or changes to the preliminary opinions below; I thus reserve the right to supplement this report as necessary.

NARRATIVE

... On (*date*), after consideration of risks, benefits, and response to prior medications, Dr. J., Mr. B.'s psychiatrist in the program, prescribed a modest dose of a mild narcotic for Mr. B.'s pain (see below). He limited the prescription to a seven-day supply at a modest, PRN dose (Bates 2437) (see also J. deposition, pp. 55–60 and elsewhere). The record and discharge summary describe "chronic back pain ... tried on many types of pain medications, but could get no relief from them ... finally tried on a mild opiate med, ... since he did not respond to any previous pain meds."

Program progress notes and the discharge summary (the latter [*date*]; Bates 2304) indicate that Mr. B. was doing fairly well in the (open residential) program until "he began to miss sessions." On (*date*), Mr. B. left the facility unauthorized, with "four other veterans, obtained and consumed

216

alcohol, which is prohibited, returned the middle of the next day." At some point, as he tried to sneak back onto the residential unit, he also got into an altercation with another patient (discharge summary; J. deposition pp. 76, 78).

A treatment team meeting was called at which staff concluded that Mr. B. would be discharged on (*date*) "in order to preserve the unit milieu." He was administratively discharged and referred to a nearby substance abuse program that accepted veterans. The other veterans involved were also discharged.

. . .

About two days after discharge, on the morning of (*date*), Mr. B. was found deceased in a _____ motel. Autopsy and laboratory results indicated the presence of several prescription and street drugs in his body, and established the cause of death as "toxic effect of (those drugs)." Police reports and interviews indicate that Mr. B. had been taking various drugs with several other people for several hours before his death. One of them, _____, stated that she was with him until early on the morning he was found, and that they had been using drugs together. She stated that they fell asleep; she was awakened when others knocked on the motel room door, and she got up and left in the dark, leaving Mr. B. in bed and—she thought— asleep. It is not clear whether or not he was alive when she left, but the record indicates that he died around that time. The room lights and air conditioner were off when police arrived. No note or other communication from Mr. B. was found, or any indication that his death was intentional. The death certificate records the manner of death as accidental.

FINDINGS AND OPINIONS

The following opinions are offered to a reasonable degree of medical or psychiatric probability, based on the national standard of care in same or reasonably similar circumstances, given the information available to me at this time, and assuming that information is an accurate representation of the facts in this matter.

1. **The manner of Mr. B.'s death on (*date*) was much more likely to have been accident than suicide.** I found no psychiatric evidence that Mr. B.'s drug-taking on (*date*) constituted a suicide attempt or suicide. In addition, the police investigation records and witness reports (Bates 2386–2452) are very consistent with "ordinary" drug-taking behavior leading to accidental death (see Narrative above), and the _____ County death certificate states "accidental drug overdose" (Bates 0444). There is a *possibility* that Mr. B. committed suicide, but the facts represented by the record do not suggest *probability*.

   Mr. B.'s substance abuse carried substantial risk. He was aware of those risks, and often took large amounts of narcotics in spite of the obvious dangers (see Narrative). During treatment, it is reasonable and important to explore whether or not overdoses such as those for which he was hospitalized in (*year*) were actually suicide attempts, but, <u>absent much more direct evidence of suicidal intent, engaging in high-risk behavior which impairs judgment (e.g., substance abuse) should not be *per se* construed as a suicide attempt</u>.

2. **Mr. B.'s immediate cause of death included, but was not limited to, _____ toxicity.** I am not a toxicologist and cannot opine about the relative contributions of _____ and other substances to the immediate cause of Mr. B.'s death; nevertheless, the autopsy record names three other drugs in his system which were apparently involved in his death (see autopsy toxicology findings and coroner Dr. _____'s finding of multiple drug toxicity as the immediate causes of death; Bates 0445–448).

   _____, which was never prescribed by the VA, is a much more potent narcotic than _____, and was present at a level more than five times that of the _____ (0.46 mg/L v. 0.078 mg/L). In addition, there were significant levels of _____ and _____, which he had abused in the past, neither of which had been prescribed by the VA.

3. **The record strongly indicates that Mr. B.'s death on (*date*) was not caused, directly or indirectly, by any action or failure to act by the VA or its employee clinicians** (see below).

4. **Whether or not any or all of the _____ in Mr. B.'s body at the time of his death came from medication prescribed or dispensed by the VA is not known, and is not reasonably knowable.** Most, possibly all, of the drugs found in Mr. B.'s body after death were obtained from some source other than the residential facility or Dr. J. Mr. B. may have had a few days' supply of _____-containing pain medication (up to 10 tablets) in his possession when he was discharged (*date*) (assuming he had not taken pills while absent from the program). Any additional pills would apparently have been acquired illicitly.

   Regardless of whether or not any of the _____ he took came from the facility, Mr. B. could easily get any of the drugs found outside the VA, and appears to have done so.

5. **The _____ program in which Mr. B. was a resident was a <u>residential</u> rehabilitation program, and not one designed, intended, or represented to be a "hospital" or psychiatric hospital program.** It was properly described to Mr. B. and others as a setting which combined personal responsibility with focused efforts to help residents deal with their personal and social post-traumatic symptoms. Its rehabilitation model was/is based on substantial professional and VA rehabilitation experience with combat veterans in dozens of similar programs (and other settings) within the VA system. (See e.g., program handouts, Dr. J. deposition.)

6. **Mr. B. was properly accepted into the ____ program.** There is no reasonable indication that he required, on admission or at any time during his residency in the program, inpatient psychiatric hospitalization. (See, e.g., his admission workup, depression screening, mental status exam, and other notes.)

7. **Dr. J.'s and the ____ treatment team's decision to discharge Mr. B. was reasonable and not negligent.** Dr. J. and the treatment team properly considered Mr. B.'s individual case as well as its impact on the other rehabilitation clients and the program itself. They considered appropriately developed program policy. Although there was known risk that he would return to abusing drugs and/or alcohol at some point, there is no indication that safety issues in his case should have outweighed the reasons for his discharge. The discharge decision was clinically appropriate both for Mr. B. and for the interests of other residents and the program itself. Other veterans who engaged in similar rule-breaking behavior were also discharged (Bates 2005, 2110; Dr. J. deposition p. 83).

8. **There is no indication in the record that Mr. B.'s condition at or just before discharge required more assessment than was provided, or that the applicable standard of care required transfer to a psychiatric unit or hospital, or that he was a reasonable candidate for transfer to a psychiatric unit or hospital.** Mr. B. was terminated from the program because of his *behavior*, and the effects of that behavior on his rehabilitation, other veterans who were trying to get help, and the program as a whole. He was appropriately given responsibility for that behavior, as reasonably expected of him according to the rules and treatment philosophy of the program.

   There was no known, or reasonably knowable, indication of substantial suicide risk, or of the presence of a psychiatric disorder with symptoms that warranted hospitalization, at the time of discharge. Assessments around the time of discharge, and earlier in his stay, were reasonable for the situation.

   Further, (a) there is no indication that Mr. B. would have been eligible for acceptance by an inpatient unit at the time of his discharge. (b) There is no indication that he would have agreed to referral to an inpatient psychiatric unit if such a referral had been offered (note that he had refused psychiatric admission in the past, and his purpose in leaving included drug and/or alcohol use, which would have been made more difficult were he to be hospitalized). (c) The record does not suggest that he would have been eligible for emergency/involuntary hospitalization if he had refused voluntary referral.

9. **The ____ discharge follow-up recommendations were reasonable and adequate.** According to the contemporaneous discharge

summary, follow-up was recommended "at _____ mental health center according to prior instructions from _____," and he was cautioned to abstain from alcohol and drug abuse. He was instructed to contact a physician as necessary. The record indicates that he was adequately assessed for suicide risk at the time of discharge and was advised to call 911 or go to an emergency room if suicidal thoughts occurred. He was familiar with the area and with most or all of its relevant nearby resources. (See _____ notes and discharge summary; Bates 1410–16.)

10. **Dr. J.'s prescribing of _____-containing pain medication was within the applicable standard of care.** First, the record and Dr. J.'s deposition indicate that Dr. J. considered the risks and benefits of prescribing the medication, noted Mr. B.'s inadequate response to trials of other medications, prescribed low doses (one tablet three times a day as needed) and relatively few pills (21, a 7-day supply) (Bates 1480), and monitored Mr. B.'s response (e.g., with pain charting), all consistent with the applicable standard of care. Second, controlled drugs were apparently prescribed for many patients within the _____ program, as indicated by safety procedures such as the "lock-box" requirement for keeping them in a resident's possession.

Third, to the extent Mr. B. left the _____ program with any medication, it was routine and well within Dr. J.'s purview to allow him to take his remaining pills with him upon discharge. Dr J. stated that Mr. B. filled only one prescription at the VA pharmacy: the one given on August 14. Contrary to Dr. O's remark ([*date*] plaintiff's expert report) about giving him "a loaded gun," had Dr. J. not allowed Mr. B. to keep his remaining medication (apparently about 5 days' supply {15 pills}), one would question why the patient was deprived of his property. Note also that Mr. B. apparently left without any additional prescription (see e.g., Dr. J. deposition pp. 91–92).

There is no indication that any member of the rehabilitation team, or any other person associated with the _____ program, raised any issue or concern about any of Dr. J.'s prescriptions.

11. **It is unreasonable to blame any of Mr. B.'s drug abusing behavior, or his death after leaving the VA program, on Dr. J.'s prescription.** Mr. B.'s behavior following discharge (and, indeed, while he was in the program, as per the rules and rehabilitation philosophy of that program) was voluntary and his own responsibility. There is no psychiatric or psychological indication that Dr. J.'s prescription, his discharge order, the treatment team's discharge decision/recommendation, or any other aspect of the VA treatment and rehabilitation efforts somehow rendered Mr. B. unable to control his behavior or drug intake, or meant that he was more likely to die in a

drug overdose after discharge. Finally, the record clearly indicates that Mr. B. did not need, nor did he rely upon, any VA prescription in order to obtain and use the drugs which led to his death.

12. With regard to plaintiff's allegation that the VA's overall treatment of Mr. B. in the several months prior to his death was inadequate and contributed to his death, **the record indicates that Mr. B. was afforded good opportunity for care of his various post-traumatic symptoms (including depression and substance abuse, whether or not related to military service). Nothing the VA did, or failed to do within the months and years before (*date*), contributed to his death.**

Mr. B. had two VA hospitalizations and several other VA contacts during the year before he entered the _____ program. His depression was recognized and treated to the extent he would allow before declining care or requesting discharge. Efforts were made to deal with the difficult-to-untangle interweaving of his substance abuse, PTSD, depression, and personality traits. Involuntary hospitalization was duly considered but not warranted. The issue of self-imposed risk from substance abuse (e.g., taking large amounts of narcotics without adequately considering the risk to one's life) vs. intending suicide was addressed insofar as reasonably feasible. Several treatment recommendations were made (which he generally declined) for further treatment. His "noncompliance" with treatment is well documented in the record (q.v., and see Narrative above).

Mr. B. was offered, but often declined or failed to follow, outpatient, inpatient, rehabilitation, and 12-step services. Even before the government changed his discharge status to "honorable for VA purposes," the VA extended help to him as a "humane emergency," though he was not entitled to services. The treatment and rehabilitation efforts offered were at least as good as, and in my experience often far more sophisticated than, most of those in the private or non-VA public sectors. Based on the information available to me, the _____ program itself is among the best post-trauma rehabilitation programs I have ever encountered.

13. With regard to plaintiff's allegation that the VA "chose to hire inadequately trained and incompetent medical staff" (paragraph 9 of the complaint), particularly in any way associated with Mr. B.'s death, I found nothing at all in the record to support such an allegation.

SOURCES RELIED UPON AND FOUNDATIONS FOR THE ABOVE OPINIONS

- Written materials as follows, provided by your office and represented as complete and all relevant records available
  (*list*)
- My background, training, and experience in medicine, psychiatry, forensic psychiatry, and mental health administration

QUALIFICATIONS AND PUBLICATIONS

. . .

CASES IN WHICH I HAVE TESTIFIED DURING THE PAST FOUR YEARS

. . .

R16

REPORT: DEFENSE, DEATH IN CUSTODY

RE: **PRELIMINARY REPORT**: _____, *as Personal Representative of the Estate of A.B., v. _____ Department of Corrections and C.D., M.D., et al.* No. _____, U.S. District Court, _____ District of (*State*)

You have asked for a report which summarizes my findings after review of the materials you provided. I am able to supply the opinions and comments below, based upon those materials and my training, background, and experience. The methods used and materials reviewed are those routinely relied upon by forensic psychiatrists in matters such as this. Any additional information received in the future may or may not suggest additions or changes to the opinions below; I reserve the right to supplement this report as necessary.

FINDINGS AND OPINIONS
The following opinions are offered to a reasonable degree of medical certainty, given the information available to me at this time and assuming that information provided is an accurate representation of the facts in this matter. Please note that they may not be exhaustive.

1. The death of inmate A.B. was not caused by any psychiatric or psychiatrically related action by Dr. D. Please see below.
2. Dr. D.'s professional conduct with regard to A.B. between (*dates*) was within the applicable standard of care. Please see below.
3. Both the setting in which Dr. D. saw Mr. B. and Dr. D.'s refusal to interview Mr. B. outside the presence of security personnel, were reasonable and were within the applicable standard of care, reasonably expected clinical behavior, and apparent jail policy for this and similar situations. (a) There is no question that close security was required in order reasonably to protect persons carrying out the examination. (b) Psychiatric examinations in this and similar situations often include a chaperone, even when close security

is not required. (c) The psychiatrist in such situations is not obligated to accommodate an examinee's wish for a private interview with the psychiatrist, especially when there is a reasonable belief that such an accommodation might threaten the safety of the psychiatrist or others, might create a security breach, might create some other form of liability (such as accusations of improper conduct), or might not be in the patient's clinical interest. (d) The jail policy for situations comparable to Mr. B.'s and Dr. D.'s situation, described by Mr. E. at deposition, dictated the kinds of cautions that were employed, regardless of whether or not Dr. D. might have wished to act otherwise.

4. **The two interview suggestions raised by plaintiff in some of the depositions – interview with the door ajar and interview by "telephone" through heavy glass or plastic – are either unreasonable or not required by the applicable standard of care, or both.**

    (a) Any direct contact with Mr. B. in the absence of immediate security carried a substantial risk of injury, hostage-taking, and/or an escape attempt. It was entirely reasonable <u>not</u> to use a "door-ajar-and-guard-just-outside" approach.

    (b) Interviews by "telephone" through heavy glass or plastic barriers in the inmate visiting area are often inadequate. A psychiatrist <u>may</u> use them, but there is no <u>obligation</u> to do so under the standard of care applicable to situations such as this. Further, Dr. D. had no duty to use such an alternative in the midst of Mr. B.'s unreasonable behavior and demands. In addition (in my experience and without personal knowledge of the visiting area itself), such "telephones" often can be monitored by corrections staff, and inmates usually know that they should not expect privacy when using them.

    Finally, there is a reasonable probability that Mr. B.'s demand for privacy during the interview was not really prompted by a wish for clinical confidentiality but by motivation to escape, to take a hostage, to harm Dr. D. or others, or simply to play a sort of manipulating "game." It is not at all certain that <u>any</u> interview setting would have led to a more nearly complete examination.

5. **Dr. D. considered alternatives and appropriately exercised clinical judgment when making decisions about Mr. B.'s interview, stopping his medication, prescribing other medication, etc.** Dr. D. (a) reviewed available information about the patient, (b) took advantage of clinical information gathered by others during earlier screening and interviews at the jail, (c) reasonably attempted to interview and examine the patient, (d) reasonably encouraged the patient

to behave in such a way that the interview/examination could be carried out, (e) appropriately weighed various alternatives, (f) discussed the situation with the nurse who accompanied him, (g) weighed the risks and potential benefits of the various medications, (h) considered possible and reasonable causes of Mr. B.'s presentation and behavior, and (i) gave clinical orders reasonably expected to promote Mr. B.'s safety and well-being. In particular, Dr. D.'s decision not to continue Mr. B.'s antidepressant prescription considered the possibility that he was showing early signs of mania (for which antidepressant drugs are usually contraindicated).

6. The <u>extent</u> of Dr. D.'s (*date*) assessment attempt was reasonable and within the applicable standard of care for the circumstances. The standard of care did not require that Dr. D. make even more attempts to calm Mr. B. during or after the efforts to examine him, or further to prolong his efforts. Even if Dr. D. had done so, there is no indication that such efforts would have been successful, or that they would have prevented Mr. B.'s death on (*date*).

7. There is no reasonable suggestion that any pharmacologic effect of changing or stopping the medications led to Mr. B.'s suicide. (a) There is no reasonable expectation of a significant withdrawal syndrome from any of the medications that were stopped, and certainly not one that would produce a substantial or reasonably foreseeable risk of imminent suicide. (b) The antidepressant medications that were stopped on (*date*), less than 24 hours before his death, (*drug names*), would reasonably be expected to retain whatever pharmacological effect they were producing for a few days. (c) (*drug names*) are not "narcotics" or otherwise federally controlled drugs (i.e., for which addiction or a significant withdrawal syndrome might be expected).

8. The theory offered by Dr. F. (plaintiff's expert) that a "placebo effect" of Mr. B.'s medications was present and was so strong that stopping the medications created some nonbiological condition that led to his death seems odd to me, and is not supported by any legitimate professional or scientific literature of which I am aware.

9. Mr. B.'s anger at the jail and other entities, to the extent that he may have been willing to die in order to punish them (see his letters), is a rare, but not unheard-of, motivation for actual suicide. The applicable standard of care does not require that a psychiatrist such as Dr. D., in a situation such as this, recognize such anger as a substantial suicide risk factor (to the extent that any increased risk existed at the time). To the extent that anger may have been a substantial part of the behavior that led to his death, it seems unlikely that Mr. B. would have communicated any suicide plan to Dr. D. regardless of interview setting (to the extent that there was one at the time he saw Dr. D.). In addition, there is no indication in the available record that Mr. B.

communicated any suicide plan or impulse to the nurse who examined his rash a few hours before he died.

10. **Mr. B.'s suicide was not foreseeable by Dr. D. at any time prior to Mr. B.'s death, and the applicable standard of care did not require an order for "suicide precautions."** Although everyone, patient or not, has some risk of suicide, there was no reason for Dr. D. to consider Mr. B. a high suicide risk. Contrary to the deposition comments of the plaintiff's expert, Dr. F., Mr. B.'s behavior described in the record of (*dates*), and particularly during Dr. D.'s interview, given his reasonably available historical information, <u>did not</u> mandate suicide precautions or an assumption of substantial suicide risk in order for Dr. D. to meet the applicable standard of care. Even if Dr. D. had had further opportunity to interview and examine Mr. B., there is no indication that he would have, or reasonably could have, discovered substantial suicide risk, or indeed that such risk would even have been present at the time of the examination.

Note that Mr. B.'s letters to his relatives and former girlfriend, assuming they were written within a few days of his death, suggest significant risk of suicide or some other untoward and dangerous behavior. There is no indication that Dr. D. could reasonably have been aware of those letters, but if he was aware, or reasonably should have been aware, of their content prior to Mr. B.'s death, then he had a duty to take some action to protect Mr. B.

SOURCES RELIED UPON

Written materials as follows, represented as all those relevant, complete, and available:

(*list*)

QUALIFICATIONS AND PUBLICATIONS

. . .

COMPENSATION

My compensation for expert consultation and/or testimony in this matter is at the rate of _____, plus expenses, subject to the details outlined in the fee agreement previously supplied.

EXHIBITS

I have not prepared, nor do I anticipate preparing, any exhibits for trial.

CASES IN WHICH I HAVE TESTIFIED DURING THE PAST FOUR YEARS

. . .

R 17

AFFIDAVIT: DEFENSE REBUTTAL, DEATH IN CUSTODY

NOTE: Forensic experts are often asked to critique the work of other experts. It is ethical and reasonable to do so, provided any opinions are reached and expressed in an objective, not ad hominem,[1] manner.

AFFIDAVIT

STATE OF TEXAS
COUNTY OF LLANO

COMES NOW, William H. Reid, M.D., M.P.H., who having first been duly sworn, deposes and says:

1. That I make this Affidavit based upon my personal knowledge of the facts of this case, the matter of A.B. (deceased), as you have supplied them, and render my opinions as a Board certified forensic psychiatrist. I have never issued an opinion that has been disqualified pursuant to _____ Statutes §_____, nor have I ever been found guilty of fraud or perjury in any jurisdiction.

2. That I am now, and was at all times material to this action, a duly licensed physician and psychiatrist, Board certified in general psychiatry and in forensic psychiatry. A copy of my current *curriculum vitae* is attached as Exhibit "A."

3. That the methods used to arrive at the opinions expressed in this affidavit are those routinely relied upon by forensic psychiatrists in matters such as this. All statements made below are intended to refer only to facts and issues which lie within my areas of expertise (generally psychiatric and/or mental health topics and those associated with the

---

1 Personal rather than objective.

227

provision of mental health services). Note that additional information could change or add to these opinions; should that become the case, I will communicate promptly with the counsel who retained me.

4. That for the opinions expressed in this affidavit, I have reviewed and relied upon the following materials, supplied by your office and represented to be all of the currently available, relevant records, . . . and have relied as well on my training, background, and experience in the fields of clinical psychiatry, forensic psychiatry, and mental health administration. A copy of my current *curriculum vitae* is on file in your office, for inclusion with this affidavit as required.

5. That I am in virtually complete disagreement with Dr. C.'s criticisms leveled at _____, as providers of mental health services to the _____ Jail (hereafter the Jail), and with his criticisms as they apply, or may apply, to clinical activities of the Sheriff's office or Jail itself, as expressed by Dr. C., plaintiff's expert, in his (*date*) pre-suit affidavit. Specifically,

   (a) In item 11 of his affidavit, Dr. C.'s statement that "the records demonstrate that the screening and evaluation fell below the applicable standard of care" is without foundation in the records I have reviewed. I cannot find any substantiation for them.

   (b) In item 12 of his affidavit, Dr. C.'s statement that "the evaluation was inadequate to detect indicators of suicide, and insure that such persons are closely monitored and restricted to avoid suicide" (*sic*), is both illogical and unreasonable as applied to the concept of potential negligence in this matter.

   First, Dr. C. appears to refer in this item to some broad, generic concept of "risk," and does not differentiate between *any* "indicators" (i.e., all persons have some suicide risk, and most have one or more "indicators") and risk which is both sufficiently substantial and sufficiently knowable through reasonable screening to require, as a matter of the standard of care, detection and subsequent protective action beyond that which was ordered and provided for Mr. B. (e.g., the special needs housing and every-15-minute monitoring which <u>were</u> ordered and provided at the Jail). <u>There is no indication in the record of such substantial and knowable risk at the times relevant to Mr. B.'s intake and screening</u>.

   Second, the applicable standard of care does not require that the evaluation process for persons such as Mr. B., under the circumstances in which he was seen at the Jail, "detect" more indicators of suicide risk that they found in this case (to the extent that any additional or knowable substantial risk actually existed at the time of his intake and screening). <u>The record contains no reasonable</u>

indication of substantial and knowable risk that might have required care or monitoring beyond that which was ordered and provided at the Jail. In addition, there is no indication, and no reasonable basis for inference, that such substantial risk actually existed, knowable or not, at the time of the screening. There is a significant likelihood that Mr. B. had no "hidden" plan or strong impulse for suicide when he was screened, and thus there was no suicide plan or impulse to discover in the first place. Mr. B., like hundreds of thousands of similar persons in the U.S., was known to have mental problems, but that is not, and should not be construed to be, tantamount to some level of suicide risk that required protective measures beyond those which were ordered and provided by the Jail.

Third, I found nothing in the record to suggest the presence of any so-called indicators of suicide (*sic*, Dr. C.) for which the applicable standard of care would require additional protective measures beyond those ordered and provided. Dr. C. does not name any of the "indicators" he alleges should have been found, and thus it is impossible to know exactly what he means; nevertheless, no such items are found in the record.

(c) In item 13 of his affidavit, Dr. C. alleges that "the Sheriff's Office and Corrections Department should have been aware of Mr. B.'s medical and mental health history." In fact, the applicable standard of care does not require that outside or archived medical and mental health records of an arrestee such as Mr. B., as he appeared in the Jail on (*date*), be obtained and reviewed by clinical staff by the time of his initial screening/evaluation, or during the small number of hours that passed before the hanging (note that Mr. B. arrived at night and was found hanging in his cell early the next morning). The screening person knew that he had been in the "special needs" section of the Jail in the past, and gathered information about his condition during his screening. That person adequately considered the information that was available and reasonably knowable (contrary to Dr. C.'s assertion that his prior history "was not considered"), and exercised good judgment with regard to placement and monitoring.

(d) In item 14 of his affidavit, Dr. C. alleges that Mr. B.'s "background information gave warning signs to the Sheriff's office." In fact, (i) nothing in the known or reasonably discernible history should have created any "warning" for which the applicable standard of care would have required more protections than were ordered and provided. In addition, (ii) even if the screening person had known more about Mr. B.'s psychiatric history, nothing in the records I have reviewed suggests that additional Jail protections would have been required by the applicable standard of care. To state that "this . . . fell below the standard of care" is simply erroneous.

(e) In item 15 of his affidavit, Dr. C. states that "it is <u>possible</u> (underlining mine) that the training provided by the Sheriff's office and the Corrections Department . . . was inadequate and fell below the standard of care . . . ," then adds that "further information . . ." would be necessary in order for him to "definitively comment on the training." Such a statement, in my opinion, cannot be taken as even an allegation of negligence, since Dr. C. himself says that he does not know whether or not the training met, or was required to meet, some standard. Dr. C.'s statement does not show, or purport to show, either relevant negligence or any causing of Mr. B.'s hanging.

(f) In item 16 of his affidavit, Dr. C. repeats his allegations, without citation or substantiation, that the Corrections Department and Sheriff's office were negligent and Mr. B.'s psychiatric evaluation fell below the standard of care, because he (Dr. C.) says it did. Once again, (i) Dr. C. does not iterate what makes up the applicable standard of care in the first place; (ii) he does not purport to describe or cite in any adequate detail how the potential defendants failed to meet it; and (iii) he does not adequately substantiate the purported difference between the potential defendants' actions and what he (Dr. C.) might consider adequate ones. Separate from my view that Dr. C.'s allegations are without foundation in the record, the Court is apparently expected to accord credibility to his allegations simply because he asserts them, without any citation or explanation.

(g) In item 16 of his affidavit, Dr. C. states that "this negligence resulted in Mr. B.'s death." <u>I can find no evidence in the record to support such an allegation of causation</u>. Further, Dr. C. gives absolutely no explanation or indication of *how* such vaguely alleged negligence may have caused Mr. B.'s death. His affidavit appears to say that causation exists simply because he says it is there, without any substantiation, description, or explanation.

(h) Item 17 of his affidavit implies that the earlier items in Dr. C.'s affidavit support his opinions to a reasonable degree of medical and psychiatric probability, and that there are reasonable grounds to support claims of medical and psychiatric negligence against the _____ Corrections Department and the _____ Sheriff's office. Based on my own review, training, background, and experience, and within my own expertise, the available record <u>does not</u> support any such claims.

6. It is my opinion, to a reasonable degree of medical and psychiatric probability, that the screening, medical and mental health care, and other clinical and protective services which lie within my areas of expertise and were rendered by _____ Correctional Department to A.B. were appropriate and did not deviate from the applicable standard of care, and that neither those services nor any alleged omission of services was a cause of Mr. B.'s death.

FURTHER AFFIANT SAYETH NOT.

R18

REPORT: WORKPLACE STRESSORS ALLEGEDLY CAUSING SUICIDE, EXPERT REPORT REBUTTAL

RE: **REPORT:** *B. v. _____ (Company), Inc.*

You have asked for a report which summarizes my findings after review of the materials you provided in the above matter. I am able to supply the comments and opinions below, based upon those materials and my training, background, and experience. The methods used and materials reviewed are those routinely relied upon by forensic psychiatrists in matters such as this. Any additional information received in the future may or may not suggest additions or changes to the opinions below.

FINDINGS AND OPINIONS

After review of the materials provided, I am able to provide the following opinions in response to the questions you have asked. Each opinion is offered to a reasonable degree of psychiatric certainty ("more probable than not") given the information available to me at this time.

1. **Was Mr. B.'s onset of major depressive disorder in (*year*) the result, in whole or in any material part, of cumulative exposure to workplace stressors?**
   No. So far as I can ascertain from the records, and without implying that I am an expert in Mr. B.'s occupation or specific working conditions, the cause of onset for his major depressive disorder was internal to him, not external. Work may be stressful and "depressing" at times, but the onset of Mr. B.'s severe major depressive disorder should be attributed to biological factors, including genetic ones, not his job.

   It may be added that reliable data in the professional literature shows that major depressive disorder occurs in people of all backgrounds and occupations at, on average, roughly the same rate and severity. No one is immune as a result of occupation, nor is the onset usually hastened by occupational factors.

232

2. Did workplace stressors aggravate either a pre-existing major depressive disorder or the major depressive disorder after diagnosis?

    No. Although truly unusual job stressors may aggravate depression and other emotional conditions, and without implying that I am an expert in Mr. B.'s occupation or specific working conditions, I do not see in the record significant evidence of truly unusual stressors after his diagnosis, or that his major depressive disorder was present before it was recognized in (*year*). Indeed, there is evidence of (*company*) attempts to accommodate his condition.

    Having said the above, persons with severe depression (including symptomatic major depressive disorder) often inaccurately <u>perceive</u> their environments to be unusually stressful, untenable, pessimistic, or hopeless. Depression, by its nature, often causes people/patients to view the world through "black glasses" (as contrasted with the metaphor of "rose-colored glasses"). Thus, for example, perceptions of overwhelming difficulty, criticism, hopelessness, helplessness, etc., are likely to be based in the patient's view through depressive "lenses" rather than in reality.

    This significant cognitive (thinking) factor in one's experience of depression (that is, erroneously pessimistic thinking caused by the depression) can feed upon itself, so that failures in the workplace and elsewhere—for example, failing in attempts to return to work—make one feel worse. Nevertheless, the cause lies in the depression and the way depression affects thinking, not in the environment. Patients with very supportive environments experience the "black glasses" phenomenon just as do those with non-supportive ones.

    Finally, it goes without saying that some work and working conditions are "stressful" or "depressing" for some employees. Job-related depressed feelings and other symptoms that do not reach severe levels are common. They may coexist with disorders such as major depressive disorder, but should not be confused with Mr. B.'s illness.

3. Was Mr. B.'s suicide the result of "volitional insanity" (irresistible impulse)? That is, did Mr. B., more probably than not, *choose* to end his life even though such a choice is not likely to be rational? Although his decision was almost certainly guided by impaired insight and judgment related to his depression, Mr. B. "chose" to end his life in the narrow sense that there is no indication that he was acting on immediate and irresistible impulse or in some "automatic" way that controlled his behavior. Without having been present and known what was in Mr. B.'s mind when he committed suicide, one cannot say exactly what he was thinking, feeling, or intending at the time; however, the record and a body of established

professional knowledge about illnesses and behaviors similar to his allow a number of reliable inferences.

Mr. B. waited for his family to leave, then carried out logical and deliberate steps in order to effect his death. The record clearly indicates that Mr. B. knew what he was doing, knew that his behavior would likely end his life, and knew that his suicide might be prevented if someone were with him, and acted accordingly. Further, there is no indication that he might somehow have believed he would survive his obviously lethal actions (e.g., in some magical or "psychotic" sense).

4. **Please summarize any criticisms or concerns you may have with regard to Dr. C.D.'s report to E.F.**

   Dr. D.'s report contains important points for the Court to consider, but it appears to (a) contain errors or misinterpretations of the record, (b) misinterpret or overstate the psychiatric and epidemiological literature as it may apply to Mr. B., and (c) misunderstand the meaning of some clinical and research information in the context apparently contemplated by the Court's issues, as I understand them.

   (a) Contrary to Dr. D.'s implication, Dr. H.'s conclusion in his notes, letters and deposition is that he <u>does not</u> believe Mr. B.'s actions in committing suicide were "automatic" (in the sense of arising from a person totally deprived of the mental power to restrain himself).[1] The record indicates that Mr. B. wrestled for years with severe depression and thoughts of killing himself, but there is nothing that tells us what he was thinking during his final minutes of life, and very little to suggest his inner thoughts at any time prior to his death. Similarly, there is nothing in the record that indicates that Mr. B.'s suicide was "impulsive" in the sense of being carried out with an absence of planning or intentional, deliberate conduct. Indeed, the fact that he waited until his family left, chose a particular method and location, and then went through a several-minute process to kill himself suggests the opposite.

   Dr. D. misquotes (or incompletely quotes with the effect of misquoting) Dr. H.'s (*date*) letter to Mr. J. (q.v.), which was intended to clarify an earlier statement (see also H. deposition, pp. 22, 24, 30).

   Dr. D. appears to assume inappropriately that Mr. B.'s job was extraordinarily stressful (and causatively so, a further, separate

---

1 These and other statements and documents by Dr. H. or others are best clarified by the individuals themselves.

assumption) without noting that the record indicates that (i) Mr. B. had worked in the same or a similar job for many years without notable psychological consequences; (ii) he expressed a strong wish to continue at his job (cf. H. deposition p. 26); and (iii) his work environment was significantly adjusted to accommodate his condition. In addition, (iv) my impression from the record (given that I am not an occupational expert) is that, over the years, his work involved both periods of very long hours (during particular projects) and periods without very long hours. (v) Nothing in the records I reviewed indicated that Mr. B.'s job was significantly different from that of other persons in his field. Finally, when Dr. D. speaks of Mr. B.'s description of his work setting (e.g., to his wife), Dr. D omits the important fact that significantly depressed individuals routinely misperceive their environments in a negative way.

Dr. D. mentions that _____ and _____ are "antipsychotic" medications, and appears to cite this to imply that Mr. B. was delusional at the time of his suicide. To the extent that this was Dr. D.'s intent, she appears not to consider the inference, supported in the record and common in psychiatric practice, that those medications were not being prescribed for "psychosis" at all (Dr. H. averred that Mr. B. was not psychotic), but actually for anxiety (cf. Dr. H.'s [date] note), as antidepressant adjuncts, and/or as mood stabilizers.

Dr. D. cites Dr. H.'s and Mrs. B.'s statements that Mr. B. did not <u>appear</u> acutely suicidal in the days or weeks before his death as evidence that his suicide was due to an impulse that arose precipitously on or just before (date) (cf. D. opinion 3). Neither the record nor relevant psychiatric knowledge supports that contention. It is very common for patients such as Mr. B. to keep their suicidal thoughts and plans to themselves.

One cannot know what was in Mr. B.'s mind, but it is more likely than not that he thought of suicide often and was able to resist that thought (i.e., refrain from attempting or committing suicide) between (date) and (date), after his family had left the house. In addition, without regard to how long he thought about suicide before carrying it out or exactly what was in his mind, the record indicates that, more likely than not, the suicide itself required several minutes of deliberate behavior. There is no indication that it was the result of some very rapid, immediately uncontrollable, "automatic" circumstance[2] (see also Dr. H. [date] letter).

---

2 That is not to say that Mr. B.'s mental illness was not a very important influencing, and causative, factor in his "choosing" a tragic death. Rather, the record and relevant psychiatric knowledge indicate simply that his death should not be viewed as a result of some immediately uncontrollable impulse.

(b) Dr. D.'s use of three citations from the medical literature appears to exaggerate the conclusions in the papers cited. In addition, those articles reflect only a small part of the overall professional literature on possible relationships between occupational stress and depression or other mental illness.

Many more comprehensive reviews, exemplified in a 2008 analysis by Bonde,[3] conclude that (i) the effect of stress generally on the precipitation of "major depressive disorder" (see definition below) is small, with an effect size of 0.5 to 1.5 across studies; (ii) the definition of "stress" or "stressor" is quite variable across studies and often appears idiosyncratic to individuals (cf. the frequent use of "perceived" stress in studies rather than more objective measurement), and (iii) the evidence for causation at any level must be viewed as "circumstantial."[4]

(c) It is important to note that the simplistic application of epidemiological or statistical findings to individuals, even to the extent they may be applicable to large groups, is scientifically improper. The mere fact that there may (or may not) be an increased prevalence of severe depression in workers who experience extraordinary job stress should not be construed to imply— and certainly not "more probably than not"—that an individual with severe depression developed it because of his or her work environment. Such fallacious *post hoc ergo propter hoc* reasoning is made worse by the fact that even the most suggestive studies report that the prevalence of major depressive disorder in people with very stressful jobs (whatever the definition) is under 10%.

This may be compared with the 5–12% lifetime prevalence of major depressive disorder in males in the general population (10–25% in females), to which 150%–300% increased risk is added for people of Mr. B.'s family history of major depressive disorder and suicide, plus additional risk for persons of his age as of (*date*).[5]

It must also be noted that "depression" is not the same as "major depressive disorder, severe" (Mr. B.'s usual diagnosis). Many situations, including work situations, are "depressing" or precipitate depressed feelings. Many studies of work stress refer simply to "depression" and other feelings or symptoms. None of these should

3 Bonde, J. P. (2008) Psychosocial factors at work and risk of depression: a systematic review of the epidemiological evidence, *Occupational and Environmental Medicine* 65(7): 438-445.

4 Ibid.

5 American Psychiatric Association (2000) *The Diagnostic and Statistical Manual of Mental Disorders*, 4th Edition, Text Revision. Washington, DC: American Psychiatric Association, pp. 372-373.

be construed as "major depressive disorder," which is a specific clinical disorder with clear diagnostic criteria. In addition, it should be remembered that Mr. B.'s type of disorder was unusually severe and resistant to treatment. It is inaccurate and scientifically inappropriate to imply that a statistical suggestion of stress-related "depression" is equivalent to causation of Mr. B.'s severe mental illness.

SOURCES RELIED UPON

- Written materials as follows, represented as all that are relevant and available:
  (*list*)
- My background, training, and experience in medicine, psychology, psychiatry, and forensic psychiatry, and health-care administration

QUALIFICATIONS
. . .

CASES IN WHICH I HAVE TESTIFIED
. . .

R19

REPORT: PRIVATE INSURANCE DISABILITY APPEAL (COMPLEX)

NOTE: Social Security disability reports are short and often follow a structured outline. Military or VA ones are a bit longer. Private insurance appeals can be much more detailed (and usually involve a lot more money). This one was related to a high-income claimant's appeal of termination of payments from a policy that paid only if he could not practice his specialty. The company requested a very detailed report.

ABC Insurance Company
Att'n. _____, Disability Specialist

RE: Disability Report: **A. B., M.D.**
                          ABC No. _____

Dear Mr. _____:

You have asked for a report which summarizes my findings after review of the materials you provided, examination of Dr. B., and interviews of his wife and his treating physician, J. K., M.D. I am able to supply the opinions and comments below, based upon those and my training, background, and experience. The methods used are those routinely relied upon by forensic psychiatrists in matters such as this.

HISTORY AND EXAMINATION
Dr. B.'s <u>psychiatric, medical, family, and social history</u> through about (*year*) is adequately summarized in earlier reports and is generally consistent with information received from him and collateral sources. Some portions will be recounted but the overall history will not be detailed here. (Please see Dr. F.'s [*date*] report to ABC and other documents.)

Since his last evaluation, Dr. B. and his wife have separated. He continues to live in the same house, and his daughter G. continues to live nearby. He is seeing someone socially but states that the relationship is not an intimate one.

According to Dr. B. and his wife, much of his time is spent sculpting, exercising, and doing things with G., whom he currently supports and sees regularly. Although apparently quite accomplished, Dr. B. does not think of his sculptures as "professional"; he has not exhibited or sold his works.

Recent/additional psychiatric history indicates that Dr. B. is still seeing Dr. K. and taking antidepressant medication much as described in the record. He had a major depressive episode a few years ago (see below). He stopped seeing his psychotherapist, Dr. Y., some time ago.

Additional medical history indicates that Dr. B. has undergone preventive checks for such things as cancer and cardiovascular health (see family history below), all of which have been generally within normal limits. He says he does not worry excessively about his own death ("I don't feel a dark cloud over me"), but see Dr. K.'s comments, below.

Additional family history includes his statement that his adult daughter G. is apparently seeing a counselor and taking an antidepressant for what he describes as a "mood disorder." He is concerned about her. A son is taking the same medication, apparently for depression and/or mood instability. Dr. B.'s only grandchild is G.'s daughter from a youthful affair.

Dr. B.'s father died after a long, deteriorating course of dementia. There is some concern in the record, from Dr. B. and others, about his own memory and concentration. He thinks about the possibility that he may become demented, but does not worry excessively about it, saying that his father had risk factors he lacks, such as smoking and coronary artery disease. Dr. B.'s mother and a maternal aunt and uncle died of _____ cancer. Dr. B. has had tests for signs of that cancer, and says he is not particularly concerned because the other victims had premonitory signs or risk factors which he lacks.

Dr. B. has several siblings, one of whom had severe social problems. Dr. B. tried to help him in a number of ways, but, after many sad and frustrating years, he died from complications of substance abuse. Dr. B. still feels badly and guilty about this, becomes emotional when thinking of him, and is bitterly disappointed that he couldn't/didn't save his brother. (Dr. B. misspoke twice when tearfully speaking of that brother, mistakenly saying his daughter's name instead of his brother's. When I mentioned this, he was a little surprised but readily saw the parallel between the two.)

Further information from his estranged wife, R. B. Although they had not lived together for many months at the time of our conversation, Ms. B. stated that she sees the claimant at least once a week, when seeing their adult daughter, etc., and that they interact frequently. She corroborates his preference for social isolation for as long as she has known him, recalling that he is nervous and had/has "anxiety around other people" except when working with patients. "He can't deal with people." He was a good clinician, proud of his work, but intolerant of others' foibles. His practice and his sculpture got all of his attention. As time went by, he "couldn't leave work at the office . . . [or] enjoy life." He has always been happier at home in his studio, working in the yard, etc., which she finds very sad.

When asked about his ability to practice (*specialty*) now, she said "(h)e loved practicing," diagnosis and treatment, but not working with the people. He "can't focus under any kind of pressure . . . gets paralyzed by decisions . . . can't get past things that happened years ago." She firmly denied that any of his symptoms are "voluntary," saying that he worked very hard to develop his skills, has a strong work ethic, and would be working if he could. When asked how he might react if he were "forced" to practice, she said he would be "a nervous wreck . . . it scares him . . . he couldn't do it . . . . But I'd never have said that five years ago."

She described Dr. B. as very depressed, not letting go of past problems and moving on, not being able to enjoy things, "something holding him back." She views him as an "emotional cripple," hanging on to, and being chronically overwhelmed by, problems from the past and his inability to deal with them (including family problems with his deceased brother and their daughter, past marital problems, etc., not simply the practice problems). She corroborates the fact that his brother's ashes are still in his den; he can't bring himself to dispose of them and feels extremely guilty that he couldn't rescue the brother (an unreasonable expectation).

When asked what might happen if Dr. B. were no longer receiving disability payments, she said he might be O.K. if he didn't have to make important clinical decisions (cf. medical practice problems and peer reviews of his cases and judgment); "he's lost *faith* in himself."

When asked whether or not she has noticed any symptoms of dementia, she says she has not. She was surprised when I told her some of Dr. B.'s erroneous answers from our interview. She assumes he takes his medication regularly ("it's his nature"). She agrees that he has been intoxicated a few times in the past, but doesn't believe he has an alcohol or drug problem. She corroborates the family psychiatric history described elsewhere in this report (dementia, depression, mood problems, some drug abuse). She does not believe he has any serious health problems. She says he may be worried about dementia because of his father, but says he is not particularly hypochondriacal.

Further information from treating psychiatrist, Dr. J. K., indicates that the primary recent improvement in Dr. B. has included his continuing symptom remission and his developing acceptance of the necessity to follow a different lifestyle in order to avoid relapse. His life after medical practice "is like negotiating a minefield" in which he carefully avoids stress and controversy. The hospitals at which he practiced treated his problems as solely behavioral, ignoring the psychiatric issues and simply being punitive. He was never referred to a hospital physicians' health committee. Dr. K. described what he believed were Dr. B.'s sincere and prolonged efforts to continue his practice, including appeals to hospitals that had curtailed his privileges, followed last year by an unsuccessful practice trial.

Dr. K. says that he (Dr. K.) was wrong about Dr. B.'s ability to work last year. At that time, he supported Dr. B.'s efforts to return to practice, where he failed because of impaired judgment, not his skills. Dr. K. disagrees with Dr. B.'s statements to me that defended his work, and believes they are defensive rationalizations by a person who must see himself as practicing good medicine in spite of others' reviews and criticisms (cf. some bad case outcomes in [year] and the hospital staff demanding that he resign in [year]). Dr. K. agrees that he knows of no episode of physical violence in the hospital, and that, so far as he knows, the day-to-day behavior problems reported were verbal expressions.

Dr. K. noted much of the history and presentation described elsewhere in this report and the record, and in addition highlighted what he believes is Dr. B.'s fear—a greater concern than Dr. B. voiced to me—about the possibility of inheriting his father's dementia. (Note the family history of _____ cancer as well, and Dr. B.'s extensive preventive workup for coronary and vascular disease.)

Dr. K. expressed no doubt that Dr. B. is disabled with respect to practice, citing his diagnosis and personality characteristics, the symptoms and behaviors that led to his practice problems, his failed attempt to return to practice, and his currently adequate but somewhat limited adaptation to life (e.g., difficulty with close relationships, limited social functioning, non-salvageable marriage). He states that Dr. B. could not adequately organize a re-entry to (specialty) practice, and it would "work against him healthwise," in part because of his lack of mental stamina, reserve, and concentration. Dr. K. was concerned when I told him of the erroneous answers to fairly simple "testing" questions. At a later visit to Dr. K., Dr. B. had said he was "tired" when the questions were asked (and may have been rationalizing what he thought was a poor performance). He agreed that comprehensive neuropsychological testing may be indicated.

When asked about secondary gain, Dr. K. says that Dr. B. is *surprised* that he feels better outside the practice environment. He notes that Dr. B. fought hard not to be extruded from his work and profession and that, although he is coming to grips with his disability and the need to decrease the stresses that exacerbate his depression and anxiety, he doesn't like it at all.

Interviews of Dr. B.

Dr. B. appeared a little early for his appointment, neatly dressed and kempt, polite, and cooperative as he described his situation and condition.

He mentioned that he had driven his rental car to my neighborhood the night before, in order to be sure he could find the office easily. He tolerated the two interview sessions well (nearly 5 hours in all), never appearing physically uncomfortable or particularly tired. He did not ask for additional breaks.

Dr. B. presented himself in a reasonably favorable light during most of the interview, not appearing to highlight or exaggerate any disability (but making it clear, when asked, that he could not tolerate return to his former practice). When asked about his disability, his demeanor was that of a person who was still distressed at not being able to continue a career he valued and which allowed him to do very productive work, but he appeared to accept the premise that changing his activities and lifestyle was the only way for him to avoid a return of severe mental and behavioral symptoms. He said, as did Dr. K. and his estranged wife in separate interviews, that he had spent many months trying to salvage his career, rebutting the concerns of credentialing committees and the state licensing agency, and attempting to return to practice, before coming to the realization that he could not function as a physician. He states that he has restrictions on his license, and that Dr. K. provides the licensing agency with reports. He discussed other kinds of practice (e.g., administrative, hospice), but said that if his disability payments were cancelled he would not return to acute care (see Dr. K.'s comments).

Dr. B.'s mental status appeared free of psychosis, severe depression, or other symptoms or signs of acute, severe mental disorder. He appeared to be in fair remission with respect to his ongoing diagnoses, but there were some areas of concern. His facies and demeanor were consistent with current mild to moderate depression. He sometimes became tearful, for example when speaking about the loss of his brother several years ago and his associated guilt.

Some unexpected findings appeared late in the interview, when I tested several aspects of ordinary brain function. Assuming that Dr. B. at one time had the intelligence and general knowledge usually expected of a physician, he performed well below expectations. I do not believe his performance is likely to have been significantly affected by depression, poor motivation, or fatigue (although he did appear a little dulled at some points and later mentioned to Dr. K. that he felt tired after the interviews), or that he was consciously feigning. It may be noted that his tearfulness when speaking of his deceased brother was not considered necessarily a symptom of neurologic lability, but it may have been. Although my questions should not be construed as an adequate test of his neuropsychological functioning, or of any deterioration thereof, they raise concerns which should be considered in his disability evaluation. Several specific examples of both accurate and inaccurate answers are quoted below. Potentially positive findings are underlined.

Orientation: Complete in all 4 spheres

Immediate/reflex memory: Generally remembered 7 forward (cf. a telephone number)
Consistently failed at 4 backward (cf. Dr. F's finding of 4 forward and 3 backward)

Recent memory: Recalled three objects at 5 and 15 minutes (cf. Dr. F's finding of 2–3 items)

Remote memory: Fair in some respects; fair to poor with regard to general knowledge. Recent presidents accurate only back to George Bush, Sr.; knew V.P. Cheney. Needed multiple choice to name Secretary of State. Didn't know V.P. Gore's home state and chose wrongly (saying he was pretty certain) when given multiple choice.

Concentration and persistence: Serial 7s from 100 contained two early errors; serial 7s from 80 O.K.; serial 3s from 40 O.K.

Abstracting: Good interpretation of "rolling stone gathers no moss."

Very simple math story problems: O.K.

Spelling: Got two fairly simple words correct, but misspelled two others ("Springfed" for Springfield (Illinois capitol) and "Minepolis" for Minneapolis)

General knowledge (also a test of remote memory):
Largest city in Illinois (he lives in the upper midwestern U.S.)? "Chicago." Approximate population? "100 million." (He persisted in this answer in spite of repeated queries.) When I asked him the approximate population of the U.S., he said "3–4 million," then corrected himself and said "maybe a billion." When I then asked him again about Chicago, he said "maybe not 100 million; maybe 50 million."
Most populous country? "China." Four cities in China? "Hong Kong, . . . Singapore, Shanghai . . ." (failed to name a fourth, and Singapore is not in China) (cf. Dr. F's "list" task findings)
Name a few U.S. cities over a million people? "Los Angeles, New York City, Chicago, Miami, Dallas." (The largest city in the U.S.?) "Probably L.A." Population of L.A.? "Over 60 million." Population of Minneapolis metro area? "10 million." Capitol of

Minnesota? "St. Paul." (Largest U.S. state in land area?) "California." When asked about Texas, he said "maybe Texas." When asked about Alaska, he said Texas is larger in land area than Alaska. (I carefully clarified this question, and he persisted in his answer. He was stationed in Alaska for several years.)

Most recent state admitted to the Union? Hawaii.

He recounted the events of September 11, 2001, accurately.

Two cities in India? New Delhi, "Bangladesh," Calcutta.

Three famous authors? Updike, Hemingway, Sinclair Lewis. Books by Hemingway? (named two). Books by Sinclair Lewis or Updike? Unable to name any (not considered a deficit). Three famous modern artists (he is an artist)? "Kadensky" (sic), Pollock, Ebencom (I don't know this artist, nor how to spell his name, but he described his work). Was able to accurately describe the work of both Pollock and Kandensky.

Knew a medical school acronym for naming the cranial nerves (well known to most U.S. physicians). Did not immediately know where the original Mayo Clinic is located (guessed Nebraska), but knew that have a branch in Arizona. Volunteered that Johns Hopkins is in Baltimore.

Current News Knowledge ("What's been in the news lately?"): Troop withdrawal from the Middle East ("What country?") Iran (eventually corrected to Iraq after prompting). Hillary Clinton candidacy for President in 2008. Recent Tsunami. ("Where?") Pacific Rim. ("What countries?") Some islands. Thinks Korea. Not sure of islands.

This performance is consistent with (but does not prove) the premise that Dr. B.'s (*date*) performance on Dr. P.'s tests was, for him, abnormal (contrary to Dr. P.'s interpretation). That is, for example, that some of his "average" results on several tests and subtests may reflect deterioration from earlier higher functioning. Dr. S.'s findings of some three years ago suggest significantly better neuropsychological functioning than Dr. P.'s more recent testing indicates. The older (*year*) results were more consistent with those expected of a practicing physician than were Dr. P.'s (e.g., Dr. S.'s earlier [*year*] findings of "superior" and "very superior" on the WAIS, although there is a *caveat* about the use of an early version of that instrument). (Dr. B. provided a copy of Dr. S.'s [*year*] report and allowed me to include those results in this report.)

FINDINGS AND OPINIONS

NOTE: I have noted elsewhere in this report what I believe to be suggestions of mild dementia. I am not a psychologist or neuropsychologist; however, I am concerned that although Dr. P.'s (*date*) "neuropsychological" report reflects inadequate assessment of some neuropsychological functions, her (*date*) testing did not include any of the complete neuropsychological batteries commonly associated with comprehensive neuropsychological assessment (such as either a Halstead–Reitan or Luria Nebraska battery), and she used abbreviated Wechsler intelligence and memory scales (in addition to several other instruments). I thus do not consider her (*year*) evaluation to be neuropsychologically complete.

Dr. F.'s disability report of (*date*) relied in part on Dr. P.'s testing and findings, and apparently did not review or independently consider Dr. S.'s report or other, more comprehensive, neuropsychological testing.

Specific Questions Asked by ABC Insurance

1. Current Psychiatric Diagnosis(es)
   Axis I: Major depressive disorder, moderate, without psychotic features, in fair remission, with dysthymic and ruminative features.
   R/O mild dementia, type unclear
   Axis II: No diagnosis. Obsessive compulsive and avoidant traits.
   Axis III: R/O source of mild dementia, type unclear.
   Axis IV: Moderate stressors at present (family concerns, concerns about disability payments, remaining malpractice litigation).
   Axis V: Current GAF about 55, based on social and vocational function. Highest in past year at least 60, perhaps higher.

2. Supporting Current Clinical Signs and Symptoms
   Continuing depression, occasional sadness, depressed facies, tearfulness in interview; describes chronically decreased libido; persistent thoughts of helplessness to rescue brother; persistent (but gradually decreasing) feelings of loss regarding medical career and the way he was apparently treated by colleagues; continuing embarrassment about the reasons for losing his practice; decreased concentration in some tasks; poor sleep when off antidepressants; anxiety when contemplating practice situations; relying significantly on obsessive/compulsive traits to structure his life and improve day-to-day functioning; similar symptoms described by estranged wife and treating psychiatrist; antidepressant medication (_____, _____) and clinical support are required to alleviate some symptoms.

   Possible symptoms/signs of mild dementia, which may also be pseudodementia related to depression, include apparent deterioration of both measured and functional I.Q., based on limited recent psychometric testing and some erroneous responses on brief oral testing of knowledge and cognition during my interview.

3. Relevance of Clinical Signs and Symptoms to Work Duties
    The depressive, obsessive, and social-avoidance/intolerance symptoms, signs, and traits significantly affect medical decision-making, professional interactions, practice organization, eligibility for licensure and privileges, etc. The symptoms and signs of dementia, whether organic or "pseudodementia," significantly affect clinical judgment and decision-making as well as eligibility for licensure and privileges.

4. Current Functioning Level
    When he is able and allowed to control his environment to prevent general and idiosyncratic stress, Dr. B. appears to function adequately, but not optimally. He modifies his life significantly to accommodate his psychological needs. He apparently has not had to function very much outside those modifications during the past couple of years, but when he attempted to do so some two years ago (by attempting to return to practice) he was professionally and psychologically unsuccessful.

5. Historical Interest In, and Ability To Perform, Job
    The history prior to about (*year*) indicates strong interest in returning to his former work, although he was unsuccessful when he tried to do so. Prior to about (*year*), his practice abilities and related performance were apparently adequate. (Please see early reports.)

6. Situational vs. Psychiatric Barriers to Return to Work
    The psychiatric barriers described above are substantial, and appear chronic, with regard to (*specialty*); they are less substantial with regard to some relatively nonclinical medical settings (e.g., administration, hospice). Situational barriers include waning of skills due to not practicing for several years, license restrictions related to diagnosis, and probable difficulty getting hospital privileges.

7. Claimant's Outlook About "Getting Better"
    The claimant appears currently to "want" to get better, in the sense of accepting his social/vocational situation. He does not want to return to medical practice, fearing that he will not be able to tolerate it (see "Secondary Gain," below).

8. Secondary Gain
    The claimant freely admits that he no longer wants to return to medical practice, and particularly not to (*specialty*) or other forms of

practice that require rapid decisions. On one hand, his disability payments support that conscious preference. On the other hand, that preference appears to reflect a realistic appraisal of his psychiatric condition and ability to tolerate, and succeed at, medical practice. The history from both the claimant and others indicates that he has reluctantly come to accept his inability to work in this field, earlier forcing himself to keep trying to return to practice regardless of the obstacles. Dr. K., his treating psychiatrist, believes that this acceptance is a good thing, a personal rationalization to help him accept not being the doctor and caregiver he pressed himself to become many years ago. I believe Dr. K.'s view is reasonable.

9. Adequacy of Treatment Plan; Recommendations for Changing Treatment Plan
At this point, I believe the treatment plan is adequate. I do not believe that one should expect any other feasible form of treatment to alleviate Dr. B.'s symptoms more efficiently or to change his personality traits.

10. Other Contributing Medical and/or Non-Medical Factors
None not already outlined above.

11. Presence of Brain Dysfunction, Based on Neuropsychological Testing.
There is sufficient evidence of brain dysfunction to warrant further testing (see details in my history and interview). This claimant should be offered comprehensive neuropsychological testing, by a qualified neuropsychologist, and the results weighed in the context of Dr. B.'s earlier functioning, before being removed from disability status. In my opinion, the (_year_) testing done by Dr. P. is not sufficient to address this need.

Having said the above, my impression of Dr. B.'s behavioral or cognitive impairment is that current findings are consistent with, but do not prove, organically based mild behavioral and cognitive impairment, with concern about future deterioration. My impression of his memory, based solely on limited oral testing and Dr. P.'s testing results notwithstanding, is that his immediate memory is impaired in some respects; his short-term memory appears adequate; and his long-term memory for certain things appears impaired. I cannot speculate on the extent of any deficit, if one exists; neuropsychological testing is recommended.

SOURCES RELIED UPON

- Written materials, represented as everything relevant and available from your office:
  (*list*)
- Neuropsychological testing report (Halstead–Reitan, etc.) by K. S., Ph.D., (*dates*)
- Extended psychiatric examination (*date*) (two sessions, 4 hours, 50 min. total)
- Collateral telephone interviews (with permission)
  (*list*)
- My background, training, and experience in medicine, psychiatry, and forensic psychiatry

QUALIFICATIONS

. . .

R 20

REPORT: EMPLOYEE EMOTIONAL INJURY, TREATER–EXPERT CONFLICT

NOTE: This is a longer federal report that includes criticism of a treater–expert conflict.

RE: **PRELIMINARY REPORT ("Rule 26"):** *A.B. v. C., Inc., et al.*
      U.S. District Court, _____, No. _____
      Your File No. _____

You have asked for a report which summarizes my findings with regard to several topics after review of the materials you provided. I am able to supply the opinions and comments below, based upon those materials and my training, background, and experience. The methods used and materials reviewed are those routinely relied upon by forensic psychiatrists in matters such as this. It should be noted that I have not personally examined Mr. B. or any other party to this action, and that although I am a medical doctor, my comments herein are generally limited to the field of psychiatry. Any additional information received in the future may or may not suggest additions or changes to the opinions below.

FINDINGS AND OPINIONS

The following opinions are offered to a reasonable degree of medical or psychiatric certainty, as I understand the meaning of that phrase, given the information available to me at this time.

A. Mr. B.'s Psychiatric (Mental Health) History Prior to the (date) Accident ("the Accident")

1. There is a great deal of evidence in the record, from a number of sources, that Mr. B. had substantial mental illness, psychiatric symptoms, and reasons for psychiatric symptoms, prior to the accident. The record indicates that he did not respond well to the various treatments offered, sometimes cooperating with them but often missing appointments (but getting prescriptions) and working sporadically with his

treaters, and was chronically unable to function well in work, personal life, and relationships before the accident.

2. The record reflects a great deal of psychiatric treatment and emotional dysfunction over at least 12 years (or "far back as he can go in his memory" [D. evaluation, {*date*}]), including thoughts of suicide and reactions to personal stresses, all prior to the accident. These are documented, for example, by Drs. D., E., F., G., H. (mentioned in Dr. G.'s records), and Veterans Administration clinicians. Dr. D.'s various notes from the year ___, for example, document severe and chronic "major depressive disorder," including no energy, appetite, or motivation, not wanting to leave the house, and "difficulty with reality" (*date*), as well as alcohol abuse or addiction and past abuse of, or addiction to, street drugs (heroin, cocaine, marijuana, LSD, PCP, and sniffing spray paint) and abuse of federally controlled prescription drugs. The latter, except for alcohol and prescription drug abuse, were said to have occurred primarily many years before. (See Dr. D.'s records from (*dates*) and his deposition statements [e.g., pp. 32–34]). Dr. G.'s records from (*dates*), for example, contain many notes of severe personal stressors, marital and child custody problems, depression, and suicidal thoughts (see, e.g., G 044–112). His symptoms are sometimes described as improved, but his participation in treatment is generally sporadic, with visits to many different physicians and mental health professionals.

    Dr. D. states that he does not recall giving Mr. B. any diagnosis of Post-Traumatic Stress Disorder ("PTSD") while seeing him prior to the accident (deposition p. 35). Mr. B. mentioned military service in the general history, but he apparently did not highlight it during treatment. When speaking of his impressions after the accident, however, Dr. D. states (pp. 35–37) that Mr. B. was exposed to significantly threatening situations in the Army and "experiencing his buddies in combat being seriously injured or killed" (but agrees that he has never seen any of his patient's military records). Nevertheless, Dr. D. now states that Mr. B. has PTSD from his Viet Nam experience (D. [*date*] report; deposition p. 38).

    With the exception of acute reactions to the accident and leg problems and PTSD diagnoses which generally appear <u>after</u> the accident, Mr. B.'s overall <u>pre-accident</u> level of psychosocial function (often appearing in the record as "global assessment of functioning" or "GAF"), symptomatology, and diagnoses are generally similar to, and occasionally worse than, those which appears in the record after the accident (especially after the amputation). Dr. D., for example, estimates his GAF on (*date*) as about 50 (100 being best), the same functional level he estimated in his initial post-accident report (which he changed to "40" in a report addendum signed (*date*) (D. deposition, p. 51). VA clinicians estimated both his acute and chronic ("highest in past year") functioning as 55 (VAMC 121). In deposition, Dr. D. explains the similarity of the GAF estimates as indicating that Mr. B. was very symptomatic on (*date*), then improved, then worsened because of the accident and its sequelae, and is not expected to improve again (p. 56). It should be noted, however, that Mr. B.'s GAF was often (but not exclusively) documented as low before the accident.

The lowest GAF I found in the <u>post-accident</u> records the accident was 40, entered by a counselor (*date*) (F 008). The next day a psychiatrist, Dr. I., estimated the GAF as "41/50," apparently indicating 41 at that moment, with the highest in the past year—which would include the two months before the accident—being 50 (F 024). Other post-accident estimates are 50 or above.

The psychiatric medications prescribed in the years before the accident were similar to—and sometimes at higher doses than—those prescribed after the accident. His pre-accident dosage of _____, an anti-anxiety medication, for example, was generally higher than his post-accident dose (see, e.g., Dr. E.'s (*date*) evaluation at E 003).

3.   The considerable substance abuse in Mr. B.'s past is likely to have had a permanent adverse effect on his brain and cognition. In particular, even a few weeks of prolonged "huffing" (sniffing to intoxication) of aromatic hydrocarbons such as spray paint is likely to have damaged his brain. There is no pre-accident neuropsychological testing in the record, which makes it difficult to verify any additional effect from the accident by means of post-accident testing. One should also note Mr. B.'s pre-accident head injury from a (*date*) assault and his abnormal MRI and CT scans at that time. (<u>Note</u> that, although I am generally familiar with some neuropsychological principles, I am not an expert in neuropsychological testing or interpretation.) Finally, a handwritten autobiographical statement apparently written in early (*year*) suggests below average verbal intelligence (K 043), although it should not be considered a complete test of verbal ability. (See discussion of psychological testing, below.)

4.   Mr. B. was sometimes considered disabled, and apparently psychiatrically disabled, at some times before the accident. He was not working at the time of the accident. Dr. D. refers to "disability money" in early (*date*) (apparently actually worker's compensation). Dr. E. drafted a letter for Mr. B. supporting some sort of psychiatric impairment on (*date*) (G 154).

5.   Contrary to the plaintiff's statements about his extensive pre-accident recreational activities, Dr. D.'s (*date*) evaluation states that there was nothing he enjoyed and he had no interests. Similarly, VA medical records of (*date*) indicate that Mr. B. said he " ... used to play golf, fish, (but) doesn't do anything now ... " (VAMC 067).

6. The record indicates that Mr. B. had substantial problems with interpersonal relationships before the accident. In particular, he appears to have had great difficulty in his marriages and in parenting his children. He appears to have abandoned custody of one child (*name*), lost custody of several others, was accused of molesting a daughter, and was told by an adult daughter that she wanted nothing to do with him (see, e.g., Dr. D.'s interviews [*dates*]; updated report [*date*]; G 078). (Note that the molestation allegation was described by Mr. B. as occurring in the context of a child custody battle [e.g., at S 012]; there are no details or corroboration in the records available to me.)

    In addition to the implication that pre-accident psychiatric problems interfered with parenting and relationships, divorce and child custody battles are often cited in the pre-accident records as sources of great stress and psychiatric symptoms (such as depression).

7. Mr. B.'s pre-accident psychiatric diagnoses and symptoms are sometimes (but not always) recorded as more severe than those after the accident. For example, Dr. E.'s diagnoses in (*date*) include "Major Depressive Disorder, recurrent, severe," compared to Dr. J.'s (*date*) (J 014) "Major Depressive Disorder, recurrent, moderate" (plus adjustment disorder and pain disorder associated with both psychological and physical factors) and Dr. D.'s post-accident billings are simply for "Adjustment Disorder." Dr. J. diagnosed him as having "??? BPD Depressive, severe . . . " among other diagnoses in (*date*).

    There are extensive pre-accident records of chronic anxiety and panic attacks, sometimes associated with substantial psychosomatic complaints (e.g., "tremendous problems with anxiety . . . profound anxiety with features of panic . . . overwhelming fear of having a cardiac event or having a stroke . . . " G 053) for which he was given moderately large doses of _____.

8. There are other, nonpsychiatric conditions which predate the accident and would be expected to cause social and/or psychiatric problems regardless of the accident and its sequelae. In particular, Mr. B.'s had (and still has) hepatitis C, a very serious liver condition. His levels of general stressors were often documented as "severe" before the accident, worse than, or comparable to, those following his physical recovery after the accident (excepting perhaps the loss of his leg) (see, e.g., E 004).

B. Likelihood of conflict of interest when a treating clinician (such as Dr. D. or Dr. K.) offers opinions (especially expert opinions) about his patient

There is a great deal of potential for conflict of interest—both conscious and unconscious—when a clinician such as Dr. D. performs a "forensic" evaluation and offers opinions about someone whom he has treated within a doctor–patient relationship, and whom he may anticipate treating after the legal matter has been resolved.

First, the doctor–patient relationship itself creates a strong duty to the patient (to act solely in the patient's interest), which conflicts with and arguably exceeds one's duty of objectivity to a court. Dr. D. treated Mr. B. for some time, both before and after his accident, in a somewhat intimate setting of psychiatric treatment and psychotherapy.

Second, the doctor–patient relationship implies an element of mutual trust between clinician and patient, and often an acceptance of the patient's statements at face value. Relying substantially on that trust to provide accurate information, which treating clinicians often do, is inappropriate when assessing a person who reasonably may have motivations other than (or in addition to) an ordinary request for care (such as in this lawsuit). In addition to the strong <u>potential</u> for such a conflict, there is evidence that this actually happened in both Dr. D.'s report (see below) and his accessions to Mr. B.'s request for support in previous DUI litigation.

Third, treating clinicians rarely have access to the broader picture of their patients' litigation, and they may not realize the need for additional, corroborative information and/or may not provide a court with disclaimers and caveats about its absence.

Other elements of potential conflict exist, and are described in the professional literature.[1]

C. Validity Concerns Raised in Plaintiff's Post-Accident Assessments and Reports

1. <u>Treater–evaluator and treater–expert conflict</u>. (See discussion above.)
2. <u>Reliance on Mr. B.'s own statements, including credibility and subjectivity issues</u>. Many of the opinions and other comments made by plaintiff's witnesses to support damage and causation in their reports, and at deposition, appear based in the plaintiff's own statements rather than in objective or corroborated data. In the absence of caveats or disclaimers regarding the possibility (or likelihood) of erroneous,

---

1 See, e.g., Strasburger, L. H., Gutheil, T. G., and Brodsky, A. (1997) On wearing two hats: role conflict in serving as both psychotherapist and expert witness, *American Journal of Psychiatry* 154(4): 448–456; Reid, W. H. (1998) Treating clinicians & expert testimony, *Journal of Practical Psychiatry and Behavioral Health* 4(2): 121–123; Shuman, D. W., Greenberg, S., Heilbrun, K., and Foote, W. E. (1998) Special perspective: an immodest proposal: should treating mental health professionals be barred from testifying about their patients? *Behavioral Sciences and the Law* 16(4): 509–523; Gutheil, T. G., and Hilliard J. T. (2001) The treating psychiatrist thrust into the role of expert witness, *Psychiatric Services* 52(11): 1526–1527.

incomplete, or misleading information, such reliance is often below the professionally accepted forensic practice standard.

Mr. B. has considerable experience with mental health professionals. It is likely that he knows many of the symptoms of the mental disorders in his records. It is fair to say, without impugning Mr. B.'s honesty unless his statements are actually purposely misleading, that the highly subjective nature of the symptoms of PTSD, of many symptoms of depression and anxiety, and of many other psychiatric damages he alleges makes it fairly easy for plaintiffs to mislead evaluators who rely substantially on their statements.

Having said the above, it should be added that not all <u>inaccurate</u> information from patients or evaluees indicates <u>dishonest</u> information. Patients and evaluees may misunderstand their symptoms and past histories, their memories may be flawed, and/or their psychiatric conditions may impair their ability to be accurate.

Further comments on questions regarding Mr. B.'s credibility are found elsewhere in this report.

3. <u>Dr. D.'s</u> (*date*) <u>report and its</u> (*date*) <u>addendum</u>. Dr. D.'s report appears unusual to me. For example, parts of it refer to Dr. D. in the third person (e.g., "data from his current evaluation by Dr. D.," "evaluative sessions of Dr. D."). Much of the wording seems unusual for a psychiatrist (e.g., incomplete titles of diagnoses, erroneous title of the *Diagnostic and Statistical Manual of Mental Disorders*). The signature lines on the two addenda are unusual for a communication from a psychiatrist. Although there is little doubt that he signed the report himself, it seems likely that some or all of it was composed by someone else, perhaps the plaintiff's attorney. If that is true, it would appear that Dr. D. did not review the report carefully before signing it.

4. <u>Dr. K.'s psychological assessment and testing</u>. I am concerned that Dr. K.'s assessment is largely subjective, omits important evaluation elements, and is subject to error from inaccurate answers by Mr. B., absence of exploration of important topics, failure of corroboration by other reasonably available sources, and misinterpretation of some of the instruments.

Several of the sessions Dr. K. conducted with Mr. B. were completely undocumented (K. deposition pp. 7, 16, 24, etc.)—a significant problem when one attempts to use the information gathered to establish or support facts and opinions in a lawsuit. Dr. K. did not contact other treating professionals for additional history or corroboration, and said at deposition that he had not reviewed any of Mr. B.'s psychological, psychiatric, or medical records (pp. 35, 44). Mr. B. apparently did not describe his extensive pre-accident psychiatric history except in the brief intake form, and Dr. K. apparently didn't ask very much about his past (cf. K. deposition pp. 7–9, 21, 22, etc.). Without representing that I am an expert in psychological testing, it is obvious that much of the assessment simply consisted of asking Mr. B. what his problems were and relying on his answers, even though Dr. K. knew he was engaged in litigation.

Mr. B.'s (*date*) Minnesota Multiphasic Personality Inventory (MMPI-2) scores indicated problems with testing validity (e.g., that Mr. B.'s answers tended to overestimate his symptoms) (K 038). However, the computer-generated interpretation said that the assessment profile was "valid" and that "there may be some tendency on the part of the client to . . . exaggerate his symptoms in an effort to obtain help" (033) (underlining mine). It must be noted that further examination of the assessment reveals, however, that the computer apparently came to that conclusion ("in order to obtain help") because Dr. K. failed to enter the assessment *setting* into the scoring program. The program erroneously assumed that Mr. B. was an ordinary patient rather than an evaluee engaged in litigation (035, 040). I recommend that the psychological testing be reviewed by an independent clinical psychologist who has expertise in use of these instruments in forensic matters.

Dr. K. appears to misunderstand or misstate some concepts related to Post-Traumatic Stress Disorder (PTSD). For example, he states that the "basic PTSD diagnosis comes from . . . Viet Nam" (deposition p. 38) (it does not). His definition of a PTSD "flashback" (p. 46) is inaccurate (see actual definition, DSM-IV-TR, p. 464). There is some suggestion that Dr. K. expected Mr. B. to have PTSD based simply on his statements that he had seen combat in Viet Nam).

Dr. K.'s estimates of prognosis and future treatment need appear highly speculative. First, he does not separate prognosis or treatment of Mr. B.'s chronic pre-accident conditions from that of any accident-related conditions or symptoms. Second, Dr. K. appears to give little o no consideration to the likelihood that (a) physical improvement, (b) resolution of the lawsuit, and (c) passage of time will have positive effects on Mr. B.'s psychiatric and psychosocial symptoms. (Physical improvement is documented in the more recent record.)

Third, he relies on a speculation that "real intensive psychological treatment" will "dramatically" improve Mr. B.'s symptoms (deposition pp. 54–56). In fact, however, Mr. B.'s pre-accident history indicates that psychological treatments have met with limited success. Most of his psychological problems—both pre- and post-accident, and excluding acute problems of accident-related pain and adjustment to his amputation—appear based largely in his pre-existing personality style or disorder (cf. E 005), chronic depression and chronic anxiety, and perhaps mild brain damage, which all existed before the accident. Dr. K. fails to mention that Mr. B. chose not to participate actively in most of the treatments offered, and that persons with Mr. B.'s background, measured intelligence, and treatment history are usually considered poor candidates for what Dr. K. recommends as "very intensive outpatient psychotherapy . . . meeting several times a week."

This is not to say that efforts at appropriate psychological support and development of improved coping styles and skills, as alluded to in Dr. K.'s deposition, p. 46, would necessarily be fruitless, assuming a motivated patient. A focused cognitive-behavioral approach could be useful as well.

5. Dr. D.'s prognosis and estimates of treatment costs. I must be similarly critical of Dr. D.'s comments about the costs of future psychiatric care. Predictions that a patient will need, much less benefit from, "13 years of weekly sessions" appear to be complete speculation. I can see absolutely no basis for estimating the time of his return to work as six years hence. The estimate of medication need and costs, and the method apparently used to arrive at it, appears completely invalid to me (e.g., speaking with a local pharmacist about the cost of current medications). Dr. D. notes that these are "estimates," and "recognize[s his] limitations"; however, such unfounded statements, in my opinion, do not belong in a report that one expects to be relied upon by a jury.

6. Dr. D.'s billing records for the treatment sessions after the accident (*dates*) gave a diagnosis of Adjustment Disorder, Predominant Symptoms Unspecified (DSM-IV-TR 303.90) rather than PTSD. Dr. D. also specifically stated in the insurance forms, on each occasion, that the condition being treated was not related to an auto accident. Similarly, although the accident is mentioned in a pain workup, Dr. K.L.'s (*date*) _____ billing claim form states that the condition being treated was not accident-related.

7. Other psychological and neuropsychological testing. Although I am not a neuropsychologist, I am concerned about Dr. M.'s conclusions and his estimates of pre-accident function, especially in the absence of a complete neuropsychological battery and pre-accident baseline neuropsychological testing. I recommend independent review of Dr. M.'s (*date*) testing and report by a certified neuropsychologist with forensic experience.

Dr. M.'s testing was interpreted as indicating, among other interpretations, that Mr. B.'s current intellectual functioning is somewhat lower than his "estimated premorbid (i.e., pre-accident) ability" (undated report from (*date*) evaluation, p. 6). However, when the two are compared (admittedly superficially, since the raw data are not provided and I am not an expert in psychological testing), Dr. M. states that the "estimated" pre-accident intellectual functioning ranged from "average" to "borderline" and actual post-accident test performance indicated a low-average verbal IQ and a borderline performance IQ.

Mr. B.'s post-accident deposition performance appears inconsistent with Dr. M.'s opinions about his post-accident verbal intellectual functioning. Mr. B.'s deposition answers, comments, and vocabulary appear to be those of a person with roughly average verbal intelligence. (See, e.g., B. deposition pp. 8, 24, 44, 51, 66, 102 on [*date*], and pp. 34, 36, 39 on [*date*].)

D. Issues of Mr. B.'s Credibility to Clinicians and the Court

I am concerned about the credibility of some of Mr. B.'s statements. There were, and are, psychiatric damages related to both the loss of his leg and the long process through which the loss occurred. However, lawsuits such as this one necessarily involve motivations that compete with accuracy and honesty. There are opportunities for gain such as personal attention, financial benefit, establishment of disability, and lessening of unpleasant personal responsibilities, as well as resolution of unconscious psychological conflict separate from the effects of the accident and pressures to meet the expectations of others (including one's spouse and even one's attorney). As a jury attempts to come to the truth of this matter, it is fair to consider the following.

1. The record indicates that Mr. B. has presented his social and psychiatric symptoms in different ways to different people. Much of what he describes is poorly verifiable in the records available to me.

2. There is evidence that Mr. B. has been dishonest in important ways at some times in his past, for example in his drug abuse and other behavior. While this does not prove that he is being dishonest in the current case, it is reasonable for either an evaluator or a jury to consider those factors when assessing his credibility.

3. There is evidence that at least some of his doctors have been concerned about Mr. B.'s abusing addictive medications prior to the accident, and that he tried to manipulate his physicians into prescribing more than they believed appropriate. (See below, Dr. D.'s records, Dr. E.'s records at P-E. 004-007.)

4. Dr. D.'s records prior to the accident indicate situations in which Mr. B. appeared to try to manipulate him in order to get things he wanted (such as additional _____ without coming in to the office, when Dr. D. was concerned about the amount he was taking). In particular, Mr. B. appears to have talked Dr. D. into writing a letter to help him defend against either one or two DUI charges (B. deposition p. 90), blaming medications he was taking that he claimed made him appear intoxicated (some of which, I believe, were not even prescribed by Dr. D.). Dr. D.'s (*date*) progress note states that he and the patient reviewed the wording of the letter together before it was sent (as contrasted with Dr. D.'s writing it himself). Dr. D. apparently

changed some of the wording before finalizing it, and Mr. B. "was upset" about the alterations and "wanted an explanation" for the doctor's not writing exactly what Mr. B. wished.

5. Without meaning to diminish the actual impact and damage of the accident, Mr. B.'s description of the accident to post-accident treaters and plaintiff's experts suggests a more severe crash than apparently occurred. He generally describes the C. truck as a "semi" (e.g., in Dr. J.'s (date) evaluation [J 004] and the _____ intake (date) [006]). He gives the impression that the truck hit him at a high rate of speed.

   It is my understanding, however, from available reports (the N. analysis and _____ Police report) that the truck was much smaller, such as a "delivery truck"; it pulled into his lane soon after having stopped (or almost stopped) at a stop sign; it was traveling fairly slowly; and Mr. B. was driving at neighborhood speeds. The police report indicates that the box truck hit the front right corner of Mr. B.'s van after swerving to try to miss it. The N. analysis suggests that the C. truck was already in the intersection as Mr. B. approached. The police report states that Mr. B. was not wearing the shoulder portion of his seat belt. Mr. B. says at deposition that he remembers unlatching his seat belt after the accident. I have not seen the initial T. analysis. (Note that I am not an expert in accident reconstruction or investigation.)

6. Mr. B.'s statements about his military service and the traumas he says he experienced in Viet Nam appear inconsistent in the record. Sometimes the records suggest that he mentioned his service almost in passing (e.g., Dr. D., (date); at other times he apparently stated that he experienced various forms of combat (e.g., Dr. J., [date], which implies "combat [for] two years" [J. 0022]).

   He states that he was "drafted into the service" during "my senior year" of high school (autobiography, K 021). However, so far as I know, high school students were never drafted during the Viet Nam conflict.

   On several occasions, Mr. B. told clinicians that he was an Army clerk-technician (e.g., K 033, in which he said he was drafted, assigned to the Army, and served as an "E1 to E3"). However, he wrote on his (date) _____ Psychiatric Services intake that he had been a boiler technician in the Navy (_____ 010). He told Dr. J. that his military occupation (MOS) was artillary (an Army MOS) (J 044). (Note that servicemen may have a combat-related MOS in addition to their primary one.) He states that he received an "honorable" discharge, but does not describe the type. He stated on Dr. K.'s intake form that he had problems while in the military and was reduced in rank at least once (K 004).

Mr. B. stated at various times, largely or entirely after the accident, that he saw combat in Viet Nam. He implies, at different times and to different clinicians, that his main Viet Nam trauma was (a) some sort of landmine locating duty in which he saw many comrades blown up doing such work, (b) being bayonetted in the leg during a medical rescue mission, and (c) "killing a woman and child" (_[date]_; _____ 015).

Available VA records list his symptoms as "NSC," which I take to mean "non-service-connected." Those records do not mention any Viet Nam service, combat service, or PTSD symptoms or diagnosis.

Neither clinical nor forensic evaluators in this case appear to have questioned Mr. B.'s statements about military service and trauma. Dr. K. avoided exploring his service history altogether during a lengthy evaluation because Mr. B. "preferred to focus on his leg." Dr. K. listed three "problems" on (_date_): his leg, his divorce, and "Viet Nam issues," but omitted Mr. B.'s hepatitis C status, finances, losses of his children, pre-existing depression and anxiety syndromes, and medication/drug problems. (See, e.g., Dr. M.'s [_date_] report; Dr. K. at K 010; K. deposition p. 37.)

Without meaning to unnecessarily impugn Mr. B.'s statements or his service traumas if they actually occurred, it must be said that individuals' reports of military combat, injury, and other trauma are often exaggerated or fabricated in the interest of personal gain, and that inconsistency of statements is one sign of fabrication. The above comments should not be construed as opinions that Mr. B. did not serve in Viet Nam, serve in combat, and/or experience the traumas he has described, but they raise reasonable questions about his statements. I have been told by counsel that Mr. B.'s official military service records (such as military occupation, theater assignment, records of injury, disciplinary record, circumstances of discharge, and early VA records)—not merely statements found in medical records—are not yet available for review.

7. Mr. B.'s allegations that the accident and resulting injury have rekindled and worsened post-traumatic symptoms from his stated Viet Nam service are not supported by the available VA records. Indeed, there is no mention of Viet Nam service in the available VA records. Although early VA records (presumably psychiatric ones) exist but are not yet available (VAMC 012), VA records of (_date_) (prior to the accident) state that his psychiatric problems were "NSC," which I take to mean "non-service-connected" (VAMC 012, 051). In other words, the VA clinicians, who are generally very sensitive to service-connected post-traumatic symptoms and disorders (such as those which might occur during combat service in Viet Nam) documented no such history in Mr. B.'s case.

8. Mr. B. appears to have omitted significant facts from some of his interactions with both treating clinicians and evaluators. For example, when focusing on damages <u>after</u> the accident, he generally fails to mention pre-accident complaints that he was severely assaulted ("mugged") around (*date*). At that time, he described significant head trauma, although the doctors whose records I reviewed did not document details. MRI and CT scans revealed old, apparently minor, brain abnormalities (a lacunar infarct deep in the brain) and noted recent damage to one eye socket and a sinus (including, according to Mr. B.'s statement to Dr. O. when he called to request pain medication, a facial fracture). There is no mention of any police report or direct documentation of the assault. (See, e.g., Dr. G.'s [*date*]; notes at G. 033, 036, 043; Dr. O. at G. 100).

9. A _____ Psychiatric Clinic intake document, apparently completed by Mr. B. himself around (date) (10 months after the [*date*] accident), described many "emotional, behavioral, or interpersonal problems," including "cancer" in remission (not mentioned previously in the record <u>and for which there is no evidence found in my review</u>). He also listed "immune problems" (apparently not noted elsewhere in the record) and says he "can't make it to bathroom in time" (no mention of urinary or fecal urgency or incontinence was found elsewhere in the record). He lists a number of items that may contribute to his problems, in the following order: "ex-wife, lawsuit papers, IRS, not seeing my children, not being able to walk, dealing with attorneys, don't trust attorney or doctor."

   The same intake form indicates that he drinks "14 cups" of coffee a day, has stopped alcohol and illegal drugs (as listed), and that "I'll go into detox (for highly addictive prescription painkillers) when this goes away" (see also _____ 006). (High caffeine intake is commonly associated with significant anxiety.) Later on the same form, when asked to describe serious or longstanding illnesses he has had, he states "depression, unhappiness, going to Viet Nam @ 18 yr. old & killing woman & child, not knowing how to act after the war, who to trust, insecure, bad dreams, liver disease, not equal to other people, panic attacks, reflux."

10. There is indication in the post-accident record that some treating clinicians are confused or frustrated by Mr. B. and/or his apparent clinical presentation. For example, Dr. P, an orthopedist, states in a (*date*) office evaluation that he is concerned about the unusual course of the patient's recovery, his continuing requirement for high doses of oxycontin, and that Mr. B. "has been fired or released from the care of Dr. Q." (J 019), a psychiatrist. (I have not been provided with Dr. Q.'s records, and have no further information about whether or not the patient was "fired"; however, such a comment is very unusual in my experience of record review.)

11. If Mr. B.'s descriptions of his symptoms are exaggerated, those exaggerations (to the extent that they exist) are not restricted to post-accident statements. Over a decade before the accident, in a cardiac consultation by Dr. R., Mr. B. apparently described specific and severe cardiac symptoms treated in an emergency room. <u>When Dr. R. reviewed the actual hospital record, he found that there was no such serious event</u>, although Mr. B. was seen there (G 220–222). (Note that the motivation for this exaggeration or misrepresentation, assuming it occurred as documented, is not clear, and may be related to anxiety and overwhelming health concerns; there is no indication of personal gain in the record reviewed.)

PREPARED EXHIBITS
None anticipated.

SOURCES REVIEWED/RELIED UPON

- Written materials as follows, represented to me as all available from your office:
  (*list*)
- My background, training, and experience in medicine, psychology, psychiatry, and forensic psychiatry

QUALIFICATIONS AND PUBLICATIONS
. . .

MY COMPENSATION
. . .

CASES IN WHICH I HAVE TESTIFIED DURING THE PAST FOUR YEARS
. . .

R21

REPORT: PROFESSIONAL LICENSING AGENCY REVIEW

NOTE: The format was dictated by the requesting agency.

RE: A.B., M.D.; (*Medical Licensing Agency*) case file no. _____
   Physician consultant review

I have reviewed all of the materials received regarding the above case (see list below). Following is my report.

A. **Qualifications**. I am a general and forensic psychiatrist with experience in clinical, forensic and administrative psychiatry. I am certified by all relevant U.S. Boards or organizations in general, forensic, and administrative psychiatry. I have worked with many _____ (*medical licensing agency*) (MLA) matters, both as an agent of (*the agency*) and as an agent of licensee attorneys. A copy of my current *curriculum vitae* is attached to the transmittal email for this report.

B. **Issues**. Patient C.D. accused Dr. B. of prescribing mistakes.

C. **Material Reviewed** (from the MLA file for this case).
(*list*)

D. **Academic Sources**. None consulted.

E. **Facts**. Based on the materials reviewed, Dr. B. saw the patient several times, performed an evaluation on the first visit and diagnosed significant depression, and prescribed treatment. Dr. B. scheduled subsequent follow-up visits, at which her condition was reviewed, treatment adjustments were made, and antidepressant medication (among other medications) prescribed. The prescriptions were communicated to the patient's pharmacy. The patient sometimes did not schedule appointments as recommended. Late in her care, perhaps associated with confusion involving the pharmacy and/or Dr. B.'s office, the patient complained to the MLA that Dr. B. had made a prescribing error. She added that Dr. B. sometimes did not remember her and had to consult her records. She apparently rescinded or recanted that complaint to his office (but perhaps not to the MLA). Dr. B. contends that the pharmacy admitted fault in dispensing. The patient contacted Dr. B. for an additional prescription after the above events and allegations. There is no allegation that the patient was injured in any way as a result of any prescription or prescribing behavior of either Dr. B. or the pharmacy. There is no allegation that Dr. B. abandoned or was disrespectful to the patient.

F. Standard of Care. The statutory reference for this case is 164.051 (a) (6) (referring to practice inconsistent with the public health and welfare. The specific issue is "care/treatment and medication dosage confusion for patient C.D . . . in (*month, year*)."

The standard of care requires adequate evaluation, treatment, follow-up, and documentation, including, when medications are prescribed, appropriate prescribing of medication and communication to the dispensing pharmacy.

G. Application of the Standard of Care. The record available to me describes adequate evaluation, diagnosis, treatment (including prescriptions), and follow-up, as well as Dr. B.'s comments about the patient's condition, potential concerns, demeanor, and treatment compliance.

H. Conclusions. The materials supplied to me indicate that the standard of care was not violated in this case. Nothing in the materials received, other than the complainant's original statement, suggests otherwise. In addition, there is no indication that the patient was injured in any way as a result of any prescription or prescribing behavior of either Dr. B. or the pharmacy. There is no indication that Dr. B. mistreated, abandoned, or was disrespectful to the patient.

R22

REPORT: PROFESSIONAL LICENSING AGENCY REVIEW

RE: **REPORT: Matter of A.B., M.D.**

You have asked for a report which summarizes my findings after review of the materials you provided in the above matter, with regard to the following question: "Would allowing Dr. B. to practice medicine or surgery in (*state*) treaten the health or safety of patients or the public."

You have noted that some of the Agency staff's concerns (and their bases) include (but may not be limited to) Dr. B.'s failure to comply with a (*medical licensing agency*) (MLA) requirement to see Dr. C.D. (his monitor assigned by MLA), and increasing concerns for Dr. B.'s mental fitness and/ or stability as manifested in emails, recent criminal charges, and what you describe as a preoccupation with a conspiracies against him.

I am able to supply the comments and opinions below, based upon all the materials you provided and my training, background, and experience. The methods used and materials reviewed are those routinely relied upon by forensic psychiatrists in matters such as this. This report refers in part to apparent symptoms, signs, and the behaviors and communications that appear associated with them, but should not be construed as a complete evaluation of the individual or his medical practice.

Disclaimer. One should note that I have not examined Dr. B. personally, nor have I reviewed any direct records of his own psychiatric care (other than letters from his psychiatrist to the MLA, which may or may not have been composed in collaboration with Dr. B.), office notes of monitoring psychiatrist Dr. D., any of Dr. B.'s patient care records, or statements from persons such as family or office staff who may be in a position to describe his behavior under various relevant circumstances. I have not seen any deposition or other sworn testimony by either Dr. B. or relevant clinicians (other than a purported draft "affidavit" and "motion" which Dr. B. apparently composed and sent to various persons). I do not offer any specific diagnosis of Dr. B.

FINDINGS AND OPINIONS

After review of the materials provided, the following opinions are offered to a reasonable degree of medical or psychiatric certainty given the information available to me at this time, and assuming the general accuracy and representative nature of those materials.

1. Many of the behaviors illustrated in the materials available to me are highly consistent with substantially impaired judgment, insight, impulse control, and/or reality testing (ability to interpret situations using objective comparing of an emotion or thought against real life) (see below). Dr. B.'s behavior often suggests misperceptions or delusions of persecution or grandiosity which interfere with his ability to assess at least some relevant situations accurately.

2. The extent of the impairments indicated in the available record is sufficient to generate significant concern about danger to the health of Dr. B.'s patients or the public because of reasonably foreseeable acts or omissions by Dr. B. That is, the record indicates a number of instances of poor judgment, limited insight, significant misperception of situations, and the like, which, although not all taken from patient care settings (see below), suggest substantial risk that those characteristics are or will be present in patient care. It is not my role to decide as a matter of fact or law whether damage to patients has occurred or will occur, but it is my opinion that there is substantial risk (see below).

3. The characteristics described in the record are highly consistent with symptoms of Delusional Disorder (DSM-IV-TR 297.1), a condition that generally interferes markedly with some aspects of a patient's life but often much less with others. Although some people with delusional disorder do not have serious problems with the law or injure others, it is not a benign condition. It is very difficult to treat, it interferes substantially with judgment and insight, and the associated delusions and inappropriate behaviors routinely incorporate additional people or situations over time.

4. Some of the characteristics described in the record are also consistent with other conditions and/or situations, including, but not necessarily limited to, (a) personality or behavior change due to medication effect or substance abuse, (b) Bipolar I Disorder (296.7), and (c) personality or behavior change associated with a general medical condition.

    (a) Dr. B. has taken illicit psychoactive drugs in the past, many of which (e.g., _____, _____) can cause or precipitate paranoia and other serious psychiatric symptoms. Drug-related psychiatric symptoms, when they occur, may be limited to the presence of the drug in the body or may be "kindled" by the drug and remain long after its elimination. The record is not entirely clear with regard to current or very recent substance abuse.

(b) Bipolar Disorder, manic or hypomanic phase, is often associated with paranoia, grandiosity, hypersexuality, and/or irritability, but there is routinely a broader panoply of symptoms and a different disease pattern and course than appears in the records available to me.

(c) <u>Personality or behavior change associated with a general medical condition</u> can be difficult to recognize, but the general medical condition (or its association with psychiatric symptoms) usually becomes more obvious over time (cf. thyroid conditions, vascular dementias, cerebral masses). The record mentions, but does not expound upon, some past and present general medical conditions and their treatments.

5. Some of the behavior and communication in the record is consistent with simple misbehavior (including illegal behavior) which, although incorporating some psychiatric traits, may be more accurately viewed as antisocial or asocial rather than something "clinical." Not all irritating or allegedly illegal, harmful, bullying, threatening, misrepresenting, or confused behavior is related to a "psychiatric" diagnosis.

During appointments with his monitor, Dr. D., Dr. B.'s explanations for his many inappropriate letters and emails appeared to indicate poor judgment and lack of foresight at the least, and an apparent intent to besmirch the reputations of the people about whom he wrote. Dr. D. said in his (*date*) report to MLA: "overall, he (Dr. B.) realizes he does not have actual solid evidence for his various claims ... [he says that] what evidence he does have is sometimes 'hidden' ... he also said at one point that even if some of his vitriolic statements about these people aren't true, they still 'deserve whatever they get'." In that record, Dr. B. said the emails (which I have not seen, but which were summarized by Dr. D.) were "poking fun" or "a form of political satire" (all quotes from Dr. D.; Bates 57–77 [*date*]); however, the content appeared deliberately accusatory and hurtful to the persons named.

Having said the above, **the overall description of Dr. B.'s behaviors and communications available to me suggests some form of mental impairment, either alone or in addition to nonpsychiatric conditions.**

6. The record indicates that Dr. B. may have violated basic tenets of patient confidentiality, which, if true, suggests poor judgment, difficulty adhering to that requirement of ethical patient care, and/or simple malice.

For example, (a) the record describes Dr. B.'s discussing one of his patients with another patient; (b) he used the appellation "patient" along with names and other identifying information in several multi-recipient emails to nonclinicians, and (c) he described various named people as patients or former patients in communications complaining about political issues. Although the facts are very persuasive, it is not absolutely clear to me whether or not each of these persons (except "_____") was really Dr. B.'s patient (rather than someone else's), had consented to identification as a patient, or was actually represented by a pseudonym.

7. **The record indicates that Dr. B. may have violated basic tenets prohibiting patient exploitation, which, if true, suggests inadequate judgment and/or difficulty understanding and adhering to a requirement of ethical patient care.** For example, the record indicates that he asked "_____" to "pay for my [Dr. B.'s] theatre tickets and hotel" (for a political fundraiser) "as payment for medical services given."

    The record indicates that Dr. B. sometimes attempted to wreak some sort of punishment on patients who irritated him. For example, he apparently told Dr. D. that he arranged for one of his patients to "flatten the tires" of another of his patients who had "pissed him off" (see Dr. D.'s report).

8. **The record contains no indication that Dr. B. has been seen by C.D., M.D. (his monitoring psychiatrist) since (*date several months before*), in spite of MLA requirements to be seen at least monthly.** Dr. D.'s communications to MLA, and MLA records, indicate that Dr. B. is well aware that he is required to see Dr. D. at least once a month, but has not done so.

SOURCES RELIED UPON

- Written or recorded materials as follows, represented to me as all which are relevant and available from your office:
  (*list*)

- My background, training, and experience in medicine, psychiatry, and forensic psychiatry

QUALIFICATIONS

. . .

R23

OPINION LETTER: PROFESSIONAL LICENSURE

NOTE: This is a letter to an attorney who asked if I could support his advice to his physician-client that a licensing agency settlement offer was in his best interest.

RE: **Dr. A., Matter of license restriction**

You have asked for my comments or opinions after review of the materials you provided (below), as well as two conversations with you about Dr. A.'s situation. I can provide the comments below, with the understanding that they are based upon the materials available to me and my background, training, and experience. I am not a (*respondent's specialty*). My comments are related to clear inferences of behavioral or psychiatric problems. As you know, I have not interviewed Dr. A., nor do I have personal experience with the (*state physician licensing agency*); my comments are based in part upon past work with other medical licensing agencies and with physician licensees/defendants, both on behalf of the agencies and on behalf of the physicians.

<u>I believe the offer made in the unsigned settlement agreement which I reviewed is very generous</u>. It is not easy to receive Board discipline, or to accept the several restrictions in the pending Agreement. They would significantly limit Dr. A.'s practice options. However, I agree with the Board that those restrictions are necessary. They are likely to be the minimum acceptable to the licensing authority and the public. The information available to me strongly suggests that many (perhaps most) similar Boards would already have revoked his license.

I am not an attorney, nor am I Dr. A.'s advocate, but should he decide to refuse the pending Agreement and carry his case further it seems to me that he runs a grave risk of losing his license altogether. Were I asked to participate in such a physician's case before a licensing board, and assuming the facts are reasonably represented by the materials I have seen, I would very probably testify that he cannot be relied upon to practice safely and competently within the foreseeable future, that treatment programs may or may not adequately restore his ability to practice, and that he should not be allowed to practice (unchaperoned in any event) unless or until he is deemed free of substantial risk by clinicians experienced in working with impaired physicians.

Please note that the above comments separate behavioral problems and impairment from "educational" issues. I have no expertise in (*respondent's specialty*) competence *per se*. In my view, based on what I have reviewed, Dr. A.'s main difficulties do not stem merely from educational need (e.g., training in taking sexual histories).

The materials reviewed included
  (*list*).

Thank you for the opportunity to comment.

R24

REPORT: CIVIL CAPACITY, CONTRACTING

RE: *X.B., as Guardian of... A. B... v. ___, dba ABC Petroleum, et al.*

You have asked for a report which summarizes my findings after review of the materials you provided. I am able to supply the opinions and comments below, based upon those materials and my training, background, and experience. The methods used are those routinely relied upon by forensic psychiatrists in matters such as this. *It should be noted that I have not personally examined A.B.* Should additional information become available which changes or adds to the opinions below, I will communicate with you promptly.

FINDINGS AND OPINIONS
The following opinions are offered to a reasonable degree of medical and psychiatric certainty, given the information available to me at this time.

1. It is my understanding from reviewing the conveyance documents and speaking with attorney ___ that the contract transaction at issue in this matter was fairly straightforward (assuming no misrepresentation by the buyer), and included primarily Mr. A.B.'s knowing what he owned, that he wished to convey it, and that he was able to determine its then reasonable value to him.

2. There is little reasonable indication in the record that Mr. B. lacked the capacity to understand the nature and effects of the (*date*) transaction in which he conveyed various ___ rights and royalties.

    I have no reason to contradict the record's or Dr. H.'s characterization of Mr. B. as having a chronic, longstanding, serious mental illness best described as ___, sometimes complicated by ___ addiction. That being considered, however, the great majority of people with _____, particularly those who have adequate treatment available, are competent for most purposes, most of the time. Exceptions may occur during acute symptoms, severe or morbid depression, or acute intoxication.

In addition, persons with this condition who lack insight or judgment in one area often have capacity in other areas. For example, in general psychiatry practice, statute usually establishes that even patients who are so ill that they must be hospitalized against their will are assumed to retain the capacity to consent to, or refuse, medication unless and until a court of appropriate jurisdiction finds otherwise. In Mr. B.'s case, when he was a psychiatric inpatient prior to the events in question, his capacity to execute various hospital documents, consent to various treatments (and hospitalization itself), etc., was affected, or at least was not questioned by those who were examining and treating him.

The record indicates that Mr. B. carried out ordinary business and social activities, apparently in a competent manner, during almost all of the days, weeks, and months prior to and soon after (*date*). This is not to say that he was "competent" for all things at every moment, but rather that, except for the brief period during which he was severely ill in (*month*), there were very few or no times during which he was out of touch with reality in ways that interfered substantially with, for example, his work as a _____, maintaining his finances, and the like.

Around (*date*), Mr. B. took an overdose of prescribed medication (_____). That overdose and its neurological sequelae rendered him confused and out of touch with some aspects of reality for about a week (as described in the medical record). His recovery was complicated by his psychiatric disorder. Although he describes himself as being "in a "coma for a week" (see his deposition, p. 45), the medical record indicates a somewhat shorter period of unconsciousness, then requiring assistance with walking and writing. After being clinically approved for discharge from the general medical part of the hospital, he was transferred to a psychiatric unit on (*date*), where he was, on that date, described by one clinician as still "rather disorganized." His sensorium and other symptoms improved rapidly, however, and a (*date*) clinical note stated that psychosis was "absent" and he was judged ready for discharge. He was discharged to his home on (*date*) without any instructions for special care except outpatient follow-up.

The fact that he was discharged from inpatient care strongly suggests that Mr. B.'s psychiatrist and the treatment team believed on (*date*) that he could safety and competently carry out the ordinary responsibilities of his life. His own judgment was relied upon to call if he had problems. **There was no proscription (or even a recommendation) regarding his ability to work, drive, or do anything** else one might foresee for an ordinary person living at home. It would be expected that any such recommendations or proscriptions would be well documented if they had been indicated; yet there is no such documentation in the medical record.

After discharge, Mr. B. followed up with outpatient psychiatry clinic visits. Such a clinical setting or experience does not in itself indicate any condition of incompetence, and in fact suggests the opposite: that, although therapy was recommended, the patient was able to function acceptably on his own outside the hospital.

The records from (*dates*) of that program indicate that he was alert and coherent, with no mention of psychosis (lack of contact with reality) in the group notes. One note mentions "a couple of odd manners" which are not described further. That phrase does not, in itself, indicate any condition of incompetence.

Mr. B.'s Global Assessment of Functioning ("GAF"), a broad and nonspecific numeric estimate of overall functioning, was recorded three times around the time of the document signing—twice by his psychiatrist and once by a nurse-clinician. On (*date*), _____, M.D., estimated his functioning as "60," a level associated with moderate problems but not generally with the incapacity alleged. The nurse-clinician entered "62" on (*date*). On (*date*), Dr. _____ wrote in a discharge summary that Mr. B.'s GAF upon discharge was "62."

These and other considerations (see below) leave one with the conclusion that there is no indication—and certainly no indication to a reasonable degree of medical certainty—that Mr. B. had psychiatric symptoms which would reasonably be expected to render him "incompetent," in the sense contemplated by this lawsuit, on the day he signed the documents in question (*date*), some nine weeks after his overdose.

3. Plaintiff's theory that Mr. B.'s mental illness and/or his overdose nine weeks before the conveyance rendered him mentally incapable of understanding those things necessary for a legal conveyance (as I understand the requirements and they have been explained to me) is flawed. There is no indication in the record that either the drug he took in overdose or the medications he was given to help his thinking before and around the time of signing had any adverse effect on his capacity to execute the conveyance on or about (*date*).

Although the immediate effect of the _____ overdose was very serious, the medication he took (_____) would have been expected to be "out of his system" long before the date of signing the conveyance (*date*). In the absence of any lasting brain damage from the overdose, his thinking is not likely to have been significantly impaired as a result of the overdose by the time he was discharged on (*date*). There is no indication in the record of lasting brain damage from the overdose. Further, his medications for _____ disorder would not be expected to limit his capacity on the date of signing.

4. Mr. B.'s (*date*) deposition statements are striking in their support of his capacity at the time of his signing the documents. He stated emphatically, on several occasions, that he understood that he was conveying _____, and particularly that he intended to convey _____. He clearly described understanding at that time what he owned and what it meant to convey it. He described prior experience with _____ fees, interests, and related matters. He stated clearly that he understood at that time that, once conveyed, his ownership and royalties would stop forever. He gave adequate reason for wanting to convey some of his property, and gave indication that he knew the general value to him of those interests. He understood that he was free to consult with others about the transaction, and said that his brother, assistant, and associates knew about the transaction.

The position reflected in his testimony appears simply that he alleges being cheated out of his property, and that he had not intended to convey certain parts of it. He does not allege that he was incapable of understanding the transaction, or that he did not understand it. (See, e.g., A.B. deposition pp. 54–61, 66–76, 96, 98–103, 111, 159–161.)

Although considerable time has passed since the transaction, and memory can be inaccurate, there is no indication in the record that one should consider his memory substantially flawed at the time of the transaction. That is, for example, there is no indication in the available record that he was intoxicated at the time, or that any of his medications would have been expected to impair his ability to remember the events, and no indication that his condition or medications at the time of the deposition would be expected to interfere substantially with his recall or ability to testify.

Mr. B., in his deposition, essentially accused ABC *et al.* of cheating him out of property that he did not wish to convey, implicitly suggesting that his signature was forged on additional documents. He did not contest, and actually supported, his competence or capacity to enter into a conveyance in the first place. (Note that my opinions herein do not address whether or not any party to this transaction was untruthful at the time it took place, or any matter of behavior outside the fields of medicine and psychiatry.)

273

5. **Dr. H.'s (*date*) opinions that Mr. B. lacked the relevant capacity on (*date*) are largely without credible support.**

Dr. H. misstates the date of the overdose, placing it much closer to the contract execution on (*date*) than was actually the case ("[*date*]," rather than the actual overdose date of _____). When one considers that the conveyance took place some nine weeks after the overdose, the likelihood of overdose-related intoxication having an effect on Mr. B.'s competence is remote.

Dr. H. apparently accepted at face value A.B.'s (or his representative's) statement that Mr. B. had "very little recall of the signing itself due to his brain impairment . . . (and) does not remember conveying any of the relevant properties." To the contrary, Mr. B. appeared to remember the events fairly well at his deposition, especially given the time that had elapsed. Whatever the case with regard to the accuracy of his memory, however, it should be noted that **the record contains no independent corroboration for any statement that he does not remember the events. Further, absence of memory for events that took place several years ago should not be considered evidence that he was incompetent at the time they occurred.**

Dr. H. implies that Mr. B.'s medication would have had adverse "cognitive effects" on him. That statement is contradicted by the great majority of the psychiatric literature which cites _____ as an agent to *improve* mental stability, contact with reality, competence, and cognition in patients with _____ and similar conditions. Except for Mr. B.'s deposition statement that he was "'way out of it" and his statement that his taking _____ indicates that he was psychotic at the time (deposition pp. 89–90, which misstates or misunderstands the purpose and effects of the medication), there is no indication in the record that Mr. B.'s medication had any such adverse effect on him. (It may be noted that hundreds of thousands of persons in the U.S. take _____ and similar medications daily, for various conditions. Many are essentially symptom-free, and the majority are competent for most purposes most of the time.)

Dr. H. points out that he did not examine Mr. B. at the time of the signing (nor did I), but then states that he does not believe that "a person just released [*sic*, and erroneous] from a mental hospital would be competent to execute legal documents." Such a statement rests on fallacious reasoning, is without clinical foundation, and creates broad and inappropriate bias against persons discharged from psychiatric hospitals. Most such patients have psychiatric diagnoses but are not considered "incompetent" in most senses of the term. **Discharge from a psychiatric hospital *per se* should not be taken to indicate** any level of incompetence, and certainly not incapacity to execute some broad range of "legal documents."

SOURCES RELIED UPON

- Written and video materials, represented as everything relevant and available from your office:
  (*list*)
- My background, training, and experience in medicine, psychiatry, health-care administration, and forensic psychiatry

QUALIFICATIONS

. . .

R25

REPORT: CAPACITY, GUARDIANSHIP (COMPLEX, CONTESTED)

NOTE: Most guardianship evaluations are much shorter than this one, for which the attorneys requested substantial detail because of a large and vigorously contested estate. Some of the detail has been omitted.

RE: **Report of Competency/Guardianship Evaluation: A.A.**
You have asked for a report of my evaluation findings in the above matter, to clarify and supplement the usual "Physician's Certificate" (which is enclosed), with particular reference to the following questions from your letter of (*date*):

1. (a) What activities can Mr. A. perform by himself?, (b) What activities (if any) must be performed in conjunction with a guardian?, and (c) What activities (if any) must be exercised solely by a guardian on his behalf?
2. Can he enter into contractual obligations of large magnitude?
3. Does he have the capacity to modify his will and/or his trust?

FINDINGS AND OPINIONS

Noting that my evaluation is generally limited to Mr. A.'s mental condition and performance, I am able to supply the opinions below, to a reasonable degree of medical certainty, based upon materials reviewed, interviews, and my training, background, and experience. The methods used are those routinely relied upon by forensic psychiatrists in matters such as this. Should additional information become available which changes or adds to the opinions below, I will communicate with you promptly.

1. **Mr. A.A. is an incapacitated person as described in the accompanying Physician's Certificate.** His incapacity is substantial, although the extent is not always superficially noticeable (please see below).

2. **Mr. A.'s incapacity is a result of a chronic dementia.** His condition is not expected to improve significantly, although it may vary

somewhat from time to time. It is likely to worsen over months or years.

3. With regard to the specific questions posed in your (*date*) letter: What activities can Mr. A. perform *by himself* (at the time of my examination)? Some ordinary activities of daily living, such as dressing, maintaining a reasonably clean environment, and getting along adequately with others in a relatively straightforward and conflict-free setting. He is likely to do best in a somewhat structured setting, with monitoring by a responsible person or persons.

He does not appear capable of complex shopping for himself. He would have to depend on others for transportation, as well as to assure he did not become lost in unfamiliar or confusing places. His deficits preclude driving or traveling beyond the sight of his residence alone. He is not able to organize and carry out fully independent living. Although he may be able to parrot some basic principles of protecting himself and his assets, he is generally unable to do so without supervision, and he is very vulnerable to exploitation by others (see below).

What activities can Mr. A. perform *in conjunction with* a guardian (e.g., with a guardian providing information but not making decisions for him)? Activities in which Mr. A. may wish to engage that are unlikely to significantly threaten his interests or well-being. In such matters, a guardian or similar person would be expected to help Mr. A. achieve his reasonable wishes (such as amenities, recreation, communication, information, and transportation).

Mr. A. might, for example, be provided with some amount of spending money or spending discretion, with larger amounts or purchases being controlled by a guardian after consultation with the ward.

The mere providing of information to Mr. A. is generally insufficient to allow him to make competent decisions in more complex matters. His deficits (particularly memory deficits) render him unable to collate such information or work with it accurately.

What activities should be exercised *solely by* a guardian on Mr. A.'s behalf after considering his interests and reasonable wishes? Activities for which errors in judgment are reasonably likely to significantly threaten his interests or well-being. For example, a guardian is necessary for activities involving substantial portions of the assets on which he depends, many activities involving significant aspects of his health or safety, and those for which careful weighing of risks and benefits is necessary.

With regard to contractual obligations: While there may be a few exceptions, I do not believe Mr. A. can generally be expected accurately to assess the information, risks, potential benefits, and/or reasonably likely consequences of large or complex contractual obligations, or to be able to come to reasonable decisions about them. He is very likely to misunderstand such issues and/or quickly forget important aspects of them.

With regard to the capacity to modify his will and/or his trusts: The above comments apply to some extent. Mr. A.'s knowledge appears simplistic, often incomplete, and vulnerable to his memory problems. He is aware that he has substantial assets, but **his appreciation of the** *extent* **of his assets is limited and inaccurate** (or at least markedly fluctuating).

Mr. A.'s knowledge and appreciation of his relatives who might be the natural recipients of his bounty after his death (such as his children) is limited, although he is aware that they exist. Upon inquiry and testing, his knowledge and appreciation of close relatives appeared quite limited and compromised by his memory problems.

Mr. A. is quite vulnerable to the influence of others in matters such as his trusts or will.

4. I specifically disagree with many of the statements made by Mr. A. in his Application for Modification of Guardianship. Mr. A. is not able to perform most or all of the functions mentioned with the "assistance and oversight" of a guardian (except to the extent that such a guardian would simply act for him in many of the functions). For example, for reasons detailed elsewhere in this report, he would not be expected reasonably to consider the issues, responsibilities, and complete consequences of marriage; he cannot be expected to operate a motor vehicle on public streets without significant danger to himself and others, as well as substantial probability of becoming confused and/or lost; his ability to contract or incur significant obligations, and understand/or remember important details of those obligations, is significantly impaired; his ability to manage property independently or rationally to make substantial gifts or distribution of property is significantly impaired; his ability to maintain an unmonitored independent residence safely and reliably is substantially impaired; his ability to understand, remember, and independently and reliably deal with large amounts of money and substantial financial obligations is significantly impaired; his ability to consider reasonably, then participate in and benefit from, educational services is impaired (at least to the extent that his memory for new information is markedly impaired); he cannot be expected to manage his financial affairs reliably; he cannot be expected to make accurate and reliable judgments about many of the implications of discharge from supervisory residential placement.

I am aware that some of Mr. A.'s capabilities have not been directly tested (e.g., by observing his driving or returning control of his finances to him). Such testing may be feasible in some instances; however, my extrapolations from direct examinations, other interviews, and record review are reasonable. I believe it would be foolhardy, and often dangerous, to assume his competence and simply offer him an opportunity to fail.

5. **Mr. A.'s ability to make simple choices and follow routines is substantially affected by the roteness and familiarity of those routines and his environment.** In a familiar and predictable setting, he is currently able to do such things as follow schedules (e.g., a meal schedule), monitor and self-dispense some (but not all) of his medications, and take care of his room. On the other hand, he is unable to do other, fairly simple new tasks with words or memory (see below). If his familiar environment or situation should change significantly, he would be very vulnerable to confusion and mental deterioration.

6. **In addition to difficulty with new or unexpected situations, Mr. A.'s performance on tasks requiring mental ability, mental agility, and memory were affected by minor pressure to perform** (e.g., trying to make a good impression on the examiner), although the examination was conducted with care and efforts were made to minimize evaluation stress.

7. **Mr. A. is vulnerable to exploitation and/or influence by others.** He appears superficially to be able to express preferences and say who is treating him well; however, his impaired memory (which appears to be worsening over time) and other characteristics almost certainly render him unable to cope adequately with changes in his situation, to weigh important information adequately in his own interest, to differentiate reasonably between accurate and inaccurate information (or judge the accuracy of information), and in some respects even to appreciate basic facts about himself (e.g., the extent of his deficits), some of his relatives (e.g., their names and relationships to him), and his environment (e.g., what has happened to him from day to day or week to week). It is noteworthy that Mr. A. appears not to appreciate the fact that substantial costs of current and past litigation, evaluations, etc., are borne by his trust and deplete his funds somewhat.

8. **Specific significant mental deficits found which are relevant to the questions posed for this evaluation include, but are not limited to, the following:**

   (a) The results of a formal "Mini Mental State Examination" (MMSE) during the first interview, and a complete mental status

examination during two interviews, indicated substantial deficits, particular of memory and memory-related functions (such as
general knowledge). Most parts of the MMSE were repeated during the second interview (particularly those on which he had done
poorly earlier), with similar results. In spite of having a calendar
in his room, he did not know the day or date (initially saying a
Friday—erroneous—in August, but also knowing it was actually
Spring). When told the correct date several times, he later
remembered only part of it. He failed the weekday and day of the
month on the second testing as well (after earlier having been told
both clearly and asked to remember them).

Mr. A. knew his complete location during the first testing, but
twice mistook the city for "_____" (a town about 50 miles away)
during the second interview. His immediate memory was tested
in many ways, always with marked deficit. For example, he failed
to remember any of three simple objects for 3–4 minutes (after
clearly being told their names and that I was testing his memory),
and failed to remember my name (after having it repeated many
times and being asked to remember it). Some other portions of
the MMSE were performed fairly well.

He responded poorly to some other standard mental status
items, such as questions about common news stories and television programs. For example, he said he watches television often
but could not immediately recall the names of any programs
except "Nova," the current or immediate past president, or
current or past governors. He suggested I "ask...about New
York" (where he did business for many years until fairly recently),
but he was able to name only ex-governor Rockefeller.

Some of his responses were very similar to common responses
by other patients with dementia—that is, often offering vague,
nonspecific comments but upon further questioning being unable
to provide real answers. For example, when asked what has been
in the news lately, he said "uprisings in foreign countries." When
asked to be more specific about what and where, he paused and
said "the Middle East and the Far East." When asked where in the
Middle East and Far East, he mentioned Iran, Iraq and Sudan,
most prominently Iran, later mentioning "the war in Iraq."
When asked about the Far East, he said "I'd hate to take a
guess."[1]

---

1 Note that many responses contained inconsistencies and unreasonable rationalizations
for Mr. A.'s memory difficulties. He gave answers, or reasons for answers, that superficially appeared logical but upon further examination were illogical or insufficient.

Mr. A. did fairly well with immediate concentration, attending to the interview questions and simple serial calculations. He was able to interpret some (not all) simple proverbs. He appeared to have limited insight into his deficits, although he seemed aware of, and a bit embarrassed by, some memory problems.

(b) I spent considerable time asking Mr. A. various relatives' names, locations, relationships, and the like. The questions were ones he would be expected to be able to answer, and to which he knew the answers at one time. The accuracy or inaccuracy of his responses was corroborated with _____, Mr. _____, and the available record.

Mr. A. was often confused, inconsistent, and/or completely unable to name relatives such as his deceased wife's parents, other relatives of _____, his first wife, or to give his daughter's current last name. He was a bit uncomfortable with some of the questions, apparently being upset that he was confused at times and could not supply the answers.

Mr. A. first told me that his daughter "_____" lives in _____. When I asked if he was sure, he corrected himself to "_____" (a different state), and later to "_____ or _____" (also incorrect); his daughter has never lived in those states. (She corroborated the information by telephone.) He was not sure whether or not he has grandchildren, saying "I suppose my daughter has children...I never hear from her." (In fact, his daughter and her children have recently written to him and sent him drawings; that family visited him a month prior to my examination.) He did not know his daughter's last name, saying "I'd like to know myself."

When I asked further about Mr. A's younger son, he appeared to misunderstand and began talking about a nephew, but confusing him with a grandson. I asked carefully if _he_ had a son, to which he replied "No . . . yes. We're estranged . . . ." He said at one point that his children were colluding to take his money.

Although Mr. A. is indeed estranged from some of the relatives discussed, his deficit appeared much more severe than would be expected from simply being out of touch.

(c) When asked about his assets, Mr. A. was a bit inconsistent but generally said he had _____ million dollars or more in a trust, which he believed was at "_____ Bank" (an error). He often accused his son of taking control of his money and various assets, and repeatedly said no one would give him information or explain what was going on with the assets or trust. At one point he said all of his assets had been taken by his son and if he were to leave the current facility he would have to "start over." When asked about the proceeds from the recent sale of his house, he said he hoped and/or believed they were now part of the trust.

Although the overall amount is apparently fairly accurate, much of what he told me in this regard changed a bit from conversation to conversation and, more important, was inconsistent with the available record and statements to me by counsel and relatives. The trust is actually at _____ (and has never been at "_____ Bank"); it apparently is not under his son's control.

Mr. A. said he had never received any information about the trust, any statements from the bank, any explanations from his son, etc., and said several times during the interviews that he wanted someone to tell him what was going on with his money, the guardianship, etc. Mr. _____ and Mr. _____ (attorney) state that this is not true. They have told me that, although Mr. A. does not receive copies of trust/financial documents (for fear his personal information would fall into others' hands at the facility), (1) Mr. _____ from the trust institution (who manages the trust and has known Mr. A. for many years) reports to Mr. A. in person as a courtesy about twice a year, and stands ready to meet with him at any time. Mr. A. has Mr. _____'s telephone number in an address book, which he keeps in his bureau. (2) _____ sent Mr. A. a lengthy letter around (*date*), with detailed information about the trust and guardianship, and (3) _____ (his son) has often tried to explain the situation to his father. He agrees that, so far as he knows, no one has sent Mr. A. actual trust statements by mail, saying he is concerned about private information such as his social security number falling into inappropriate hands.

(d) With regard to the current guardian and guardianship proceedings, Mr. A. knows that _____ is his guardian and has considerable control over his life, but misunderstands his son's relationship to his assets. He said several times (even after clarifying statements from me) that his son had not visited for many months, and that he last saw him at the original guardianship proceeding years ago. Although questioned several times about it, he never acknowledged the recent hearing (a few weeks prior to our interviews), or seeing his son at that hearing, or any of his son's recent visits (_____'s name appears in the facility visitor log at least three times over the past three months). Mr. A. recalled being taken to _____ by _____ to see a psychiatrist (apparently Dr. _____) some time in the past.

(e) When asked what he might need to do in order to live on his own, Mr. A. began with getting a place to stay, such as an apartment. He said he would need about $350–400 for rent (but admitted that rents vary), about $60 a week for food, and would have to deal with other bills such as those for laundry, doctors, transportation and (with some hints) utilities. When asked where he might live, he said it would be a choice between being near his brother in _____ or near his nephew in _____. His discussion of how he might go about these processes was limited (although, in fairness, the question was posed to him somewhat suddenly).

(f) Mr. A.'s day-to-day activities are quite limited by his condition, in spite of a number of opportunities and general freedom. He apparently wishes or needs to keep his environment simple, sometimes saying that the facility activities are not interesting to him. The facility nursing director says he is a very private fellow who prefers to sit alone on the garden patio (generally in the same chair) or in his room, but that he is sometimes observed at activities standing in the back of the room. Mr. A. said his son "left orders that I'm not allowed out," but the nursing director and facility notes indicate that the son allows, and encourages, outside activities and trips with facility staff.

Mr. A. said he doesn't walk to a nearby store because he has no money. When asked about spending money, he initially says he has none, but a few minutes later says he has about $40 but doesn't want to spend it. He said he has had that $40 "all along" (apparently meaning since he arrived, although he is unable to consistently answer questions about when or where he got it, or whether _____ brings him spending money). Sometimes he said he has no use for spending money, as there is nothing to buy; at other times, he said he doesn't want to spend the money because it is all he has. (His trust can provide whatever spending money he wants or needs, within reason; Ms. _____ has excellent access to money for him or for his expenses.)

When asked whether or not he ever takes advantage of the facility van service for shopping or other excursions, he said that he did not because (variously) "it costs $20 a trip"; he doesn't need to buy anything; they only offer the van a few times a week; or it is inconvenient and uncomfortable. (In fact, there is no charge for the van service, which operates five days a week for shopping, appointments, and other excursions.)

SOURCES RELIED UPON

- Written materials from your office, represented as everything relevant and available
  (*list*)
- _____ (facility) resident record, provided by the facility
- Background interviews
  (*list*)

- Examinations of Mr. A., (*date*), 2 hours 30 minutes (two sessions) in and near his room
- My background, training, and experience in medicine, psychiatry, health-care administration, and forensic psychiatry

QUALIFICATIONS

. . .

R26

OPINION LETTER: CAPACITY, BUSINESS, AND TESTAMENTARY

NOTE: Competency and capacity assessments are frequent exceptions to my general rule about not examining evaluees in their homes or lawyers' offices. Thoughtful attorneys know that it is often a good idea to have a forensic clinician assess capacity at the time of executing (signing) documents such as wills or contracts. Since signing usually occurs in an office or home, it is logical to do the assessment on-site, just before the event.

RE: Matter of A.B.; Competency/Capacity

On (*date*), you asked me to assess Ms. B.'s mental competency/capacity to execute various instruments related to her will and financial holdings. That having been accomplished, you have asked for a written summary of that evaluation and my opinions.

At your request, before examining Ms. B., I reviewed her medical history, spoke with her longtime internist (Dr. D.) and cardiologist (Dr. F.), and spoke briefly with Ms. B. and her husband by telephone. You provided me with an example of (*state*) jury instructions regarding the requirements for testamentary capacity. On (*date*) I met with Ms. B. at her home and evaluated her competency/capacity with respect to the purposes above. At your request, the interview was not recorded except in my handwritten notes and worksheet. I used, among other things, a list of questions I had prepared from the examples of jury instructions, checking Ms. B.'s answers against information previously provided by your office (e.g., the names of her children and other family members, the general extent of her property and holdings, and the like). The reason for choosing to interview her at home was that I believed she might be better able to demonstrate her true level of competence in that familiar setting and, further, that was the setting in which the documents were to be executed. The following is a summary of my visit.

When I arrived at the B. home, Ms. B. greeted me, nicely dressed and kempt in casual attire and appearing somewhat younger than her documented age of 84. She was friendly and socially appropriate, inviting me in, seating me, offering refreshment, and the like. We talked informally for a few moments, then her husband appeared. After several more minutes of informal conversation, some private and some with her husband present, you arrived, followed by Mr. G.

I first spoke with Ms. B. in private. She clearly understood why I was there, and showed no anxiety or concern about the proceedings. I asked her, in private, whether she preferred to be interviewed alone or in the company of her husband or others. She said that she preferred having her husband and attorneys present, and they were called into the room. It should be noted that all of those persons sat quietly out of Ms. B. line of sight. None spoke or otherwised participated in the interview, attempted to offer answers, or attempted to encourage or influence Ms. B.

During the interview, I asked the questions that were on my worksheet, among many other things. Ms. B. answered as noted on the worksheet I provided to you. She also looked briefly at some of the documents in order to refamiliarize himself with them. **Her answers, related comments, and behavior clearly indicated at least general understanding and competence to execute the relevant instruments, as I understand the requirements.**

It should be noted that (as you know) Ms. B. has some short-term memory deficit which has been diagnosed by her treating physicians and which is noticeable upon detailed testing and conversation. Nevertheless, she clearly understood the nature and purpose of the documents as she read them during my interview. She was able to explain them to me quite accurately while consulting them. When asked to explain the documents again, from memory, some 15 minutes later, her explanations were accurate overall, but she was unable to recall some details such as subsets of assets and the names of some board members. Nevertheless, she accurately provided the names of, and general information about, both the children born to her current marriage[1] and said convincingly that she did not wish to provide for them in these documents. She also said convincingly that she did not wish to provide for her husband's two children, born to his former marriage decades ago, accurately naming them as well. She firmly said that she wanted all of her property and the financial controls detailed in the other documents to go to her current husband, describing him, among other things, as her longtime (several decades) companion, helper, and friend. She said further that, should her property eventually pass to him, she understands that he may do as he wishes with it. When asked how she

---

1 The accuracy of all answers was corroborated by my earlier record review and others' statements about the family structure.

came to her preferences, she reiterated the long, continuous, and rewarding relationship she has had with Mr. B.

Following the interview, which lasted about 45 minutes, I orally, privately, communicated the above findings to you and your colleague Mr. G. You then began the signing procedure, which I observed. Neither Ms. B.'s mental state nor her physical condition appeared to change in the interim or during the signing. There was no indication of duress or exploitation, and she appeared to participate quite willingly as you reiterated your explanations of each document as you placed it before her.

Materials Reviewed
(*list*)

R27

REPORT: AUTO ACCIDENT VS. SUICIDE

NOTE: Forensic experts are sometimes asked whether or not a death can be attributed to suicide. Any such opinions should be carefully justified by specific evidence, rather than anecdote or subjective factors, and expressed in terms of probability, not absolutes. In the following case, a restaurant was sued for serving liquor to an intoxicated man who then drove his car and killed another driver. The restaurant, through its lawyers, alleged that the non-intoxicated decedent hit the intoxicated driver on purpose, in a suicide attempt which should not be blamed on the restaurant or the intoxicated driver.

RE: **PRELIMINARY REPORT: B. v. *Estate of D., E. Café, et al.***

You have asked for a report which summarizes my findings after review of the materials you provided in the above matter. I am able to supply the comments and opinions below, based upon those materials and my training, background, and experience. The methods used and materials reviewed are those routinely relied upon by forensic psychiatrists in matters such as this. Any additional information received in the future may or may not suggest additions or changes to the opinions below.

FINDINGS AND OPINIONS

After review of the materials provided, I am able to provide the following opinions with regard to the likelihood that A.B.'s death was a suicide, each of which is offered to a reasonable degree of medical or psychiatric certainty given the information available to me at this time. It should be noted that my comments come from the viewpoint of a forensic psychiatrist, not an accident reconstruction expert, and I have not personally examined the decedent.

1. There is no reasonable evidence, much less evidence that implies "more likely than not," that Mr. B.'s (*date*) death was the result of a suicide attempt.

There is no indication in the records reviewed that Mr. B. was at significant suicide risk at the time of his death. In addition, there is no indication that his known or reasonably inferred behavior immediately prior to his death suggests or indicates suicidality, other self-destructive thoughts or actions, or any condition (such as intoxication) which might reasonably cause recklessness, impulsivity, or self-destructiveness.

With specific reference to Mr. B.'s counseling experience during the year prior to his death, there is no indication in those records that he might, much less would, be at significant suicide risk on (*date*). I have seen no evidence of mental health counseling or treatment other than that with Mr. F.

With specific reference to the website, messaging, and telephone records supplied, there is no indication in those records that he might, much less would, be at significant suicide risk on (*date*).

Further, I have found no reason to argue with the findings of the law-enforcement officers and accident investigators who found Mr. B. to have been a victim of a driver who was in the wrong lane of Interstate __, and no reason to argue with the related findings that Mr. B. was driving in the correct lane and was not at fault.

2. **There is no reasonable evidence, much less evidence that indicates "more likely than not," that Mr. B. was thinking of or planning suicide <u>immediately prior to</u> his (*date*) death.**

There is no indication in the records reviewed that Mr. B. was at significant suicide risk during the minutes and hours prior to his death. In addition, there is no indication that his known or reasonably inferred behavior during that period suggests or indicates suicidality, other self-destructive thoughts or actions, or any condition (such as intoxication) which might reasonably cause recklessness, impulsivity, or self-destructiveness.

With specific reference to Mr. B.'s counseling experience during the year prior to his death, there is no indication in those records that he might, much less would, be at significant suicide risk on (*date*). I have no evidence of mental health counseling or treatment other than that with Mr. F.

With specific reference to the website, messaging, and telephone records supplied, there is no indication in those records that he might, much less would, be at significant suicide risk on (*date*).

3. **There is no reasonable evidence, much less evidence that indicates "more likely than not," that Mr. B. had been thinking of or planning suicide <u>during the days, weeks or months prior to</u> his (*date*) death.**

There is no indication in the records reviewed that Mr. B. was at significant suicide risk during the days, weeks, or months prior to his death. In addition, there is no indication that his known or reasonably inferred behavior during that period suggests or indicates suicidality, other self-destructive thoughts or actions, or any condition (such as intoxication) which might reasonably cause recklessness, impulsivity, or self-destructiveness.

With specific reference to Mr. B.'s counseling experience during the year prior to his death, there is no indication in those records that he was at during (*year*), or any indication that he might, much less would, be at significant suicide risk on during (*year*). I have no evidence of other mental health counseling or treatment other than that with Mr. F.

With specific reference to the website, messaging, and telephone records supplied, there is no indication in those records that he might, much less would, be at significant suicide risk on (*date*).

4. **In addition to the extreme rarity of suicide in persons similar to Mr. B., when such suicides do occur, it is even rarer for the person knowingly to endanger or kill others.**

    Without implying that Mr. B. may have committed suicide or was at significant suicide risk, one may say that persons who commit suicide by motor vehicle usually choose situations that do not endanger other drivers or pedestrians. Thus, while a "one-car accident" is not an uncommon method of killing oneself when suicide does occur, purposely hitting head-on another car which is driving on the wrong side of an interstate highway is extremely rare (*reference*).

5. **The relevant, peer-reviewed professional psychological and psychiatric literature overwhelmingly contradicts any implication that Mr. B.'s cause of death might reasonably (more likely than not) be construed as suicide.**

    Suicide is a well-studied topic of peer-reviewed clinical, mental health, and social science literature. Although it may be said that everyone may have some level of suicide risk at some time, that risk is extremely small for the great majority of people, and very small even for psychiatric or psychological patients (including counseling clients) (*reference*). A small minority of suicides occur without any other person being aware of significant mental illness or substantial risk factors (*reference*); however, once a suicide occurs, evidence of significant mental illness and risk factors is routinely discovered upon post-event examination (*reference*).

    Conditions such as those described in Mr. B.'s occasional counseling with Mr. F in (*year*), as reflected in his transcribed records, are not associated with significant suicide risk, and should never be construed as establishing significant risk of suicide over a year later, much less suggesting that a death should be attributed to suicide (*date*).

Messages and website postings such as those attributed to Mr. B. in the records supplied are not associated with significant suicide risk. Both clinical experience and the professional literature are clear that such postings and communications, especially when taken out of context, are quite generic with regard to any psychiatric meaning or suggestion of risk, and should not reasonably raise any assumption of significant risk or "prediction" of future suicide (*reference*).

SOURCES RELIED UPON

- Written materials as follows, represented to me as all which are relevant and available from your office:
  (*list*)
- Peer-reviewed journal articles
  (*list*)
- My background, training, and experience in medicine, psychology, psychiatry, and forensic psychiatry, and health-care administration

QUALIFICATIONS

. . .

R28

AFFIDAVIT: SUPPORTING MOTION TO STRIKE EXPERT TESTIMONY (FORENSIC PRACTICE STANDARDS)

_____ COURT

COUNTY OF _____

IN RE: _____ _____ This document relates to: *A.B. et al.* **PLAINTIFFS,** v. ____ (*Company*), ____ (*Company*), and DOES 1–100, inclusive. **DEFENDANTS.** _____	) Case No. _____) Proceeding No. ____)) **DECLARATION OF DR. WILLIAM H.**) **REID**)) Filed Concurrently with Plaintiff's Motion to) Strike Expert Testimony)) Trial Date: ____))))

I, William H. Reid, M.D., M.P.H., declare as follows:

1. I make this Declaration in support of Plaintiff's Motion to Strike Expert Testimony by Dr. ____. The matters set forth in this Declaration are of my own personal knowledge and, if called upon to do so, I could and would competently testify thereto as a witness in a legal proceeding.

2. I am a general and forensic psychiatrist licensed to practice medicine in Texas and _____, among other states. I am certified by the American Board of Psychiatry and Neurology in both general psychiatry and forensic psychiatry. I am a past president of the American Academy of Psychiatry and the Law. I am a clinical or adjunct professor at three medical schools and teach regularly in training programs and continuing education settings on forensic matters and practice standards. I have published a number of books, book chapters, and peer-reviewed articles on forensic and clinical topics. My forensic experience includes the performance and interpretation of psychiatric independent medical examinations (IMEs).

3. A true and correct copy of my *curriculum vitae* is attached to this Declaration as Exhibit A.

4. I am not an attorney, and do not intend for the contents of this Declaration to be construed as an interpretation of legal (as contrasted with "forensic psychiatry") issues.

5. I am not a neurologist or a neuropsychologist, and do not intend for the contents of this Declaration to be construed as an interpretation of the practice standard for forensic neurology or neuropsychology.

6. Typical practice standards for independent medical examinations (IMEs) in forensic psychiatry.

    (a) The recording of IMEs is common, and often recommended. Reasonably qualified and prudent forensic psychiatrists understand both the utility of recording and its potential drawbacks. Many experienced forensic psychiatry practitioners and teachers recommend recording when feasible.

    (b) When unexpected procedural problems or issues arise during an IME performed at a lawyer's or court's behest, it is common practice to try to resolve the issue by contacting the retaining lawyer, especially when proceeding without such contact involves foreseeable risk of legal or clinical problems.

    (c) The practice standard requires that a forensic psychiatrist reasonably recognize tasks which may be outside his/her area of expertise, and either decline the IME or discuss limitations, *caveats*, and/or disclaimers as professionally and ethically appropriate.

7. The concept of "consent" in forensic psychiatry IMEs such as those envisioned in the hypothetical.

(a) With regard to the examination itself, and without meaning to address applicable law, it is my view that participation in IMEs ordered in the context of the hypothetical discussed does not require the examiner to obtain additional examinee "consent," since (i) the person has put his condition into question; (ii) his/her attorney has properly agreed to the examination and presented the client for examination; (iii) the person has voluntarily (or pursuant to lawful order) appeared for examination and expresses some level of consent or assent merely by participating; and (iv) issues being addressed by such an IME often suggest limitations of the examinee's capacity to consent in any event.

(b) Similarly, with regard to audio-recording of an examination, it is my view that routine procedures integral to the examination, including audio-recording, are not matters for consent, particularly if they are required by court order or statute *or* to effect an accurate outcome (excepting procedures which are dangerous or very uncomfortable).

(c) None of the above eliminates the need to notify the examinee and/or his agent of relevant facts about the examination, such as the reason for it, the examiner's role and agency (e.g., who has retained him/her), the uses to which the results may be put, the fact that the results may be shared within the constraints of the litigation, and the fact that the examination is being recorded (if it is). It is considered unethical in almost all settings for an examiner to record surreptitiously or misrepresent his/her role in the procedure.

8. Reasonable and prudent actions expected of an examiner when an examinee states that he/she does not want to be audio-recorded, in spite of a court order to audio-record the examination, and assuming that the examiner understands that he/she is responsible for the recording. Such examinee expressions occur from time to time and may take several forms, from simple utterances to outright refusals to proceed. If the examiner believes that recording is important *or* is procedurally required, he or she should, as a matter of the practice standard, further explain its nature and importance and encourage the examinee to cooperate with it. If that effort is unsuccessful,

(a) If the examining forensic psychiatrist is aware that a court of proper jurisdiction has ordered "recording" (and understands that to mean audio-recording), and the examinee persistently refuses to proceed unless recording is stopped, then the customary procedure is for the examiner to stop the process and contact the person who retained him/her (e.g., a retaining attorney) for clarification and/or instruction. The option simply to cancel the IME is also within the practice standard, especially if the relevant lawyer is not easily available. However, to proceed with the examination without recording and without guidance from the attorney or court would be outside the agreed (and ordered) parameters of the IME, may affect the legal usefulness of the result, and is probably outside forensic practice standards.

Forensic psychiatrists know or should know that proceeding without authorization and clarification is outside usual routine, is often inappropriate, is likely to be questioned during the legal process, and may alter the results of any future "make-up" examination. (There may be exceptions to these principles, such as an examinee who presents with a clinical condition that requires immediate attention, but I cannot think of one that is relevant to the hypothetical as I understand it.)

(b) If the examining forensic psychiatrist is not aware of a particular court order but has been informed by the attorney who retained him/her that the IME is to be audio-recorded, and has agreed that he/she will record the examination, and the examinee persistently refuses to proceed unless recording is stopped, then, as above, the customary procedure is for the examiner to stop the process and contact the person who retained him/her (e.g., a retaining attorney) for clarification and/or instruction. The option simply to cancel the IME is also within the practice standard, especially if the relevant lawyer is not easily available. However, to proceed with the examination without recording and without guidance from the attorney or court would be outside the agreed parameters of the IME, may affect the legal usefulness of the result, and is arguably outside forensic practice standards (see 8[a], above).

9. Choice of an appropriate specialist to perform an IME in order to determine the extent of a person's neurologic/brain injuries following a cerebrovascular incident ("stroke"). The primary consideration in choosing an examining expert, and in an expert's accepting an examiner role, is whether or not the examiner is adequately trained and experienced with regard to the (alleged) condition being evaluated, and with regard to other conditions that may be present or relevant to the purpose of the IME (such as alternative diagnoses and effects of current treatment on the examinee's condition).

10. In matters involving assessment of the presence and extent of neurologic/brain injuries, symptoms, and signs; involving allegations that those conditions (assuming they are present) are caused by a "stroke";

and/or involving whether or not a "stroke" is caused by some specific factor, it is important that the examiner be extensively trained and experienced in neurology and/or neuropsychology. In general (and without opining here as a neurologist or neuropsychologist), experts with those qualifications have completed lengthy, recognized specialty training, been certified by a recognized body in that field (neurology or neuropsychology), and have practiced extensively in it.

11. Some psychiatrists have substantial neurology training and experience and practice extensively at the interface of neurology and psychiatry. If such a person is qualified by education and experience to assess the neurological conditions relevant to the injuries alleged in the hypothetical, then he or she may well be within the forensic practice standard in doing so. (The specifics of those qualifications are outside my own expertise.) If, however, the issues to be assessed are outside the examiner's true expertise, the examiner should offer appropriate *caveats* and/or disclaimers about the extent of his/her expertise or should decline the IME. A forensic psychiatrist who does not comply with the above is likely to be practicing outside the standard.

I declare under penalty of perjury under the law of the State of _____ that the foregoing is true and correct, and that this Declaration was executed on _____

_____

William H. Reid, M.D., M.P.H.

_____ (Notary Block)

R29

LETTER: REBUTTAL OF EXPERT'S REPORT, FORENSIC PRACTICE STANDARDS

RE: *U.S. v. A.B. and C.D.*

You have asked for my general opinions with regard to two issues in the above matter: whether or not it is within the forensic psychiatry practice standard to offer diagnostic opinions without examining an evaluee <u>and</u> the accepted psychiatric criteria for a diagnosis of "pedophilia" with respect to the above case.

As I have stated in our telephone conversations, although I have reviewed the available records, I have not had an opportunity to examine either the defendants or the alleged victim in this matter. I have reviewed Dr. F.'s (*date*) letter/report addressed to AUSA G.H., and her *curriculum vitae* received with the records you provided.

1. Dr. F.'s report states that she has "concluded" that the defendants engaged in behavior that "indicates they are repetitive pedophiles." **Dr. F. appears to be making and conveying a diagnosis without performing a *bona fide* evaluation of either person, and without offering any disclaimer about her lack of examination.**

    It should be noted that there are some situations in which a qualified clinician, after appropriate and adequate review and in the absence of in-person examination, can legitimately offer a diagnosis; **however, when such an opinion is offered, the accepted practice standards generally require that the opinion be accompanied by *caveats* or disclaimers describing the potential sources of error in rendering the diagnosis without an in-person examination.** The American Medical Association *Principles of Medical Ethics* (as annotated for use by psychiatrists and published by the American Psychiatric Association [1995]) holds that this practice standard is also a matter of professional ethics. The American Academy of Psychiatry and the Law endorses that ethics position (1995).

Although she stated that her conclusions were based on the information reviewed, I found no disclaimer or *caveat* in Dr. F.'s, report.

2. Similar concerns can be raised about Dr. F.'s opinion or implication that the alleged victim is a so-called compliant victim. That condition is actually called "child abuse accommodation syndrome" in its original iteration (Summit, 1983) and, to my knowledge, has largely been discredited (American Academy of Child and Adolescent Psychiatry, 1997).

    I found no disclaimer or *caveat* about the lack of any in-person examination of the alleged victim, or about Dr. F.'s apparent lack formal of training or experience in child psychiatry (as reflected in her *curriculum vitae*), nor did I find reference in her report to the considerable professional literature which rebuts the existence of "child abuse accommodation syndrome." Since I am not a child or adolescent psychiatrist, I will leave further comment about that topic to someone with additional qualifications.

3. In order to be consistent with the professionally accepted American Psychiatric Association *Diagnostic and Statistical Manual of Mental Disorders, 4th Edition, Text Revision* (DSM-IV-TR, 2000), a psychiatric diagnosis of "pedophilia" must include at least six months of relevant symptoms and behaviors involving <u>pre-pubescent</u> children. Without expressing any opinion about whether or not the defendants engaged in criminal acts, it must be said that, if sexual acts did occur but the victim was not pre-pubescent, and the fantasies involving her did not focus on pre-pubescent children, then a diagnosis of pedophilia would appear to be clinically inappropriate.

    I reiterate that I am not offering a diagnosis or diagnostic rebuttal of persons whom I have not evaluated; however, the DSM-IV simply does not recognize pedophilia in the absence of chronic and intense fantasies/urges focusing on prepubescent victims, in addition to acting on such urges.

References

American Academy of Child and Adolescent Psychiatry (AACAP) (1997) Practice parameters on forensic evaluation of children/adolescents who may have been sexually abused, *Journal of the American Academy of Child and Adolescent Psychiatry* 36 (10 Supp.): 37S–56S.

American Academy of Psychiatry and the Law (1995 and later) *Ethics Guidelines for the Practice of Forensic Psychiatry*. Bloomfield, CT: American Academy of Psychiatry and the Law (also available at www.aapl.org).

American Psychiatric Association (2000) *The Diagnostic and Statistical Manual of Mental Disorders*, 4th Edition, Text Revision (DSM-IV-TR). Washington, DC: American Psychiatric Association.

American Psychiatric Association (1995 and later) *Opinions of the Ethics Committee on the Principles of Medical Ethics, with Annotations Especially Applicable to Psychiatry.* Washington, DC: American Psychiatric Association (also available at www.psych.org).

Summit, R. C. (1983). The child sexual abuse accommodation syndrome, *Child Abuse and Neglect* 7: 177–193.

INDEX

Note: page numbers followed by "n" and another number refer to information in the footnotes.

AAFS (American Academy of Forensic Sciences) 3
AAPL (American Academy of Psychiatry and the Law) 3, 297
ABPN (American Board of Psychiatry and Neurology) 2, 3, 75–6
ABPP (American Psychological Association's American Board of Professional Psychology) 3, 76
accents, depositions and trial testimony 60
access 77–8
accessibility, and office and office procedures 82
accident cases: auto accident vs. suicide, sample report 288–91; personal injury defense (PSTD) (with treater–expert conflict), sample report 147–52
ACLU (American Civil Liberties Union) 25
ad litem, definition 16
ADA (Americans with Disabilities Act) 12
affidavits 47–8; defense rebuttal, death in custody 227–31; drafts, discovery 51–2; format 48–51; grammar, spelling and vocabulary 52; lawyer participation in 48–9; malpractice, plaintiff pre-suit 176–8; presentation 52–3; supporting motion to strike expert testimony (forensic practice standards) 292–6
agent, experts' role as 6
ambivalence 33
American Academy of Forensic Sciences (AAFS) 3

American Academy of Psychiatry and the Law (AAPL) 3, 297
American Board of Professional Psychology (ABPP) 3, 76
American Board of Psychiatry and Neurology (ABPN) 2, 3, 75–6
American Civil Liberties Union (ACLU) 25
American Medical Association, *Principles of Medical Ethics* 157, 297
American Psychiatric Association 3, 102; ethics principles 8, 70, 157, 297
American Psychological Association 2; American Board of Professional Psychology (ABPP) 3, 76; ethics principles 8, 70
Americans with Disabilities Act (ADA) 12
amicus (amicus curiae), definition 16
appeal, definition 16–17
appearance: and courtroom presentation 96–7; depositions and trial testimony 58, 59–61; and marketing 79
appellate, definition 16–17
appreciate/appreciation, definition 17, 51
appreciation, and marketing 80
archives 82
attendants, and evaluations 41
attitude, and courtroom presentation 96, 98
attorney work products, definition 23
attorneys *see* lawyers
audio recording, of evaluations 41–3
authenticity, and courtroom presentation 97

auto accident cases, auto accident vs. suicide, sample report 288–91
availability 77–8

"bad" news 34
behavior: and courtroom presentation 96; and evaluations 43
believability 96
bias 8, 11
billing 62–5, 83–5, 110; fee sheets 65–9, *see also* fees; money
books, as information source 3
budgeting 85–6
business capacity; sample opinion letter, capacity, business, and testamentary 285–7
business cards 78–9
business client, definition 17

capacity 12; capacity, guardianship (complex, contested), sample report 276–84; civil capacity, contracting, sample report 270–5; definition 17; sample opinion letter, capacity, business, and testamentary 285–7
career directions in forensic practice 10–11
case review, typical process 27–9
cases, experts' help in assessment of 93
causation, malpractice, plaintiff pre-suit, lack of causation, letter 179–80
cause, definition 51
caveats 51
censures, avoidance of 4
certifications: for forensic practice 3; and marketing 75–6; unblemished 4, *see also* licensing
certiorari, definition 17
charge, mitigation of, sample report 137–42
children: child cases 11, 12; and evaluations 41
civil capacity, contracting, sample report 270–5
clarity, and courtroom presentation 97–8
client, definition 17–18
client files 82
clients of retaining entities: avoidance of clinical relationship with 6–7; duty to 6
clinical practice: in forensic settings 13; maintenance of 4, 101

clinicians: and ethics 71; as target market 73–4
cognitive behavior therapy 100–1
colleagues, avoidance of expert role in defense of 14
collections 62, 64, 65, 83–5
communication, with lawyers 14, 29, 38, 49
competence: and consent 18; definition 18, 51
competency 12; definition 18, 51
complainant, definition 21
confidentiality 7; employee confidentiality agreement 123–4; vendor confidentiality agreement 122
conflicts of interest 6; employee emotional injury, treater–expert conflict, sample report 249–62; friends and close colleagues 14; initial lawyer/expert contact 24–5; personal injury defense (PSTD) (with treater–expert conflict) 147–52; treater/expert witness/consultant roles 7–10
consent: definition 18; and evaluations 44–5, 293–4
conservatorship cases 12
consultants, conflict of interest with treater role 7–10
consultations 13, 33, 88
contingency fees 22, 63, 67; definition 18
continuing education 3
counter-transference 37
court orders, and payment 65
courtroom presentation, of expert witnesses 95–8
courts: duties to 6; as target market 73
credentials 2–4; malpractice, defense (facility), forensic practice standards, sample report 201–3
credibility 4–6, 83; and testimony 56
criminal cases 12; defendants 46
criminal responsibility: not guilty by reason of insanity (NGRI) 12, 35n1, 143–6; sample report 134–6
criticism, and testimony 56
cultural markers: and courtroom presentation 96, 98; depositions and trial testimony 60–1
custody staff 39, 40

daily rates 66, 109, *see also* fees

Daubert v. *Merrell Dow Pharmaceuticals* 50

death in custody cases: defense rebuttal, death in custody, sample affidavit 227–31; defense, sample report 223–6

death penalty cases 102

debts 69

deceased people, forensic work on 89

defendants: criminal defendants 46; definition 18

defense: death in custody, sample report 223–6; defense rebuttal, death in custody, sample affidavit 227–31; experience with 11; malpractice, defense (clinician) (alleged fetal damage from medication), sample report 208–15; malpractice, defense (complex, facility), sample report 195–200; malpractice, defense (facility), forensic practice standards, sample report 201–7

definitions, legal 16–23, 50–1, 52

delegation 33

deposition 104–5; definition 18; questions 94; testimony 54–8, 59–61

deposits 63–4, 66–7, 83, 110; pre-testimony deposit letter 119–20; pre-testimony deposit worksheet 118

depression cases: workplace stressors allegedly causing suicide, expert report rebuttal, sample report 232–7, *see also* suicide cases

diction, and marketing 79

disability cases 12; insurance company reviews 29, 64; private insurance disability appeal (complex), sample report 238–48

disclaimers 51

discovery 32; definition 19; and record review 31–3; recordings of evaluations 43; reports 51–2

discovery depositions 57; definition 18, *see also* depositions

DOJ (U.S. Department of Justice) 25

dress: and courtroom presentation 96, 97; depositions and trial testimony 58, 59–61; and marketing 79

duces tecum see subpoena

duPont v. *Robinson* 50

duties of forensic practitioners 6–7, 8; and liability 87

electronic records 31

Elements of Style, The (Strunk and White) 52

email communication 27, 82; discoverability of 32; security of 81, *see also* office/office procedures

emotional injury, employee emotional injury, treater–expert conflict, sample report 249–62

employees: employee emotional injury, treater–expert conflict, sample report 249–62, *see also* staff

errors of law 17

ethics 2, 4, 8, 64, 70–2, 83, 104, 297; clinician–patient sex, plaintiff, sample report 153–62; unethical practice 7

ethnicity: and courtroom presentation 96, 98; depositions and trial testimony 60–1

etiquette, and marketing 79

evaluation, notification of treatment need discovered during 114–15

evaluations 35–7; consent and notifications 44–5; criminal defendants 46; evaluation appointment letter 112; evaluee failure to appear/cooperate 37–8; evaluee information sheet 113; evaluees with clinical needs 45–6, 114–15; format and behavior 43; interview style 44; jail/prison setting 39–40; lawyer presence 41–2; and outside consultation 38; parties present during 40–1; recording of 42–3; safety considerations 40, 223–4; scheduling 38–9; setting for 39, *see also* examinations; Independent Medical Examination (IME)

evaluees: clinical needs of 45–6, 114–15; definition 19; evaluee information sheet 113; failure to appear at/cooperate with evaluations 37–8; language of 37; notification of treatment need discovered during evaluation 114–15

evidence: rules of 91, 98–9; spoilation of 22, 33

examinations 29, 88; and ethics 71–2, *see also* evaluations

examinee, definition 19
expenses 66, 67, 109, 110; time worksheet 121
expert deposition, definition 19
expert witnesses 71; academic credentials 101; conflict of interest with treater role 7–10, 147–52, 249–61; courtroom presentation 95–8; definition 19; duties of 6–7, 8; and juries 90–1, 94–5; past testimony 102–3; professional experience and training 98–9; professional standing 101; recommendation by lawyers 6; relationship with lawyers 1–2, 6, 13, 14–15, 17, 24–9, 90–105; reviewing/ testifying about other professions 99–101; role of 1–2, 10; rules concerning 91–3; time-limited permits for 89

Facebook 75, 84
fact, definition 19
fact witnesses: definition 19; experts as 46, 71; rules concerning 91
factfinder: addressing testimony to 58; definition 19
families: and evaluations 41
fax machines 79
FDA (Food and Drug Administration) 212–13
Federal Rules of Evidence 98–9
fee splitting 67
feedback, and evaluations 44
fees 62–5; fee sheets 65–9, 109–10; pre-testimony deposit letter 119–20; pre-testimony deposit worksheet 118; time worksheet 121, *see also* billing; money; retainers
fetal damage cases, malpractice, defense (clinician) (alleged fetal damage from medication), sample report 208–15
fiduciary duty 8, 17; definition 19–20
files, client 82
Florida 89
"foreign" appearance: and courtroom presentation 96, 98; depositions and trial testimony 60–1

forensic client, definition 17
forensic organizations, membership of 3
forensic practice 1; career directions in private practice 10–11; duties 6–7; kinds of cases 11–13; liability in 87–9; principles of 13–14; rebuttal of expert's report, forensic practice standards, sample letter 297–9; reputation and credibility 4–6; supporting motion to strike expert testimony (forensic practice standards), sample affidavit 292–6; training and credentials for 2–4; treater vs. expert witness/consultant roles 7–10
foreseeability, definition 20, 51
"friend of the court" *see amicus (amicus curiae)*
friends, avoidance of expert role in defense of 14

gender: and courtroom presentation 96; depositions and trial testimony 60
Google 75
government contracts, and payment 65
grammar, and reports 52
gross negligence, definition 20, 51
guardian *ad litem*, definition 16
guardianship cases 12; capacity, guardianship (complex, contested), sample report 276–84

"hired gun" role 4, 6, 102
hiring practices, malpractice, defense (facility), forensic practice standards, sample report 201–3
honesty 5; duty of 6; and evaluations 43
hourly rates 66, 109, *see also* fees

impairment cases 12
Independent Medical Examination (IME) 293–6; definition 20; scheduling of 29, 38–9, *see also* evaluations
Independent Psychological Examination, definition 20
information, required from lawyer before proceeding 26–7
initial attorney letter, sample 108

insanity, not guilty by reason of insanity (NGRI) 12, 35n1, 143–6
insurance companies: disability reviews 29, 64; private insurance disability appeal (complex), sample report 238–48
insurance, for forensic practice 87
integrity 92
interest, charging on overdue bills 68, 84
Internet, as a marketing tool 74–5, 79
interpreters 37, 41
interviews 29; interview styles in evaluations 44

jail, settings for evaluations 39–40
Joint Commission on Accreditation of Healthcare Organizations (JCAHO) 202
judges, as triers 22–3, 91
juries: and experts 90–1, 94–5; as triers 23
juvenile cases 12

Keenan, Don 97
know, definition 20, 51
knowledge, and consent 18

language: of evaluees 37; legal 16–23, 50–1, 52
lawyers: participation in reports/affidavits 48–9; presence during evaluations 40, 41–2; recommendation of expert witnesses 6; relationship with expert witnesses 1–2, 6, 13, 14–15, 17, 24–9, 90–105; as target market 73
"lay witnesses": definition 19, 20; rules concerning 91
legal client, definition 17
legal education, and forensic practice 4, 10
letters: discoverability of 32; evaluation appointment letter 112; initial attorney letter 108; malpractice, plaintiff pre-suit, lack of causation 179–80; notification of treatment need discovered during evaluation 114–15; opinion letter, capacity, business, and testamentary 285–7; opinion letter, professional licensure 268–9; pre-testimony deposit letter 119–20; rebuttal of expert's report, forensic

practice standards 297–9; settlement acknowledgment 111; *subpoena duces teum* response 116–17
"letters of protection" 67–8
liability, in forensic practice 87–9
libel 84
licensing: license blemishes 4, 101; opinion letter, professional licensure 268–9; professional licensing agency review, sample reports 262–3, 264–7; time-limited permits 89; and unethical practice 7; working in states in which you are not licensed to practice 88–9, *see also* certifications
LinkedIn 75, 84
listening, to the lawyer 103–4
litigants, not target market 74
litigation consultancy 10
logs 82

malingering 133, 136, 207
malpractice cases 4, 5, 87, 100; malpractice, defense (clinician) (alleged fetal damage from medication), sample report 208–15; malpractice, defense (complex, facility), sample report 195–200; malpractice, defense (facility), forensic practice standards, sample report 201–7; malpractice, plaintiff (complex, doctor and hospital), sample report 163–75; malpractice, plaintiff (complex), sample report 181–94; malpractice, plaintiff pre-suit affidavit 176–8; malpractice, plaintiff pre-suit, lack of causation, letter 179–80; report format 50
manners, and marketing 79
marketing 73; access and availability 77–8; quality of public interface 78–9; recommendations 74–7; referrals 79–80; target market 73–4
media interviews, as a marketing tool 76
medication: accidental overdose vs. suicide, sample report 216–22; malpractice, defense (clinician) (alleged fetal damage from medication), sample report 208–15
mentoring 3

mitigation of charge or sentence, sample report 137–42

MLA (Medical Licensing Agency), professional licensing agency review, sample reports 262–3, 264–7

money 90–1, *see also* billing; fees

motivation 90

negligence: cases 12; definition 20, 51; in forensic practice 87

nonprofessional organizations, as a marketing tool 76–9

nonprofessional pursuits, and credibility 5

"not guilty by reason of insanity" (NGRI) 12, 35n1; sample report 143–6

note-taking 25–6, 31

notifications, and evaluations 44–5

objectivity 6, 14, 33, 34

office/office procedures 81–6, *see also* email communication; telephone systems

opine, definition 20

opinions 13–14, 95; courts' rules on credibility of 50; initial case review 28–9; in reports/affidavits 47, 48–9

opposing entities: duty to 6; refusal of evaluations 37

oral communication 49

overdue bills, charging of interest on interest 68, 84

package pricing 68

patients: definition 17–18, 20–1; not target market 74

payment 24

personal injury cases 12; defense (PSTD) (with treater–expert conflict), sample report 147–52; employee emotional injury, treater–expert conflict, sample report 249–62; malpractice, defense (clinician) (alleged fetal damage from medication), sample report 208–15

"phantom experts" 26, 27

physical examination of patients 195–6

plaintiffs: attorneys of 83–4; clinician–patient sex, plaintiff, sample report 153–62; definition 21;

malpractice, plaintiff (complex, doctor and hospital), sample report 163–75; malpractice, plaintiff (complex), sample report 181–94; malpractice, plaintiff pre-suit affidavit 176–8; malpractice, plaintiff pre-suit, lack of causation, letter 179–80

"possibilities" 95

post office boxes 78

pre-testimony conferences 54–5

predictability 20

pregnancy, malpractice, defense (clinician) (alleged fetal damage from medication), sample report 208–15

preliminary reports 51

presentation: courtroom 95–8; of reports 52–3

principles, of forensic practice 13–14

prison, settings for evaluations 39–40

privacy, during evaluations 39

pro bono work 64

pro se, definition 21

professional organizations: and ethics 8, 70; membership of 3

prosecution: definition 21; experience with 11

prosecutor, definition 21

prudent, definition 21

PSTD, personal injury defense (PSTD) (with treater–expert conflict), sample report 147–52

psychiatric certainty/probability 95; definition 21, 51

psychiatrists, reviewing/testifying about other professions 99–101

psychological certainty/probability 95; definition 21, 51

psychologists, reviewing/testifying about other professions 99–101

PTSD cases: accidental overdose vs. suicide, sample report 216–22; employee emotional injury, treater–expert conflict, sample report 250, 255, 256, 259; personal injury defense (with treater–expert conflict) 147–52

publications, as information source 3

quality 2, 4, 73; of public interface 78–9

reasonable, definition 21
reasonable medical/psychiatric/
psychological certainty/probability 95;
definition 21
recommendations 6
recording: depositions and trial testimony
58, 104; of evaluations 41–3
records 82; receipt of 28, 30–1; record
reviews 31–3, 35, 88
referrals 79–80
"reportable" conditions/behaviors 71
reports 47–8; accidental overdose vs.
suicide 216–22; auto accident vs. suicide
288–91; capacity, guardianship
(complex, contested) 276–84; civil
capacity, contracting 270–5; clinician–
patient sex, plaintiff 153–62; criminal
responsibility (sanity) 134–6; defense,
death in custody 223–6; discoverability
of 32; drafts, discovery 51–2; employee
emotional injury, treater–expert conflict
249–62; format 48–51; grammar,
spelling and vocabulary 52; lawyer
participation in 48–9; malpractice,
defense (clinician) (alleged fetal damage
from medication) 208–15; malpractice,
defense (complex, facility) 195–200;
malpractice, defense (facility), forensic
practice standards 201–7; malpractice,
plaintiff (complex) 181–94; malpractice,
plaintiff (complex, doctor and hospital)
163–75; mitigation of charge or
sentence 137–42; not guilty by reason of
insanity (NGRI) 143–6; personal injury
defense (PSTD) (with treater–expert
conflict) 147–52; preliminary 51;
presentation of 52–3; private insurance
disability appeal (complex) 238–48;
professional licensing agency review
262–3, 264–7; rebuttal of expert's
report, forensic practice standards 297–9;
trial competency (fitness to proceed)
(complex) 127–33; trial competency
(fitness to proceed) (simple) 125–6;
workplace stressors allegedly causing
suicide, expert report rebuttal 232–7
reputation 4–6, 74, 84

Resnick, Philip 3
responsibility, definition 51
retainers 63–4, 66, 69, 83, 110; definition
21–2
retaining entities, experts' duties to 6
risk 20
risk assessment 164–5, 184, 189
rules, concerning experts 91–3

safety: during evaluations 39, 40, 223–4;
safety violations 93
sanity *see* criminal responsibility
scheduling: depositions 54, 57; evaluations
29, 38–9
schizophrenia, trial competency (fitness to
proceed) (complex) 127–33
search engine placement 74–5
second opinions 13
secondary gain 241, 246–7
security, of office and office procedures 81, 82
security staff 39, 40
sentence, mitigation of, sample report 137–42
settings: for depositions 104–5; for
evaluations 39; jail/prison 39–40
settlement acknowledgment, sample 111
sexual relationships: clinician–patient sex,
plaintiff, sample report 153–62;
malpractice, defense (facility), forensic
practice standards, sample report 201–7
shackles 39
shredders 83
Simpson, Skip 90–105
slander 84
SOC (standard of care) 100; clinician–
patient sex, plaintiff, sample report
153–62; definition 22, 51; malpractice,
defense (clinician) (alleged fetal damage
from medication), sample report
211–12; malpractice, defense (complex,
facility), sample report 195–6;
malpractice, plaintiff (complex, doctor
and hospital), sample report 163–75;
malpractice, plaintiff (complex), sample
report 181–92; professional licensing
agency review, sample reports 263; and
safety violations 93n9
social media 75

Social Security disability reports 238
specialization in forensic practice 10–11
speech: and courtroom presentation 96; depositions and trial testimony 60; and marketing 79
spelling, and reports 52
spoilation of evidence 33; definition 22
staff 81, 103; employee confidentiality agreement 123–4; quality of 78
standard of care *see* SOC
stationery 78–9
stress cases, workplace stressors allegedly causing suicide, expert report rebuttal, sample report 232–7
strokes 295–6
Strunk, W. 52
subpoena: definition 22; and definitions 48; and records 30, 32; *subpoena duces teum* response 116–17
suicide cases: accidental overdose vs. suicide, sample report 216–22; auto accident vs. suicide, sample report 288–91; defense, death in custody, sample report 223–6; defense rebuttal, death in custody, sample affidavit 227–31; malpractice, plaintiff (complex, doctor and hospital), sample report 163–75; malpractice, plaintiff (complex), sample report 181–94; malpractice, plaintiff pre-suit, lack of causation, letter 179–80; risk assessment 164–5, 184, 189; workplace stressors allegedly causing suicide, expert report rebuttal, sample report 232–7

target market 73–4, *see also* marketing
teaching, as a marketing tool 76
telephone systems 77–8, 79, 81–2, *see also* office/office procedures
terminology, legal 16–23, 50–1, 52
testamentary capacity, sample opinion letter, capacity, business, and testamentary 285–7
testimony 90; deposition and trial 54–61; in states in which you are not licensed to practice 89; supporting motion to strike expert testimony (forensic practice standards), sample affidavit 292–6

testings 29
time worksheet 121
training 2–4
translators 41
travel expenses 66, 67
treater role, conflict with expert witness/ consultant role 7–10; employee emotional injury, sample report 249–62; sample report 147–52
trial competency (fitness to proceed): complex 127–33; simple 125–6
trial deposition, definition 18
trial testimony 54–6, 58–61
trier, definition 22–3
trust 96
truth 93

U.S. Department of Justice (DOJ) 25
U.S. Supreme Court 17

vendor confidentiality agreement 122
Veterans Administration: accidental overdose vs. suicide, sample report 216–22; disability reports 238; employee emotional injury, treater– expert conflict, sample report 250–1, 259; malpractice, defense (complex, facility), sample report 195–200
video recording: depositions and trial testimony 58, 104; of evaluations 41–3
videographers 41, 42
vocabulary, legal 16–23, 50–1, 52
voluntariness, and consent 18

websites, as a marketing tool 74–5
White, E.B. 52
witchcraft, and professional credibility 5
witnesses *see* expert witnesses; fact witnesses; lay witnesses
word of mouth 74
work products, definition 23
worker's compensation cases 13
workplace stress cases, workplace stressors allegedly causing suicide, expert report rebuttal, sample report 232–7
writ of *certiorari*, definition 17
written agreements/contracts 28